POX

POX

Genius, Madness, and
the Mysteries of Syphilis

DEBORAH HAYDEN

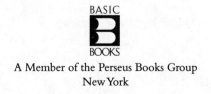

A Member of the Perseus Books Group
New York

Chapter 19: The 4 lines of poetry on page 240 from a letter of Oliver St. John Gogarty to J. Joyce are reprinted here with the courtesy of Colin Smythe Ltd. on behalf of the heirs to the Gogarty Estate.

Published by Basic Books,
A Member of the Perseus Books Group

Designed by Trish Wilkinson
Set in 12.5-point Bembo by the Perseus Books Group

Library of Congress Cataloging-in-Publication Data

Hayden, Deborah.
 Pox : genius, madness, and the mysteries of syphilis / Deborah Hayden.
  p. cm.
Includes bibliographical references and index.
 ISBN 0-465-02881-0 (alk. paper)
1. Syphilis—History. I. Title.

RC201.47 .H39 2003
615.95'13'009—dc21

2002015847

03 04 05 / 10 9 8 7 6 5 4 3 2 1

To Rudy Binion
Dear friend, ferocious editor

A zest in the ferreting out of the obscure,
a positively detective zeal in the running to earth
of this most subtle master of the dissembling art,
that is the foremost asset of the clinical syphilologist.
—John H. Stokes, *Modern Clinical Syphilology*

Contents

Cactus Flower
Portrait of a Syphilitic

A Fantasy

a sensation, touch the spot under the covers, hard like a button beneath the skin, but that was weeks ago, soft skin, maybe, yes, but the risk the terrible risk, a glass of steaming absinthe the glowing green muse, and now this blossom unfolds like a flower on a cactus stalk. bathe it in the water of the narcissus, they say. then gentle bumps everywhere, the soles of the feet, palms of the hand, a rash pale as a sweet rose. the doctor says yes, finally yes, it is the pox, the splendid pox of columbus, fruit of the new world, horror. no one must know, i will quarantine myself like a leper. such pain. my throat, and deep in the bones, fever, is this typhoid? malaria? it's like being bound hand and foot at the bottom of a deep dark well. no food, no hunger. fear. white moss in the mouth. must not kiss. must never kiss. sweet thick hair falls to the floor, gleaming patches of scalp in the candlelight. i whisper this disease to a friend, give it a name, but in the dark, please, please don't tell. the horror of life. the rash goes away, and the fever. the cactus flower withers, shrinks to a small scar. cured, yes i am cured.

again it returns. what does the blasted doctor know? salve, mercury mixed with rosewater, honey, licorice, conserve of rose petals, lard. i rub it everywhere but not by the heart, the head, the hairy parts, i glow with a blue light, smell like a fried potato. laxatives, purges, colic, sleepless nights—gigantic nuisance—, tongue like an ox. suffering. quicksilver, quacksalver, those quacks, what do they know? saliva gushes like a river, teeth rattle and rot, mercury, penis the color of slate. cured again, then again the fever,

aching bones and joints. now a pain in the heart, a sore on the finger, eyes like a vampire, bandaged at night, blindness, please not
the eyes.

years go by, so much pain, it grinds the head to atoms. vomiting again again. a green demon, health, since that first button, that
cactus flower. are there no clear skies? a dry wind plagues the
nerves. such agony of loneliness, no friend, no lover, i am poison
to anyone, poison in the blood, poisoned, poisoned. criminal. out-
cast, leper. evil, ghastly miserable and hated in society. flower of
evil. a sharp pain in the chest, always the night headache, and ears
ringing, singing, rushing, the devil lives in the ears, give him green
nut rinds or fresh horseradish on a cotton cloth, is there no part of
the body that does not grieve?

years. so many doctors, so many theories, damn them, jars and
tins of powders and pills and potions. patched with leeches,
shocks, and spas with hot water baths and cold water plunges. roast
meat, raw eggs, red wine, never eat vegetables, and the doctors say
no fresh air. walk with a cane. see through a haze. a hypochondriac? a neurasthene? no one must know i'm rotting inside. rotting
in the bones, melting like an old camembert. oozing sores now on
my shins, i bandage them, hide them. when will i find an end?

today i felt a breeze from the wing of madness.

is that how it will end? but, oh, such visions. i fall to the earth
and weep for such ecstasies. a mystical light. could there be a god?
electricity lights my brain, i am the lightning rod of god, i am a
zigzag doodle drawn by god's hand. the world will know, some
day, the world will explode, because of me. christ, buddha, all gods
in one, celestial angels sing to me, only me. when will be my coro-
nation? i fear doing harm. my fingers crab, words pile up at the
end of a line, they blotch. i fear i will kill someone. myself.

a tight jacket, i lick the wall, they will poison me, they feed me
feces, steal my fortune. i chase thoughts like colored butterflies, my
urine is full of jewels. i scream, i rage. then i play the piano, gently,
and all is well. i remember everything. my friends visit, we laugh,
and then, one day, i ask: who is that face in the mirror?

Introduction

WHEN LOU ANDREAS SALOMÉ JOINED THE FREUD GROUP in 1911, she brought with her the rich mythology of having had an intense intellectual companionship with Friedrich Nietzsche in the summer of 1882, when she was twenty-one. In utmost confidence, Nietzsche had shared with her the secret, terrifying insights that were to mold his late philosophy. Freud and his followers (including Carl Jung who was still on good terms with Freud then) were avidly interested in Nietzsche's life—including the question of the influence of syphilis on his philosophy.[1]

P. J. Möbius, the Berlin neuropsychiatrist who first revealed Nietzsche's diagnosis in 1902, wrote that he was exhibiting syphilitic euphoria, a precursor to later syphilitic madness, as early as 1881—the year before he met Lou. Freud's group, knowing of this hypothesis, would surely have interrogated Lou about Nietzsche's mental state then. But she adamantly considered conversation about Nietzsche to be off-limits. I wondered why.

What I found reading dozens of versions of the Lou/Nietzsche story was that no one knew for sure what happened during the summer they were so intellectually close or a few months later when Nietzsche viciously criticized her: If I reject you now, it will be a censure of your whole being. This sword hangs over you. According to some, Nietzsche was devastated when Lou rejected his marriage proposal. Others say that he was part of the gay

Bayreuth circle that followed Richard Wagner and that Lou was guilty of spreading rumors of pederasty. Perhaps she made up the marriage proposal. At the end of this inquiry, I published an article, "Nietzsche's Secrets,"[2] about the complex contradictions in the Nietzsche lore. But the syphilis question, and what part it played in the high drama of the summer of 1882, continued to intrigue me.

How did Nietzsche react to having syphilis—assuming that he even knew? Was syphilis one of the secrets he imparted to Lou when he said that she and their mutual friend Paul Rée were the only two to whom he could speak without a mask? Was it true, as many scholars believe, contrary to Möbius, that syphilis did not affect Nietzsche at all until 3 January 1889, when he collapsed, insane, in the town square of Turin? And Nietzsche's illnesses were legendary. He had attacks of migraine and gastrointestinal agony that in one year devastated him for 118 days. By his own admission, he was seven-eighths blind. Were any of his physical conditions, I wondered, caused by syphilis? What was known about syphilis in Nietzsche's time? What prognosis would a doctor then have given him?

The lavishly illustrated nineteenth- and early-twentieth-century medical texts on syphilis (which I began to collect) were written in language remarkably accessible to the layperson. Reading the old texts, I saw that Nietzsche's ongoing painful attacks for the ten years after he took a health leave of absence from Basel University in 1879 were typical of the misery of progressing syphilis. His profound reflections about his dreadful health are well known, and yet how often has his excruciating pain, so poignantly revealed in his remarkable correspondence and in his published work, been considered as a possible manifestation of the disease that was to send him into madness?

Nietzsche wrote to one of his physicians, Otto Eiser: "My existence is a *fearful* burden: I would have long thrown it over if I had not been making the most instructive tests and experiments on mental and moral questions in precisely this condition of suffering and almost complete renunciation. . . . On the whole I am happier than ever before. And yet, continual pain; for many hours of the day a feeling closely akin to sea-sickness, a semi-paralysis which makes it difficult to speak, alternating with furious attacks."[3]

Wondering if this same pattern could be true in the lives of others, I turned to biographies of the three best-known French writers who had syphilis—Charles Baudelaire, Guy de Maupassant, and Gustave Flaubert. Again, there were years of pain and misery and chronic, relapsing illnesses that would have sent any syphilologist running for the mercury treatment, yet syphilis, if it was mentioned at all, was rarely linked to these painful attacks. From Nietzsche and the three French writers, I began to explore others known or suspected of having had syphilis.

What I found was astonishing. At the end of the nineteenth century, syphilologist Alfred Fournier estimated that 15 percent of the population of Paris was infected with syphilis. And yet, next to nothing has been written about the experience by or about people who had syphilis, either in memoirs or in biographies. Syphilis was life's dark secret. The word was taboo, with the terrifying diagnosis at most whispered to an intimate friend, and then only with assurances of utmost secrecy. It was too shameful to record by name in a diary and was alluded to in correspondence only in code. How much, I wondered, was syphilis an unacknowledged subtext in nineteenth-century biography?

In 1907, novelist Stefan Zweig noted that in Vienna at the turn of the century, one or two out of ten young men had received the dreaded diagnosis (usually after an experience with a prostitute). Many chose the revolver over that fate. What did a young man (or older man, or woman) diagnosed with syphilis have to look forward to after hearing the bad news? First, a moral dilemma: total sexual abstinence or the risk of infecting a lover. Syphilis is highly infectious for the first two years, then progressively less so up to about year seven. The treatments of the time—toxic mercury and arsenic—had devastating side effects sometimes as bad as the disease itself. A woman with syphilis risked delivering a baby that would soon be covered with black, crusty sores. And since the disease was incorrectly thought to be hereditary, the syphilitic feared that the taint would be passed to subsequent generations and the family line degenerate as a result.

Of all the curses of syphilis, one of the most frightening was the prospect of years of debilitating illness. Infection first manifests as a sore, usually on the genitals, followed by a fever, rash, and exceptional malaise. In his 1933 text *The Modern Treatment of Syphilis*, Joseph Earle Moore of the Johns Hopkins University described what happened next: "The patient then enters a period of indeterminate length, varying from a few months to a lifetime, but averaging seven years, during which there is no outward sign of syphilitic infection."[4] But already during this latency and its apparent quiescence, beneath "the outwardly serene surface," parasites remaining in the body initiate a "mild and exquisitely chronic," slowly progressive inflammatory reaction.

Today, the Centers for Disease Control in Atlanta, Georgia, lists on its website the same information that Moore provided decades before: "The latent (hidden) stage of syphilis begins when the secondary symptoms disappear. If the infected person has not received treatment, he/she still has syphilis even though there are no symptoms. *Syphilis remains in the body and begins to damage the internal organs including the brain, nerves, eyes, heart, blood vessels, liver, bones, and joints.*" [emphasis added]

Syphilis was known as the Great Imitator for its facility in mimicking many other conditions. The clinical syphilologist had a long list of what to look for during the years of relapsing illness: excruciating headaches, pains in the bones and joints, severe gastrointestinal agony, fevers, blindness, deafness. In short, no part of the body was free of chronic, relapsing pain. Many of those who survived to the last stage could look forward to insanity and paralysis. Before then, there were years when brief episodes of uninhibited, uncharacteristic behavior presaged the madness to come. Right before madness, the syphilitic was often rewarded, in a kind of Faustian bargain for enduring the pain and despair, by episodes of creative euphoria, electrified, joyous energy when grandiosity led to new vision. The heightened perception, dazzling insights, and almost mystical knowledge experienced during this time were expressed while precision of form of expression was still possible. At the end of the nineteenth century, it was believed that, in rare instances, syphilis could produce a genius.

Syphilis carried with it the stigma of five hundred years of sexual shame, beginning with the epidemic in Naples in 1495, when the Great Pox produced grotesque sores all over the body. The disease was so frightening that it seemed as if infection could be passed by its smell alone. Even lepers protested when syphilitics moved into their neighborhoods. Stefan's Zweig's hypothetical young man had adequate reason to consider taking his own life.

Today, most clinicians have never seen a case of long-term, untreated syphilis. The texts describing the complexities of diagnosis are stored away in dusty archives of the history of medicine and are not available on-line. The characteristic features of the primary, secondary, and tertiary stages are well known, but the agonies of the middle years—those that imitate other diseases and are not easily identified as being caused by syphilis—have been forgotten. Many doctors today who have practiced medicine after penicillin was discovered to be an effective treatment for syphilis in 1943 believe that the "latency" period is a reprieve from illness, when in fact it signals chronic inflammation and insidious damage to every part of the body.

The medical investigation in *Pox* spans the period from 1493, the beginning of the syphilis epidemic in Europe, when millions died of disease on both sides of the ocean, to 1943, when the first case of syphilis was successfully treated with penicillin. The first section gives historical, cultural, and medical information about the disease and about *Treponema pallidum*, the microscopic parasite that causes it. The next sections investigate the theme of hidden syphilis through medical and literary biographies of a number of people known—or suspected—to have had it.

The reader looking for proof in the contentious cases will find none. The old syphilologists knew that the Pox was identified by the cumulative weight of many "suspicion arousers"—that is, by a preponderance of circumstantial evidence. Take, for example, the case of Guy de Maupassant. When his doctor diagnosed syphilis, he trumpeted: "I've got the Pox!" During the progressing years, he had a long list of the complaints listed in the Centers for Disease Control's summary. He died in a mental hospital with a diagnosis of general paralysis of the insane. And yet, no single indicator constitutes proof short of post mortem, and even then not all cases are definitive. Maybe his doctor misdiagnosed gonorrhea. Each complaint of the middle period by itself could have been something else. Perhaps at the end, he was schizophrenic. And yet we don't question that he had syphilis.

With other suspected sufferers of syphilis, the clues do not line up as neatly. Rumors of infection often come from disreputable witnesses. The signs and symptoms of syphilis seem to point so clearly to other diseases that syphilis is dropped from a differential diagnosis, or the sufferer died before a diagnosis could be clinched by demonstrable tertiary disease. Syphilis was often rejected for incorrect reasons—because the person was not (yet) demented, or lacked a particular eye sign, or had a masking concomitant illness. After reading the chapter on Hitler, one person asked how anyone could doubt that he had syphilis. Another reader found confirmation there that Hitler could not possibly have had syphilis. For him, another hundred pages of "suspicion arousers" would do nothing to sway the argument because he looked at each clue separately and rejected it as inconclusive.

Here is the fascination of syphilis, the disease that Carl Jung called "the poison of the darkness."

Acknowledgments

POX COULD NOT HAVE BEEN WRITTEN WITHOUT THE ONGOING encouragement of Rudolph Binion, beginning with our spirited discussions of his inspiring, infuriating psychobiography of Lou Salomé (*Frau Lou*) ten years ago. The late Dr. Eugene Farber, eminent syphilologist and past chairman of dermatology at Stanford University's School of Medicine, generously reviewed chapters along the way. Special thanks go to Dr. Ashley Robins, psychopharmacologist and Wilde scholar from Cape Town, South Africa, for a lively email debate about the philosophy of nineteenth-century medicine. I fondly remember the late Richard Webster, professor of history at the University of California, Berkeley, for his witty, irreverent historical perspective. Heartfelt appreciation to Joseph Fell for that first Nietzsche class. Thanks to medical doctors who generously answered questions and read chapters: Robert Berger, Norbert Hirschhorn, Frank Johnson, Adrienne Kane, Jonathan Mueller, and Larry Zaroff. And to all the generous readers along the way: Alice Binion, Peter Buxton, and James Jones for Tuskegee; David Brook for van Gogh; Kathleen Ferris for Joyce; Albert Jerman, Joan Chacones, and Jim Turner for Lincoln; Leonard Heston for Hitler; Lise Ostwald for the composers; David Rose for Wilde and others; Bruce Rothschild for Columbus; Bill Schaberg for many chapters; Van Harvey and Walter Sokel for Nietzsche. Thanks to Colman Jones and John

Scythes for their in-depth knowledge of pre-penicillin syphilis. Special thanks to friends: Victor Barbieri, David Bolling, Rick Buckley, Bill Dodd, Dorothy and Jim Fadiman, Diane Fischler, Carolyn Fremgen, Pat Gelband, Jeff Gillenkirk, Pam Grossman, Weslyn Hants, Paula Huntley, Peter Keville, Alan Lakein, Diane LeBold, Karen Littmann, Patrick McNutty, Jan Pehrson, Howard Raphael, Jim Simmons, and Ken Smith. Special thanks to John Lacombe for website design and to Beth Kuper for editorial assistance and moral support; to my editor at Basic Books, Jo Ann Miller; and finally, warmest thanks and appreciation to my agent, Rosalie Siegel, who first suggested the idea for *Pox*.

Anyone wishing to contact me can do so on my website: www.poxhistory.com.

PART I

The Disease

Christopher Columbus
The First European Syphilitic?

IN 1492 CHRISTOPHER COLUMBUS SET SAIL FROM SPAIN looking for a sea route to Asia. Instead he made port in paradise, the islands of the Caribbean, and brought the dubious gifts of European culture and Catholicism to the (sometimes) gentle, immunologically naive inhabitants of the luscious New World, along with disease. Measles, tetanus, typhus, typhoid, diphtheria, influenza, pneumonia, whooping cough, dysentery, and smallpox were all unknown before the arrival of the first European adventurers. Later, malaria was brought by a mosquito and trichinosis by a pig. How could a handful of invading Europeans subdue a continent? For every person viciously murdered by the guns, knives, crossbows, or attack dogs of the conquistadors, thousands died from these new illnesses. The European conquest of the New World began what has been called the most massive genocide in human history, leaving 100 million people, or 95 percent of the population, dead from murder and disease.[1]

Columbus's ships and those that followed returned to Spain loaded with gold, slaves, cigars, and exotic cuisine to tantalize the cultural elite of Europe. If the plunder brought back from the New World enriched European coffers, the gastronomic delights packed on those small vessels battling the Atlantic storms changed forever the odors emanating from European kitchens. New dishes were created from chocolate, paprika, peanuts, sweet potatoes,

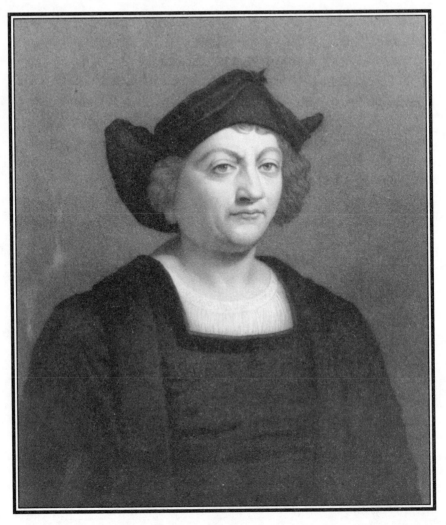

Figure I.I   Christopher Columbus: An engraver's idea of Columbus's image. (Library of Congress)

tomatoes, corn, and gorgeous sweet red pepper. In return, cooks in the Americas gained domestic animals—cattle, goats, pigs, and sheep—as well as rice, wheat, and honeybees.

Did the returning ships also harbor a microscopic stowaway, the revenge of the Americas: the pale criminal, the Neapolitan Disease, the *Morbus Gallicus*, the Great Pox, syphilis? This disease may have been a payback in kind delivered to the unsuspecting Europeans anxiously awaiting the bounteous gifts from paradise when they embraced the returning explorers. The European death toll from syphilis may have reached ten million, but what might the worldwide death toll have been? During the next five centuries, when the disease was less virulent and more discreet, the picture of the rotting, pustular, incredibly painful first manifestation remained present in the European mind.

The drama and horror of the syphilis epidemic in Europe began soon after Columbus and his crew sailed into the harbor of Palos, Spain, on 15 March 1493. Was this just a remarkable coincidence? For five hundred years epidemiologists have debated whether the causal organism was brought back to Spain from the island of Hispaniola (now Haiti and the Dominican Republic) or had already existed for centuries in Europe but mutated to a virulent form just as ships were returning from the New World. The controversy is further complicated by those who suggest that the 1495 scourge of Naples (the beginning of the syphilis epidemic) may have been caused by numerous diseases acting in concert, of which syphilis was but one.

The American position has gained the edge with the discovery by paleo-anthropologist Bruce Rothschild and his colleagues of clearly syphilitic bones on the island of Hispaniola, where Columbus and his men made camp. The only skeletons found in Europe that appear to have pre-Columbian syphilitic damage are more likely the victims of another spirochetal disease, yaws. If it is true that the returning explorers of the fifteenth century were the source of the syphilis that ravaged Europe, then their voyages of discovery not only brought about economic, cultural, and spiritual cataclysms but also introduced a disease that would change the course of history in Europe and beyond.

In 1492, with three ships and a crew of 120 men, Columbus sailed toward an uncertain horizon. Previous explorers had proven that the sailors would not fall off the earth when they reached that thin line, but beyond that nothing was known of what dangers lurked beyond the familiar. On his first of four trips Columbus noted that the native people, who would love their neighbors as themselves, had the softest speech in the world. He named their islands "The Virgins" after St. Ursula, who, according to the myth, set sail with eleven thousand virgin friends, ending their trip as martyrs at the hands of Attila and his Huns. When Columbus returned in early January 1494, landing on the northern coast of Hispaniola with seventeen ships that Ferdinand and Isabella, the king and queen of Spain, had outfitted for violence, his attitude had changed dramatically. The islanders who met the ships brought him gifts of fruit and fish; in return Columbus and his men and dogs took over the island and ruled ruthlessly, murdering, raping, enslaving, even lopping off noses and ears at whim. Many committed suicide and murdered their children rather than leave them at the mercy of the Christian invaders.

Bartolomé de Las Casas, historian of Hispaniola, deplored this viciousness: "It was a general rule among the Spanish to be cruel; not just cruel but extraordinarily cruel. . . . So they would cut an Indian's hands and leave them dangling by a shred of skin. . . . They would test their swords and their manly strength on captured Indians and place bets on the slicing off of heads or the cutting of bodies in half with one blow. They burned or hanged captured chiefs."[2] Newborn babies were thrown to the dogs.

The Spain that Columbus had left behind was already one of great carnage. Seven hundred years of warfare to take back Spain from the Moors had formed a warrior culture rooted in the values of the conquistador. The Inquisition sought out heretics and non-Christians to torture and murder at the stake or on the gallows, to burn or hang, behead or flay. Columbus, very much a man of his culture and times, used these same violent methods against the people he found in the New World.

A heroic Christopher Columbus emerges from the pages of history books, an astute and fearless explorer who set sail from Spain in 1492 to discover a new world, a man worthy of a national holiday who would inspire children to follow their dreams. Yet not everyone bows to this Columbus. There is a second powerful image of him, that of the vicious conquistador who initiated atrocities against the native people. A third image of Columbus might now be added, one found neither in history books nor in mock genocide trials in South America. This Columbus became sick in the New World and complained for fifteen years about incurable ailments. At the end of his life he believed he was on a mission from God and was spoken to by angels. This question has rarely been asked: Was Admiral Columbus himself among the first European victims of the Great Pox?

Although no likeness of Columbus exists, we know from his son Fernando's biography that he was above average height, with a florid face and red hair that turned white in his later years. Fernando also gives us insight into the onset of the illness that began his father's decline. Columbus became ill on his second voyage, which began in September 1493. In early April 1494 he experienced an intermittent fever in the village of Isabella, on the island of Hispaniola (as did many of his men). In September he came down with another fever, described by Fernando: "He fell gravely ill in crossing to San Juan; he had a high fever and a drowsiness, so that he lost his sight, memory, and all his other senses."[3] Delirium lasted for several weeks: "He lay in a stupor, knowing little, remembering nothing, his eyes dim and vitality oozing, until the little fleet sorrowfully but gladly entered the harbor of Isabella.'"[4] Five months of illness followed, including episodes during which he was unable to feed or care for himself. He slept little for thirty-three days and felt that his fatigued state nearly deprived him of his life. Unfortunately for the inhabitants of Hispaniola, it did not.

In March 1495 Columbus had recovered enough to assemble two hundred soldiers in full armor, with twenty mounted cavalry and attack dogs, and "with God's aid," he began to round up and massacre thousands, a pattern of murderous raids the Spanish would follow for the next decade. Columbus continued his reign of terror with beheadings and burnings at the stake. Bodies hung from gallows in every town on Hispaniola.

Many of his men—one-third by the count of the ship's doctor, Diego Alvaraz Chanca (former physician to the king and queen)—were ill with a scourge that left the crew eager to return home. They did so in June 1496, arriving sick and almost starved, with thirty to forty captives on board. Columbus had to be carried ashore, where he lay incapacitated for another five months.

In 1498 Columbus returned to Hispaniola on his third voyage, outfitted with an armed fleet of six ships. In his journal he wrote of having had a "grave illness" of two years' duration in Spain followed by "travails at sea . . . without parallel."[5] On the way he again experienced violent fever, fatigue, insomnia, and a severe attack of gout—or so he thought, although the inflammation was not limited to a few of the smaller joints and extremities as gout often is. He prayed to the Lord to free him from his bleeding eyes. On this voyage he began to hear voices and to think he was the emissary of God, a man of divine destiny. He believed the world would end in 150 years. When he arrived in Hispaniola on the last day of August 1498, he found 160 Spaniards, or 20–30 percent of the total there, sick with syphilis.[6] In his diary Fernando called it "The French Sickness" (*Morbus Gallicus*), which is what syphilis was called when it broke out in Naples in 1495.

Rumors about Columbus's despotic rule in Hispaniola led Ferdinand and Isabella to send a commissioner, Francisco de Bobadilla, to check up on their colony. Bobadilla reached Santo Domingo, the capital of Hispaniola, in the spring of 1499. His first sight was of gallows displaying the corpses of seven rebel Spaniards, with five more waiting to be executed for insurrection against Columbus's rule. Since murdering Spaniards was not within Columbus's mandate, he was arrested and manacled. On board his ship, Bobadilla offered to unchain him, but Columbus proudly declared he would only let the restraints be removed by royal decree. Parading through the streets of Cadiz, still burdened with shackles and chains, the discoverer of the New World aroused great popular sympathy. Royal decree did unchain him, but his monarchs also put an end to his rule in Hispaniola.

While in the brig on the return journey, Columbus had experienced fever, aching, swollen joints, and a "badly overwrought nervous system."[7] In the quaint words of Dr. A. M. Fernandez de

Ybarra, who wrote the first comprehensive medical history of Columbus in the *Journal of the American Medical Association* in 1894: "His reason was just beginning to lose its equipoise."[8] His illness brought him "very near to the realms of madness,"[9] and he exhibited bizarre, at times quite demented, behavior.

In 1502 Columbus made his fourth and final voyage to the New World, with 150 men. This time, too sick to be in charge, he assigned responsibility to a former shipmate. Ships were lost and Columbus's arthritis-like illnesses and gout incapacitated him. He had a small cabin constructed on deck so that he could keep a lookout even while lying in his bed. On this voyage, he complained that many times he lay at death's door. In the middle of October 1502 off the coast of Costa Rica, he had a vision he took to be sent by God, and he heard a piteous voice reminding him of biblical passages about trusting in the Almighty. De Ybarra paints a picture of a fifty-five-year-old Columbus on this last voyage, battling hill-like waves in desperate seas, defining himself as the chosen one to carry "the light of the true faith into the far-distant, unenlightened and pagan lands," suffering "the most excruciating pains from his old malady," [10] until he finally returned home in 1504, so sick that he again had to be carried off the ship. "His crazy and shattered little bark anchored in the harbor, with her haggard, emaciated, crippled and almost blind master aboard."[11] When the royal court moved in 1506, Columbus followed painfully on muleback, having petitioned Ferdinand for this inelegant mode of transportation rather than an Andalusian horse that he felt would be too jittery for his aching bones. By the end of the journey his legs and belly had swelled.

Medical writers have attributed Columbus's physical complaints to ailments such as typhus, rheumatic heart disease, and Reiter's Syndrome.[12] It was not until well into the twentieth century that Thomas Parran, one of the originators of the infamous Tuskegee Syphilis Study and later surgeon general of the United States under Franklin D. Roosevelt, first suggested that Columbus's death was due to syphilis: "With his whole body dropsical from the chest downward, like that which is caused by injury to the valves of the heart, his limbs paralyzed, and his brain affected—all symptoms of late, fatal syphilis—he died on 20 May 1506 in Valladolid, Spain."[13] He was draped in the gray robe of the order of St. Francis, poor, fallen from royal grace, and semi-mad. His last words were: "In manus tuas, Domine, commendo spiritum meum." (Into your hands, Lord, I commend my spirit.)

Other researchers since Parran have cautiously raised the possibility of syphilis. Christopher Wills asked: "Was Columbus himself suffering from syphilis, and does this explain his progressive mental derangement? Certainly when he returned to Spain from his final voyage at the end of 1504, he was clearly mentally ill and his legs were paralyzed."[14] Philip Marshall Dale ventured: "The sickness may have been syphilis."[15] Anton Luger concurred: "His symptoms resemble those observed in general paresis or in taboparesis, both conditions of late syphilis."[16]

But the Columbus literature is vast, and most writers pondering the origin of European syphilis have failed even to consider that Columbus and his men may have been suffering from this disease. One simple reason: Columbus's medical history had not been compiled during the first four hundred years of the debate. Fernandez de Ybarra first performed that task in 1894. Opening his discussion with adulation for his subject, de Ybarra declared Columbus's expeditions to be second only to the birth of Christ in beneficial results for humanity. "The subject of the medical history of Columbus is a barren one," de Ybarra declared, "so barren indeed that it has never been touched upon."[17] By the end of his research, however, he had managed to compile a fairly extensive medical portrait.

Although he did speculate that the fever called "the scourge" that leveled Columbus and his men in April 1494 might have been syphilis, de Ybarra did not see the full progression of the disease over decades from infection to death. It took Thomas Parran and other syphilis experts at the beginning of the twentieth century to see that pattern and raise the question of syphilis as a lifelong illness in Columbus's case. And then the question was dropped. Why? Possibly because when penicillin was discovered to be a cure for syphilis in 1943, medical writers no longer had clinical experience of the untreated disease, and thus, like many of their predecessors, they failed to see significance in the pattern.

We know from the writings of his son Fernando and other contemporaries that Columbus came down with fever and delirium while living on Hispaniola, where there was a great risk of the Pox. A few years later he experienced relapsing fever as well as many complaints associated with late secondary syphilis: inflamed eyes,[18] arthritis, and a gout-like condition. He heard voices from God and imagined himself to be God's emissary, while showing other signs of mental derangement. He had the beginnings of paralysis, and he died of heart disease with indications of damage to the valves, all typical of late syphilis. Columbus's medical picture, unavailable until de Ybarra compiled it in 1894, allowed later syphilologists to see a pattern of syphilis in Columbus's history. Was Columbus the first well-known European secret syphilitic? How fitting to set the stage for the five-hundred-year drama of syphilis with this captivating enigma.

2

The Revenge of the Americas

Nothing could be more serious than this
curse, this barbarian poison.
—Nicolas Squillacio

Alonso Pinzón, commander of the good ship Pinta,
had reason to consult a doctor upon his return from the New
World. The physician Ruiz Diaz de Isla treated him, as well as several members of the crew, for a disease contracted from women in
the West Indies and subsequently passed on to Barcelona waterfront prostitutes.[1] At least one of the men, the helmsman of the
Niña, had a severe fever and skin lesions.

This unknown malady seemingly sent by divine justice first
appeared in 1493 in Barcelona, according to Diaz de Isla. It owed
its origin to the island of Hispaniola. "And since admiral Don
Christopher Columbus, who had relations and congress with the
inhabitants of this island during his stay, discovered this island and
since this disease is naturally contagious, it spread with ease, and
soon appeared in the fleet itself."[2]

Diaz de Isla reported that in 1494 the most Christian King
Charles of France accepted many Spaniards stricken with the disease into his army, and soon many were infected: "Just as we now
talk of bubas, pains, apostemes and ulcers, so the Indians of the is-

land of Hispaniola described this sickness in ancient times. . . . It is a grave malady which ulcerates and corrupts the flesh."[3]

Stories are told of others following Columbus to the New World and returning with the disease. Antonio de Torres returned from the Americas with twenty-six slaves in 1494, and the following spring with three hundred more (two hundred others had died in passage). Soldiers "who mixed with these shameless and unchaste Indian women and behaved lewdly with them were struck down with this deplorable sickness."[4]

Early in 1495 the French army (with its infected Spaniards) invaded the Kingdom of Naples. The Neapolitans quickly gave in to the eighteen thousand French horsemen assisted by twenty thousand foot soldiers. In May, victorious Charles VIII, king of France, entered his conquered city in a chariot drawn by four white horses. The local population, who had at first accepted and even fraternized with the invaders, rebelled against their pillaging and debauchery and expelled Charles within a week.

Various groups have been identified as additional possible carriers of the Pox from Spain to Italy at that time: sailors who were with Columbus,[5] women brought from the New World, Jews and Moors expelled from Spain at that time, Ferdinand's own Spanish troops sent to help Alfonso II of Naples fight the French, and an estimated five hundred multinational prostitutes who accompanied Ferdinand's army.

Poor Charles was the first of many monarchs to fall prey to the disease. The historian of the house of Burgundy revealed Charles's malady as the Great Pox, "a violent, hideous and abominable sickness by which he was harrowed; and several of his number, who returned to France, were most painfully afflicted by it; and since no one had heard of this awful pestilence before their return, it was called the Neapolitan sickness."[6] Charles died of apoplexy three years later, at age twenty-eight,[7] after hitting his head against the frame of a low door.

The role played by prostitutes in the spread of disease comes from stories told by those who were there. The anatomist Gabrielo Falloppio recalled a story told by his father, who was in

Naples taking refuge in a fortress with some of the Spanish soldiers and infected prostitutes. Under the pretext that food was in short supply, the soldiers expelled the women, who were cheerfully accepted by the French soldiers—an early example of germ warfare. Falloppio wrote that Spanish soldiers returning to Europe from America, laden with more sickness than gold, passed the curse on to the other European soldiers in the siege of Naples.

On 18 June 1495 Nicolas Squillacio, a Sicilian doctor, observed (in vivid Latin) the worst of what the newly infected might expect:

> The purulent pustules spread in a circle, and there is an abundance of the most virulent lupus. The signs of the sickness are these: there are itching sensations and an unpleasant pain in the joints; there is a rapidly increasing fever; the skin is inflamed with revolting scabs, and is completely covered with swellings and tubercules which are initially of a livid red colour, and then become blacker. After a few days a sanguine humour oozes out; this is followed by excrescences which look like tiny sponges which have been squeezed dry; the sickness does not last more than a year, although the skin remains covered in scars which show the areas it affected. It most often begins with the private parts. . . . I exhort you to provide some new remedy to remove this plague from the Italian people. Nothing could be more serious than this curse, this barbarian poison. [8]

Those who wrote about their experiences left a gruesome literature. One of the more graphic descriptions of the Pox (the first to be published) came from scholar Joseph Grunpeck: "The disease loosed its first arrow into my Priapic glans, which on account of the wound, became so swollen that both hands could scarcely encircle it."[9] Putrid-smelling pus flowed from an abscess for months. Pustules covered his body. The external signs healed, but he was left with pain in the veins, arteries, limbs, and joints. He died at the age of eighty-one, his advanced age illustrating that syphilis did not always act in predictable ways.

Those who favor the New World origin of syphilis have used the testimony of two witnesses in addition to that of Diaz de Isla. Fernandez de Oviedo, a nobleman from Madrid who had once been page to the infant Don Juan, wrote a history of the Indes while a superintendent of the gold and silver mines of the New World[10] and was present when Ferdinand and Isabella celebrated Columbus's successful return from his first voyage with his gold trinkets, slaves, and colorful parrots. As one who had interviewed both Columbus's sailors and natives in the New World, he was in a unique position to report on the new illness:

> Your majesty may take it as certain that this malady [the bubas] comes from the Indes, where it is very common amongst the Indians, but not so dangerous in those lands as in our own. . . . The first time this sickness was seen in Spain was after Admiral Don Christopher Columbus had discovered the Indes and returned from those lands. Some Christians amongst those who went with him and took part in that discovery, and many more who made the second trip, brought back this scourge, and from them it was passed on to others.[11]

Oviedo blamed the new disease on immoral women from Hispaniola. An eighteenth-century historian, C. B. Godfrey, added witchcraft and menstrual pollution to the picture, quoting Oviedo, who wrote that "the women there from habitual nastiness, indolence, often lived on worms, spiders, serpents, bats, and on a kind of lizard palatable indeed, but poisonous to any but the natives."[12] (This was not to be the last time that women, rather than men, were seen as the source of disease.)

The second witness was Bartolomé de las Casas, known as a defender of the oppressed Native Americans. Las Casas wrote a history of the Indies confirming the existence of syphilis on Hispaniola prior to Columbus: "I, for my part, took the trouble to enquire several times from the Indians of this island if the sickness had been there for a long time, and they replied in the affirmative. . . . It is also well known that all those incontinent Spaniards who did not observe the virtue of chastity on this island were infected with the bubas."[13]

Opponents of the American origin theory object that if there had been a rotting, pustular condition on the ships, it would have been noted as such in the ship's log. The European bodies of the conquistadors in Hispaniola should have been vulnerable to the disease in the same way that the European bodies of the soldiers of Charles VIII in Naples were, and yet there was no mention of rotting, stinking sailors aboard the ships returning from the New World. Fernando's reports of the syphilitic sailors on Hispaniola tell of no such extreme illness. Hernán Cortés may have had syphilis,[14] and Pedro de Mendoza, the founder of Buenos Aires, as well; neither exhibited the ugly lesions that characterized the disease in its early days in Europe. In fact, Diaz de Isla recounted simply that: "The Spaniards had never before encountered this sickness, so when they felt the pains and other symptoms of the said malady they attributed them to the tiring effects of being at sea."[15] No one thought to attribute the dreadful, oozing, quickly fatal syphilitic lesions in Charles VIII's army merely to the tiring effects of a day's work.

Could it be that the nonpustular condition that Columbus and his men exhibited coexisted with a more virulent strain in the early days of the epidemic? Addressing the question of what the disease looked like during its first known manifestations in Europe, some quite logically ask how a sexually transmitted pathogen could spread so efficiently if it produced putrid lesions all over the body. Would anyone really have sexual relations with such an obviously diseased sexual partner? On another tack, if syphilis had existed in Europe for centuries before the Neapolitan outbreak in 1495, why did it not gain epidemic speed sooner? Like the great nineteenth-century syphilologist Sir Jonathan Hutchinson, many conclude that the causal organism must have been brought back with the sailors. Given its incredible contagion and rapid spread immediately after the explorers' return, it is difficult to believe that any previous cases would not have provoked an earlier epidemic.

According to the sixteenth-century knight Ulrich von Hutten (who had the Pox), a friend of the Dutch humanist Erasmus (who also had the Pox[16]), the new disease exhibited the gross dermatological signs for seven years only, after which it spread less rapidly and became invisible and insidious. Those who hold that the Pox had always existed in Europe suggest that it may have been caused by a relatively harmless organism known as a treponeme that suddenly mutated into a malignant venereal agent, only to mutate again to a less virulent form a few years later. Opponents of this view scoff that such a convenient seesaw evolution does not fit the treponeme.[17]

Ellis H. Hudson, a scholar of the treponeme, argued that there could have been more than one syphilis: "strains are by definition labile, capable of shift and change in response to the environment."[18] Hideyo Noguchi of the Rockefeller Institute of New York, who first discovered a spirochete in the brain of a late-stage syphilitic in 1913, claimed that he had isolated strains of *Treponema pallidum* that might account for different pathogenicity. If a non-pustular strain existed at the time of the Naples epidemic, then perhaps the pustular form did not mutate after about seven years but just was a less successful pathogen.

The observations of Nicolò Leoniceno, fifteenth-century professor of medicine at Ferrara, humanist, and specialist in the philosophy of medicine, support this view. Leoniceno met with a group of learned men in a palace in Ferrara in 1497 to conduct the first formal discussion of the dreadful French sickness, *Morbus Gallicus*.[19] His remarks are especially useful because they were based on autopsies of those who died in Naples. In these post-mortems, Leoniceno found two discrete forms of disease, one exhibiting external sores and the other causing extreme pain in the joints and nerves with no outward sign. Autopsies of sufferers free of external lesions revealed internal abscesses, the reason, Leoniceno said, for the greater torment.

Leoniceno's written record of his observations asks and answers two questions: Why do sores initially appear on the genitals? Why do some sufferers experience more torment than others? A believer in the theory of bodily humors, Leoniceno observed that the genitals were more inclined to putrefaction because of their natural heat and humidity. He linked the disease to sexual transmission, giving as a reason the additional heat during copulation. Of course, he did not know that a pathogen was responsible. In answer to the second question Leoniceno proposed that although *Morbus Gallicus* was one generic disease, it had several species (or strains).

Sexual activity was riotous in Naples in 1495, with an invading army (accompanied by hundreds of prostitutes) mixing with a citizenry that quickly surrendered and joined in the revelry. The multinational army, aided by rapidly expanding commerce, brought to the party a full complement of diseases, both new and old. Hudson listed diseases rampant at the time: pneumonia, meningitis, smallpox, leprosy, typhus, and typhoid, "any of which might have occurred coincidentally with syphilis."[20] We might add measles, dysentery, and influenza, and note in passing that this complexity of pathogens occurred without the benefit of antibiotics. Hudson suggested that the short-lived, otherwise inexplicable virulence of the early disease might have been caused by the interaction of more than one pathogen in the immunologically compromised swamp that was Naples in 1495. It was his opinion that syphilis did not become milder after the brief initial period; rather, diagnosis became more accurate. Syphilologist Lloyd Thompson agreed that the new malady was "in all probability complicated by other diseases."[21] Karl Sudhoff, twentieth-century spokesman for the anti-American origin position, hypothesized that there was a typhus epidemic in Naples that confused the diagnosis at the time. Typhoid in this context is of particular note because it, too, had just been introduced to Spain and carried to Italy by soldiers who had been fighting in Cyprus. To complicate the picture further, a papal bull in 1490 had closed all the leper colonies, putting thousands of lepers, covered with lesions, on the streets.

Typhoid and louse-borne typhus may have arrived with the nine shiploads of Jews who sailed to Naples in August 1492 after being expelled from Spain by Ferdinand and Isabella when they refused to convert to Catholicism. The first ship sailed coincidentally as Columbus was leaving the same harbor—or was it coincidence? Simon Wiesenthal has hypothesized that Columbus was himself Jewish and had chosen that day to sail to avoid being expelled.[22]

Professor Leoniceno's early postmortem observations of two manifestations of syphilis—one shockingly visible, one clandestine—provide room in the debate about the origin of syphilis in Europe for both the European and the American positions. Perhaps treponemes were present in Europe from ancient times and gradually adapted to venereal transmission in a well-clothed population where soap was used, at least occasionally. Maybe the Spaniards did bring a syphilis-causing pathogen from Hispaniola. Maybe syphilis was only one factor in the epidemic along with typhus, leprosy, and all the other diseases of the time in the mobile, multinational, promiscuous marketplace of Naples.

The debate continues. In November 1993 a conference was held in Toulon to mark the five-hundred-year anniversary of the first recorded case of the Pox in Europe and to focus on the question that had been so passionately debated for five centuries: "Pox: Before or After 1493?" There, Louis J. André of the Institute of Tropical Medicine, Marseilles, posed this provocative question: "Was 'le mal de Naples' AIDS?"[23]

Can an answer to the Columbian question be found in the bones? As the origin debate rages on, paleo-anthropologists have dug on both sides of the Atlantic to unearth bones with the telltale scrimshaw patterns and sabre thickenings on the lower legs of adults and the characteristic notched teeth (known as Hutchinson's teeth, after the nineteenth-century syphilologist Jonathan Hutchinson) of children with congenital syphilis. Bone sleuths have been looking for an answer to the dilemma of the origin of syphilis since 1877, when Dr. J. Parrot began systematic investigation of supposed osseous syphilis from the Stone Age.

Syphilitic bones located in the New World, but not in Europe, from the fourteenth century tipped the scales in favor of the

Columbian origin until a rich find of damaged skeletons in a medieval monastery known as Blackfriars, in Hull, England, reopened the debate in June 2000, when researchers from the University of Bradford published a report. When carbon dating of the Blackfriars bones put their date between 1300 and 1420,[24] the popular press paraded headlines such as: "Columbus Didn't Do It." A Public Broadcasting Service special program, *The Enigma of Syphilis*,[25] explored the ramifications of the finding of pre-Columbian syphilitic bones in Europe.

Not so fast, says paleo-anthropologist Bruce Rothschild. First, he questions the validity of the Blackfriars findings, suggesting that those bones did not conform at all to the bones of syphilitics but belonged instead to victims of yaws, a nonvenereal spirochetal disease. Second, in October 2000, a few months after the PBS special aired, Bruce and Christine Rothschild (with two other authors)[26] published the results of their studies of pre-Columbian bones turned up in the Dominican Republic, the former Hispaniola, where Columbus and his men made camp in the New World, and found what they maintain is indisputable evidence of venereal syphilis.[27]

"That's the smoking gun," says Rothschild, presenting his proof that the bones in the Dominican Republic, unlike the Blackfriars bones, can be definitively identified as syphilitic.[28] "Thus, the fifteenth century Dominican Republic clearly provided the opportunity for contraction of syphilis by Columbus's crew."[29]

Rothschild also asserted: "While findings diagnostic of syphilis have been reported in the New World, actual demonstration of syphilis in areas where Columbus had contact was missing, until now."[30] More to the point, based on his findings in the Dominican Republic, Rothschild is convinced that "if Columbus got syphilis, it was certainly from his visits to the New World."[31]

Researchers will continue to debate when and how the first spirochete discovered a venereal pathway. Epidemiologists will track the couplings of Spaniards with Native Americans in the glorious new paradise. Paleo-anthropologists will go on lobbing bones at each other across the ocean. But the admiral's own bones will not weigh into the long debate about syphilis pre-Columbus or post-Columbus. They were transported to Seville and then back to Hispaniola. Some historians believe they were moved to another resting place in Havana in 1795, although it is possible that those bones belonged to one of his brothers or his son Diego, and that the bones of Christopher Columbus still rest where Bruce Rothschild and his colleagues are searching today. Spanish scientists are considering using DNA analysis to try to identify which bones belong to Columbus. Scholars may be wary of concluding that Columbus had syphilis, but if you ask a tour guide today at the Columbus monument in Santo Domingo, "Do you know how Columbus died?" the answer is likely to be, with a grin, "Si, syphilis."

A Brief History of the Spirochete

He first wore buboes dreadful to the sight
First felt strange pains and sleepless passed the night
From him the malady received its name
—FRACASTORO,
SYPHILUS SIVE MORBUS GALLICUS

SYPHILIS IS CAUSED BY AN ANCIENT MICROSCOPIC ORGANISM, a spirochete, also known as a treponeme. University of Massachusetts biologist Lynn Margulis has proposed that one hundred million years ago it densely populated the airtight guts of cockroaches.[1] She hypothesizes a controversial evolutionary theory: that wriggling, forward-moving spirochetes are the ancestral inspiration for the whiplike structures that provide locomotion to sperm tails of humans. Her still more daring claim: axons and dendrites that allow communication between cells of the brain descended billions of years ago from spirochetes as well. Others say that a few hundred thousand years ago the spirochete was a saprophyte, a creature that lived on dead and decayed matter.[2]

According to Ellis H. Hudson, around 15,000 B.C. the spirochete found a congenial host and became a parasite of humans in some hot climate, probably in Africa, by slipping through a cut in the warm, moist skin of a playing child. A rosy rash soon spread to other children in the village, then to other villages, and eventually to the populated world. A disease of one thousand names, it has been called variously yaws, bejel, pinta (the name of one of Columbus's ships), bubas, and frambesia.[3]

However mysterious the origin of the spirochete may be, and however uncertain its early relationship to humans, history records a specific event, the invasion of Naples by the French army of Charles VIII in 1495, as the natal moment (22 February 1495 at 4:00 P.M.) of the worldwide syphilis epidemic. Mercenary soldiers of various nationalities disbanded after that military adventure and returned to their homes, spreading the Pox throughout Europe and then to much of the rest of the world. It blazed through Italy and then into France and Germany, racing across the roads of Europe just as it did through the bloodstreams of the newly infected.

Within a decade all the countries of Europe had felt the sting of the dreadful disease. India received the novel contamination before the end of the century, possibly in 1498 as a result of Vasco da Gama's trip from Lisbon to Calcutta. From there it spread to China as the "Canton rash" and to Japan in 1512 as the "Chinese ulcer." Each country blamed its neighbor for the malevolent import. In Russia it was the Polish sickness, Poland blamed it on the Germans, and the Germans called it the "Spanish Itch," while the French and Italians blamed each other. Muslims blamed Christians. Catherine the Great of Russia later blamed the Americas (with faulty arithmetic): "Two hundred years are now elapsed since a disease unknown to our ancestors was imported from America and hurried on to the destruction of the human race. This disease spreads wide its mournful and destructive effects in many of our Provinces."[4] Voltaire called this Pox the "first fruit" gathered from the New World by the Spaniards. Conquistadors with virulent syphilis even introduced it to parts of the New World where it had been unknown.

Of course no one knew what caused the Pox, but there were many theories, such as the common potato, the American iguana, or the curse of God for illicit sex. Some blamed cannibalism, others the sexual union of a courtesan with a leper. Perhaps it was wafted through the air by the breeze from the batting of an eyelash. Astrologers claimed that a conjunction of Saturn and Jupiter at 6:04 P.M. on 25 November 1484 presaged this sexual plague. Unfavorably placed Mars combined with Saturn to overcome Jupiter, they wrote; chaos on earth resulted, with floods, earthquakes, wars, famines, and the dreadful venereal plague. Once the sexual cause and effect was confirmed, couples clung together in fearful monogamy to avoid bringing home the contagious, oval, hard, oozing ulceration with the red-varnished surface that marks the first stage of the disease. Sex became an ever more dangerous business as the number of dead rose into the millions. Virginity took on new value.

In 1530 the physician Girolamo Fracastoro composed a 1,300-line Latin poem, *Syphilus sive morbus gallicus,* about the Pox. Fracastoro, a physicist, astronomer, geologist, and philosopher of medicine (and classmate of Copernicus at Padua), postulated the existence of germs when he suggested tiny invisible living things as the cause of disease. Like most others by that time, he believed the Pox came from Hispaniola. His poem told the story of a shepherd named Syphilus who cursed the sun and destroyed altars when Apollo sent a drought that killed the king's sheep. Fracastoro's germ theory was proven true when the microscope made possible the viewing of tiny pathogens. The organism that causes the Pox was finally seen with the human eye in 1905 when a twenty-five-year-old woman from Berlin, complaining of skin lesions and headaches, consulted a doctor, Erich Hoffmann, who found a genital sore on her right labium. He excised a small eroded papule and sent the specimen to his colleague, Fritz Schaudinn, a specialist in the parasites of ducks and owls, under whose microscope a pale, twisted creature appeared. (See Figure 3.1.)

Schaudinn gave his discovery two names, *Treponema pallidum* and *Spirochaeta pallida,* the first being correct from a taxonomic viewpoint, although in popular usage it is more often referred to as a spirochete. Eleven days later, he examined a specimen from a lesion of a fifty-eight-year-old widow, and again the long, thin organism appeared. By the end of the month the two doctors had found eleven such cases.

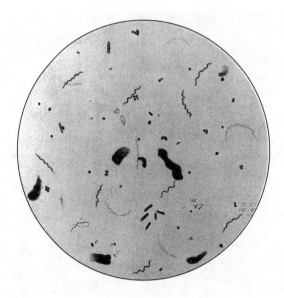

Figure 3.1 *Treponema pallidum* as first seen by Fritz Schaudinn and Erich Hoffmann in 1905 (New York Academy of Medicine Library)

The silvery organism Schaudinn observed undulating relentlessly from one side of the microscope slide to the other had a snakelike shape and was about the length of the diameter of a red blood cell, 4 to 20 microns, and .1 to .2 microns wide, with six to twenty-four evenly spaced spirals tapered at both ends. To put size in perspective, the diameter of the round retrovirus HIV is .1 micron while the E. Coli bacterium is 1-2 microns long. Beneath the outer membrane six endoflagella, its source of mobility, wind around an inner cell, giving it a corkscrew appearance. It moves three ways: with a rapid spinning motion on the long axis, with a forward and backward movement, and with a lateral bending motion. (See Figure 3.2.)

The spirochete reproduces by dividing in half lengthwise once every thirty to thirty-three hours, at least during the active infection; afterwards, it divides more slowly, perhaps only once every six months. Social historian Christopher Wills calculated that in the time it would take one spirochete to divide in the infectious period, E. coli would have reproduced itself 10^{27} times.

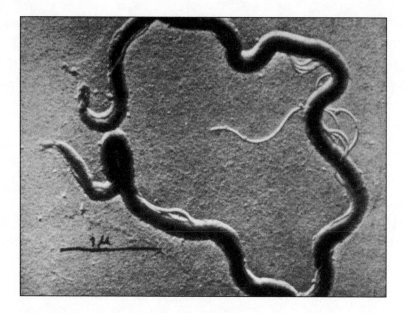

Figure 3.2   *Treponema pallidum,* the syphilis spirochete (Corbis)

Almost a century after Fritz Schaudinn first spotted the syphilis spirochete, it was revealed in even more exquisite detail. On 17 July 1998 *Science* magazine published the "Complete Genome Sequence of *Treponema pallidum,* the Syphilis Spirochete," the result of a joint project of the Institute for Genomic Research in Rockville, Maryland, and the University of Texas Health Science Center in Houston. Together the researchers found 1,138,006 base pairs containing 1,041 predicted coding sequences in the syphilis spirochete. This information gives biologists hope of someday creating a vaccine.

A definitive bone test to differentiate syphilis from yaws (a nonvenereal treponemal disease) would solve the mystery of the skeletons of the Blackfriars monks and put to rest the question of whether there were syphilitic bones in Europe prior to Columbus's return from the New World. That test may not be far away. Since the gene mapping, the Houston scientists have compared this gene with that of the organism that causes yaws and have found four areas with noticeable differences. Now they are wondering if they can isolate the bacterial DNA from the bones that Rothschild and the others have found at Columbus's original site on Hispaniola as another way of definitively identifying syphilis.[5]

Despite the scientific discoveries, *T. pallidum* remains mysterious. Little is known about it in comparison with other bacterial pathogens. It cannot be cultured continuously. Existing diagnostic tests are less than optimal. Even after treatment with penicillin some patients harbor spirochetes in "treponemal sanctuaries" such as the eye and the lymph glands. Many of the details of its life cycle remain unanswered. And the interaction of the syphilis spirochete with the more recent sexually transmitted killer, HIV/AIDS, remains highly controversial.[6] *T. pallidum* still chooses the human being as its only host. It has not become resistant to penicillin. Yet it persists.

4

Shedding Light on the Poison of the Darkness

> What you done in the dark sure come to the light.
>
> —Nurse Eunice Rivers
> quoting a Tuskegee Syphilis Study subject

In 1520, when the Pox had been spreading from the epicenter of Naples for several decades, Erasmus declared it to be the most dangerous of all illnesses: "If I were asked which amongst all the diseases kills the most people I would reply that it is this sickness. . . . It alone combines all that is dreadful in the other contagions."[1] The new sexual plague was relentless.

Occasionally a malignant syphilis with deep ulcerating lesions could still be found centuries later displaying the full visual horror and rapid progression that was seen in Naples. The nineteenth-century French poet (and friend of Charles Baudelaire) Théophile Gautier observed an unhappy French army occupying Rome:

> There is a splendid American pox here, as pure as at the time of
> Francis I. The entire French army has been laid up with it; boils
> are exploding in groins like shells, and purulent jets of clap vie

with the fountains in the Piazza Navona . . . tibias are exfoliat-
ing in extoses like ancient columns of greenery in a Roman
ruin . . . lieutenants walking in the streets look like leopards,
they are so dotted and speckled with roseola, freckles, coffee-
coloured marks, warty excrescences, horny and cryptogamic
verruccae and other secondary and tertiary manifestations
which appear here after a fortnight.[2]

But this rapidly progressing syphilis was rare. For the most
part, after the initial chancre and rash had cleared up, the disease
only showed such lesions when it relapsed during the first few
years. Other than that, it was invisible and therefore secret, and although the victim was often dreadfully sick much of the time and
complained of feeling poisoned, the aches and pains were rarely
attributed to syphilis. The successful parasite did not kill its host
quickly, and because an attractive host, one without oozing lesions, has a better chance of providing sexual transmission, it continued to find new lovers to shock with its terrifying first sign. It
was this silent disease that perplexed and fascinated the medical
community in the nineteenth century when scientific research
dedicated itself to understanding, treating, and seeking a cure for
it. Syphilology became a respectable, challenging branch of medicine.

In their eagerness and desperation to understand this disease
and find medical breakthroughs, syphilologists often suspended
conventions of medical ethics. Inoculation experiments involved
felons and prostitutes, the most likely subjects, but also servants,
and even children and infants. Harvesting mucous pus from the
large supply of readily available sores, doctors began to inject anything and everything living: themselves, their students, chim-
panzees, monkeys, horses, rabbits, cats, and rats.

Philippe Ricord, the most famous syphilologist of the mid-
nineteenth century, was one of the major offenders in this inoculation frenzy. Ricord was physician to many well-known people,
including Napoleon III. The indefatigable journal-keeper Jules de
Goncourt observed that at one Pox per medal, the row of ribbons

on Ricord's chest was not reassuring for the state of the "crowned phalluses." Baltimore-born Ricord's house on the rue de Tournon in Paris had five waiting rooms, and he boasted of the great number of syphilitics he had treated in the course of his career. He was famous for wisecracks such as: In the beginning God created the heavens, the earth, man, and venereal diseases.

Many of the rich and famous spread the disease because of Ricord's persistent denial of the infectiousness of the secondary stage, long after it had been established. When he began using the vaginal speculum (which had been used at least since Roman times), prostitutes quickly named it "the hospital's penis." Doctors were then able to find syphilitic chancres in the vagina more easily, but not in "proper" women who could not be examined unclothed. Any doctor bold enough to get on his knees and reach under a skirt risked contracting the famous "physician's chancre" on his finger and joining his patients getting rubbed with salve made from toxic mercury.

The eminent Boston physician Oliver Wendell Holmes Sr. parodied Ricord as "the Voltaire of pelvic medicine" who would have submitted even the vestal virgins themselves to a course of his little blue mercury pills. The vestal virgins might indeed have needed the little blue pills if Ricord had gotten his hands on them. One of his experiments (1835–1838) involved the inoculation of 2,500 people (including Paris prostitutes) with gonorrheal pus to prove that syphilis and gonorrhea were distinct diseases. Since syphilis often accompanied gonorrhea and since prostitutes were the most likely population to spread the disease from fresh infection, not to mention that they were quite unlikely to have been enthusiastic volunteers, this experiment qualifies as one of the more unethical in medical history. Ricord's *Traité pratique des maladies vénériennes,* published in 1838, documents hundreds of such inoculations.

Ricord's favorite student, Alfred Fournier, had a philosophy of experimentation different from his professor's. Fournier was anticipating discussion of the ethical issues of human experimentation and informed consent when he wrote: "We should not use the lancet on a healthy subject; if the doctor wishes to study and verify a scientific fact he must choose himself as the experimental subject, not a patient who entrusts himself to his care. . . . There is particular cause for concern when research has been attempted without their [the subjects] having been informed of the nature of the disease with which they were being infected."[3]

Despite Fournier's passionate admonition, physicians continued to use humans experimentally because animals remained resistant to infection, at least until 28 July 1903, when the infected clitoris of a two-year-old chimpanzee was proudly displayed to enthusiastic onlookers during a medical lecture at the Academy of Medicine in Paris. A month later she developed secondary lesions. There the experiment ended, since tertiary syphilis develops only in the human.

Albert Neisser, a dermatologist who discovered *gonococcus* as a cause of gonorrhea, set up a laboratory in Java where he successfully inoculated over a thousand monkeys with syphilis. The medical enthusiasm attending the first infected chimpanzee derived in no small part from the hope that test animals might replace humans. This would have appealed especially to Neisser, who in 1895 had injected a group of young prostitutes—the youngest was aged ten—with a syphilis serum, trying to provide immunity. When many of them showed signs of syphilis, the failed experiment became a public scandal, possibly the only inoculation project to draw public censure.

Syphilis often appeared to be cured after the initial chancre and fever passed. Infected young men often bragged as if the Pox were an initiation of sorts that would leave them in full health with at most a small penile scar as a souvenir. But most did not regain full health. Many astute physicians observed the pattern of relapsing illness that followed the first infection and surmised that syphilis was responsible.

By careful observation, two physicians finally identified syphilis as a lifelong disease and the cause of the wide variety of miseries that plagued those supposedly cured. Alfred Fournier established the full pattern of progressing syphilis when he was able to show that insanity and paralysis occurring decades after the first infection were related to the earlier chancre and fever. And Jonathan Hutchinson revealed the many illnesses that syphilis simulates, giving it a name that has lasted until today: "The Great Imitator."

An American-born French physician (like his mentor Ricord), Fournier devoted his life to the study of syphilis. In his clinical practice, he noticed over time that patients with the painful, paralytic condition known as locomotor ataxia, later named tabes dorsalis, had a history of syphilis, more than could be accounted for by chance. Although he gained acceptance in 1876 for the theory that this condition was syphilitic, when in 1879 he noted a similar pattern with paresis (general paralysis of the insane, or dementia paralytica), many psychiatrists were unwilling to take the leap because of a prejudice that the brain was impervious to syphilis. By 1884 the official dictionary of medical science listed such symptoms of tertiary syphilis as delusions of wealth and grandeur, violent fits of mania, disruption of movement, and impairment of speech. However, Fournier's published papers continued to stir up spirited opposition from those who found that the long decades between early infection and later insanity required too great a leap of faith.[4]

It may be that no one before Fournier was able to make this connection because the brain had previously been impervious to syphilis. Psychiatrist P. J. Möbius observed that in the eighteenth century no famous person died of any illness like dementia paralytica, whereas in the nineteenth century there were numerous examples. In a 1959 article, E. Hare proposed that sometime at the end of the eighteenth century, *T. pallidum* underwent a mutation that enabled it to invade the central nervous system. This new strain, he suggested, was rapidly spread throughout Europe by Napoleon's armies. On 14 September 2002, a *New York Times* article revealed a discovery of skeletons of soldiers from Napoleon's army who froze to death in Vilnius, Lithuania, after the disastrous siege of Moscow in 1812. Scientists at the site report several of these skeletons showed signs of advanced syphilis. If that is true, could these men have been carriers of Hare's hypothesized new strain of neurotropic syphilis? His well-documented article lends scientific support to the long-held popular idea that syphilis could be linked to genius in certain cases in the nineteenth century, but not before.[5]

What happened to the spirochete after the secondary infection resolved? Did it remain in the tissues? This core question was finally answered in 1913 when Noguchi made his discovery of spirochetes in a paretic brain, officially validating Fournier's hypothesized link between syphilis and paresis. Fournier, who saw syphilis as a serious threat to the human race, became eloquent in his crusade for mandatory hospitalization of syphilitics, police assistance in tracking down sexual partners, and control and treatment of prostitutes. Much of current public health policy is the legacy of his efforts to stop the syphilis epidemic.

In 1879, the same year that Fournier linked insanity to late-stage syphilis, Jonathan Hutchinson (who dedicated his text on syphilis to Fournier) delivered a speech, "Syphilis as an Imitator," to the British Medical Association. The son of a Quaker businessman, Hutchinson entered medicine as a surgeon. But having a generalist's mind and an exceptional memory, he studied other areas of medicine, specifically dermatology, leprosy, diseases of the eye and the central nervous system—and syphilis. From a lifetime of observation he was able to catalogue the many diseases that syphilis imitates and to write a textbook of syphilis using case histories and treatment protocols that was to serve for decades as a key source of information about diagnosis and treatment.

Hutchinson's speech, printed in the *British Medical Journal*, marked a turning point in the history of syphilis study and became the basis for teaching about syphilis in medical schools. Moving methodically from one organ system to another, he listed disease states for which he had found a syphilitic double, encouraging doctors to look for a history of syphilis behind symptoms that would otherwise appear to be another disease. His list of examples included smallpox, measles, psoriasis, lupus vulgaris, iritis, and epilepsy. The discovery of this "general law of imitation or simulation" gave him a clear picture of how illness manifests in various forms with no apparent connection to the primary disease. Thus he bridged the gap between initial infection and the late stages of syphilis described by Fournier, showing that the chronic pain and a wide variety of illnesses in the years following initial infection were caused by syphilis.

Six years after Hutchinson's address, R. W. Taylor published *The Pathology and Treatment of Venereal Diseases*, a meticulous catalogue of the effects of syphilis on every cell of the body. Taylor exempted only the crystalline lens of the eye from the harmful effects of syphilis during the decades after the initial infection, although he did note that secondary cataracts can occur and that the capsule of the eye is sometimes involved.

An Italian physician, Giovanni Maria Lancisi, had linked syphilis to aortic aneurysm in 1728, but the link was not firmly established until 1875, when Francis H. Welch, a British army surgeon, found that about two-thirds of the records of fifty-three cases of rupturing aortic aneurysm had a previous history of syphilis. Autopsy confirmed his hypothesis when he was able to distinguish changes in the great vessels of syphilitic patients from those of non-syphilitics.

After Jonathan Hutchinson linked the disease states occurring during the middle stage of syphilis to the early manifestations, Welch showed that syphilis caused aortic damage, and Fournier completed the picture with the paralysis and insanity of tertiary syphilis, physicians were able to expand the range of inquiry to put together the progression of the disease over a lifetime, greatly aiding diagnosis. They now were able to see visceral syphilis, cardiac syphilis, diseases of the bones and nerves, and psychiatric and paralytic complaints as part of the general syphilitic carnage.

In everyday practice, however, syphilis often evaded diagnosis. Many doctors interviewing patients with untreated syphilis did not step back to view their patients' life histories in a context that would prompt a question about a sore that might have appeared and disappeared decades before, or a fever of no apparent lasting consequence. When faced with a syphilis that seemed to be a clear case of something else—rheumatism, arthritis, gout,[6] eczema, hypertension, epilepsy, headache, stomachache, jaundice, mania, depression, dementia, schizophrenia, deafness, or just plain "nerves"—as often as not the condition presenting itself to the doctor's eye and hand was taken for the disease to be treated, and the Great Imitator lurked silently undiscovered (and untreated) in the background.

Patients would see doctor after doctor, take fanciful and often ghastly remedies, and finally humbly accept a diagnosis of hypochondriasis. Because syphilis was not infectious after the first few years (very infectious for the first two years after infection, less so after that, and rarely after five, although Jonathan Hutchinson conservatively opted for seven),[7] there was even more reason to think it had disappeared.

The nineteenth century closed with the pale spirochete still eluding detection and no cure in sight, but after Fournier and Hutchinson it was possible to see it in the entirety of its progression over decades, from chancre and rash through damage to all parts of the body, and finally to paralysis, madness, and violent cardiac death. The course of syphilis was mapped out in a way that would reveal it to those diagnosticians clever enough to see the pattern of a disease that imitates other diseases with no distinguishing signs or symptoms of its own.

Researchers at the beginning of the twentieth century accepted the premise that syphilis was a relapsing lifelong disease. Although both European and American scientists dedicated themselves to finding a cure, the Americans took the lead in collecting and analyzing data. Numerous experiments were conducted to further understand the many signs and symptoms of syphilis and to refine the treatment protocols. All this observation and tabulation would provide the clinician with guidelines for administering the toxic chemicals (early chemotherapy) that controlled but did not cure, thereby reducing the effects of the disease with minimal hardship for the patient.

Syphilis became more of an international issue when World War I accelerated its spread. Because of the false belief that it was hereditary, this proliferation caused grave concern, and Fournier's warnings that the future of the human race was at stake were taken with new seriousness. After the war, the League of Nations (precursor of the United Nations) took on the challenge of coordinating syphilis research internationally. A spin-off project in the United States, known as the the "Cooperating Clinical Group," published numerous studies between 1928 and 1942, including an early report that examined 3,244 cases of syphilis. Four U.S. universities—Johns Hopkins, the University of Pennsylvania, the University of Michigan, and Western Reserve—participated, along with the Mayo Clinic, all under the direction of the Public Health Service.

As patients filled waiting rooms and lined up around the block for their shots of Salvarsan, the new drug based on organic arsenic developed by Paul Ehrlich in 1910, clinicians kept records of the subtleties of the disease and the success of various treatments. The pooled information resulted in vast amounts of data. Textbooks full of statistics rolled off the presses, citing studies involving thousands of patients.[8]

John Stokes's lavishly illustrated *Modern Clinical Syphilology* (first printed in 1926) with its 1,332 pages of small print, was one of the more useful texts. Like Hutchinson before him, Stokes provided the clinician with a wide variety of case studies, each with its unique diagnostic challenge. In boxes set off from the text, he listed signs and symptoms followed by a brief and readable discussion, usually noting with obvious relish how he had confirmed a diagnosis missed by numerous colleagues. A professor of dermatology and syphilology at the University of Pennsylvania, Stokes was also active with the League of Nations. In 1944 he published a final edition with the collaboration of colleagues, including information about the new wonder drug penicillin[9] and data from many studies including those of the Cooperating Clinical Group.

Because patients were treated as soon as they were diagnosed, what was missing from the burgeoning scientific literature was a study of progressing, untreated disease over a lifetime. That void was filled between 1890 and 1910, when Caesar Broeck, chief of the venereal clinic at University Hospital in Oslo, Norway, withheld mercury treatment from 2,181 patients with early syphilis based on his belief that toxic medications interfered with the body's own healing power. When Salvarsan became available in 1910, Broeck attested to its effectiveness by administering treatment to those in his study who could still be found.

Beginning in 1925, Broeck's successor, E. Bruusgaard, tracked down 473 patients who had not returned for the Salvarsan treatments and compared them to the treated group. His subjects had four times the neurosyphilis and twenty-six times the bone and skin lesions, suggesting that Salvarsan, although not a cure, did improve the long-term outlook. In 1955 Trygve Gjestland published a comprehensive review, *The Oslo Study of Untreated Syphilis.* Because many of the patients had been lost for the middle years of disease and because the focus was retrospective, this widely read study understated the complex illnesses that follow the early infection.

That problem was accentuated in the next study of untreated syphilis. What was still missing in the literature was a prospective study, that is, one that observed the natural history of untreated syphilis as it developed over the long term. In 1932 the Public Health Service began a project that was originally planned to last six months, to study syphilis in the black community. It continued for forty years—the longest nontherapeutic human medical experiment in history. It was an ill-conceived bureaucratic nightmare on autopilot that would eventually blow up in the press and begin a series of discussions that would set new guidelines for human experimentation. It was called "The Tuskegee Study of Untreated Syphilis in the Negro Male."[10]

THE TUSKEGEE SYPHILIS STUDY

Joseph Earle Moore of the Johns Hopkins University School of Medicine, author of a key text, *The Modern Treatment of Syphilis,*[11] and "a giant in the exploratory field" according to his colleague

John Stokes, was an early consultant on the Tuskegee Study. (Of parenthetical note, Moore was the doctor who administered malaria treatment to Al Capone for his tertiary syphilis.) The experiment was designed to track untreated syphilis in the impoverished and illiterate rural population of sharecroppers in Macon County, Alabama, where there was an especially high rate of syphilis. Forty thousand people had been tested for syphilis in six counties; the overall rate of infection was estimated at 25 percent. In Macon County it was 36 percent.

Being male, having a positive Wassermann syphilis test, and remembering the date of the original chancre were the criteria for inclusion in the program. Excluding syphilitics who had experienced a mild initial infection (no memory of a chancre) might have been a mistake. Some syphilologists had contended for years that those who developed severe tertiary neurosyphilis often had experienced a very mild initial infection and could not recall the initial chancre, fever, or rash, whereas those who had a gross lesion and severe subsequent infection often had a milder outcome. By mandating that only those who could clearly recall the date of the chancre be included, the study may have been skewed against severe late-stage neurosyphilis. Of the final group selected, 399 had syphilis; a control group consisted of 201 healthy men. On Moore's advice, careful histories of the subjects were taken at the outset, along with chest X rays and electrocardiograms. He provided a list of fifteen signs to look for in the physical examination.

Although it was supposed to be a study of untreated syphilitics, from the beginning that claim was slippery. Some, if not all, were slathered with mercury after the project began, thus receiving more treatment than people in the community who were not in the project. Just how "untreated" these men were is made clear in a letter from Dr. Vonderlehr of the Public Health Service requesting supplies of mercury and arsenic. Three hundred patients would require mercury treatment, he said, for eighteen weeks, at fourteen doses per week. That would come to 75,000 doses, or three hundred pounds of oleate of mercury. He also asked for six hundred grams of arsenic to supplement the existing supply. Over the years, many subjects received sporadic treatment elsewhere, which may have been more damaging than no treatment at all. Anyone in the control group who became infected was just shuffled to the other side of the experiment. At thirty years into the study, 96 percent of the "untreated" subjects who were still alive had received some treatment.

The collecting of the steady stream of blood samples flowing to the Centers for Disease Control was very well organized. Groups of government public health doctors visited Tuskegee annually and took blood samples daily over several weeks. The trip to Tuskegee was called "the roundup"; one doctor even spoke of "corralling" the subjects. In the later years, going to Tuskegee was a perk of sorts for the younger public health officers, who for the most part had little clinical experience and limited knowledge of the progression of untreated syphilis.

The Tuskegee study was not based on a doctor/patient relationship but rather on a researcher/subject model. It produced blood samples and autopsy reports. Dr. John Heller, medical director of the Venereal Diseases Division of the Public Health Service, pointed out that although the doctors were concerned with obtaining the most efficient examinations possible, there were six hundred men to test: "While they tried to give each patient the personal interest he desired, this was not always possible due to the pressure of time. Occasionally the patient was annoyed because the doctor did not pay attention to his particular complaint."[12] Language was an additional problem: the local dialect was not easily understood by the visiting doctors.

A more callous statement of how little interest was taken in the men's progressing syphilis was made by Dr. Oliver Clarence Wenger, one of the early planners of the study. He complained that when Eunice Rivers, the public health nurse who was with the project for all forty years, drove down the long country dirt roads to visit the men, she was just wasting gas. To a colleague he wrote: "As I see it, we have no further interest in these patients until they die."[13]

Eunice Rivers, who was in the best position to observe the many painful conditions that her patients inevitably were experiencing over the years as a result of syphilis, had received no training in syphilology. When she was hired and expressed concern that her lack of knowledge of syphilis would be a detriment, she was told it would not be necessary for what she had to do. So the men of the Tuskegee Syphilis Study suffered the pain of a life of syphilis without medical attention or understanding. Although the gross signs of the progression of syphilis were periodically recorded, the more subtle and relapsing illnesses of middle-period syphilis were ignored.

The Tuskegee Study might have continued until the last man was dead, but in 1966 Peter Buxtun, a young venereal disease interviewer/investigator for the Public Health Service in San Francisco, overheard talk in a lunchroom about a patient who had been treated for late syphilis but should not have been because he was part of a study. Buxton requested a thick file from the Centers for Disease Control on the Tuskegee project. What he found led him to ask some tough questions about the ethics of this study, in particular, why penicillin was not administered to the men when it became available in the late 1940s. Draft boards had even been contacted to get the men exempted from enlistment during World War II so that they would not be treated. Although penicillin would not have reversed the syphilitic damage done so far, it would have curtailed further progression of the disease.

Buxtun, whose family had fled Prague in 1938 when he was nine months old, reread the proceedings of the Nuremberg War Crimes Tribunal having to do with human experimentation and took some tough questions to the Public Health Service.[14] Ignored and then rebuffed when he posed his questions, Buxtun finally took what he had found to the Associated Press in 1972. The story broke to public outrage and pandemonium. In March 1973 the experiment was officially halted, and the U.S. Senate began hearings on human experimentation. Buxtun testified before the Senate Health, Education, and Welfare subcommittee chaired by Senator Ted Kennedy.

As the Tuskegee story unraveled and became a topic of household conversation, officials at the Public Health Service were baffled and dismayed as they saw themselves compared in the press to Nazi doctors, condemned for not getting informed consent, and accused of everything from injecting patients with syphilis (as their predecessors had done in the nineteenth century) to planned genocide. Dr. Wenger had said in 1932 that the study would cover them with mud or glory when completed.[15] It proved to be an enormous mud bath.

In 1974 syphilologist Rudolph Kampmeier (author of the 1943 text *Essentials of Syphilology*) published an article attempting to put some of the issues into perspective. He pointed out that the informed consent idea was an anachronism, testily asking, who informed the 35,000 patients who took penicillin before animal studies were complete when the country was at war?[16] He observed that the inflammatory headlines "probably reinforced the ignorance of many physicians about the natural history of this chronic granulomatous self-limiting disease."[17]

Eventually, a lawsuit was filed; the final award was $10 million (each living syphilis patient received $37,500). More than two decades later, on 16 May 1997, President Bill Clinton made a public apology acknowledging the government's shame to the eight surviving subjects from the Tuskegee study. The youngest man was eighty-seven years old.

"In all, the majority of the men were unscathed by their syphilis."[18]

Unscathed?

This opinion was expressed in a 1993 article ("Deadly Medicine," by freelance writer Tom Junod) about the Tuskegee fiasco. Unless the men of Tuskegee were different from all syphilitics since the time of Columbus, they had the usual complaints of headaches, muscle and joint pain, skin lesions, iritis, severe gastrointestinal pain, and general miseries that characterize the progression of the disease. And yet, this fallacious idea that the men did not suffer from their (untreated) disease is one of the many sad legacies of Tuskegee. In 1992, Sid Olansky, one of the last of the syphilologists associated with Tuskegee, made a statement to ten million people on *Prime Time Live* television. Said Dr. Sid (smiling, perhaps nervously): "Syphilis was not such a bad disease."[19]

Based on an overview of the many syphilis studies done under the auspices of the universities participating in the Cooperative Clinic Group of the early twentieth century, as well as his own extensive clinical experience, Joseph Earle Moore concluded that *eight out of ten people* experienced the miserable relapsing progression of syphilis after the initial infection. The generally held idea that only one-third of syphilis patients progress to tertiary disease is probably a vast understatement. For example, many studies show more than 50 percent of syphilis patients at autopsy show syphilitic damage to the heart, and that is just one manifestation of tertiary disease. The statistics from Tuskegee, muddled at best, are often cited in lieu of the more carefully controlled syphilis experiments taking place at that time in the university medical centers, and the splendid old texts with their wealth of data are out of print.

In more recent times, volunteer prisoners at Sing Sing penitentiary who had previously been treated for syphilis with penicillin were reinoculated in a 1956 experiment harking back to the nineteenth century.[20] And in 1986, Dr. Stephen Caiazza, who had tested positive for HIV, experimentally inoculated himself with syphilis to provide serum as a control for an experiment. After about two weeks he had a skin lesion, followed by extreme colitis, "horrible" depression, and inability to concentrate. He was treated with penicillin.[21]

The men in the Tuskegee experiment were never told they had syphilis. The doctors used the vernacular "bad blood." But the men knew they had a venereal disease. In an interview, Eunice Rivers recalled a man who said: "'What you done in the dark sure come to the light.' . . . I sure loved the expression of those folks [laughs]. So they knew. So they knew. But the word 'syphilis' was not used."[22]

5

From Poisonous Cures to Wonder Drug (Almost)

WHEN THE POX DEVASTATED EUROPE IN THE LATE fifteenth century, physicians tried everything they could think of to alleviate the agonies of their patients using remedies that were often as bad as the ailment or worse. Charlatans promised quick cures to desperate and gullible sufferers. Inventive methods of sexual protection gave an illusion of safety to those who braved the venereal terror, and equally creative and bizarre folk remedies promised relief when protective devices failed. (See Table 5.1 for key dates in the history of syphilis.)

Men were told to be sure after engaging in risky sex to wrap the endangered organ for hours in a piece of cloth soaked in wine, shavings of guaiac, flakes of copper, precipitated mercury, gentian root, red coral, ash of ivory, and burnt horn of deer—elaborate shopping for an evening of pleasure. If a chancre did appear, the ulcerated part was to be covered with a spider's web and a band of violet fabric. Other unhelpful early remedies included binding the base of the penis to prevent the disease from traveling to the rest of the body—useless because infection becomes systemic within hours—or excising the sore. More benign remedies included bloodletting, leeches, purging, special diets, hydrotherapy, and

TABLE 5.1   Key Dates

1492	Columbus sails to the New World.
1493	The first outbreak of the Pox in Europe.
1495	Charles VIII and his army spread the disease from Naples.
1497	Mercury is first used as a treatment for the new disease.
1530	Fracastoro publishes his poem about the shepherd Syphilus.
1834	Wallace introduces potassium iodide.
1864	Rollet's glassblowers of Lyon demonstrate the infectiousness of saliva.
1875	Francis Welch discovers link between syphilis and aortic aneurysm.
1876	Fournier posits the syphilitic origin of tabes dorsalis.
1879	Fournier posits the syphilitic origin of general paralysis of the insane.
1879	Hutchinson delivers his "Great Imitator" address to the British Medical Society.
1905	Schaudinn and Hoffmann view and name *Treponema pallidum*.
1907	August von Wassermann perfects his test.
1909	Paul Ehrlich discovers the arsenical Salvarsan.
1913	Noguchi and Moore discover a spirochete in a syphilitic brain.
1927	Julius von Wagner-Jauregg wins the Nobel Prize for malaria therapy.
1943	Mahoney, Arnold, and Harris treat four cases of syphilis with penicillin.
1998	Scientists decode the syphilis gene.
2001	Rothschild et al. confirm syphilis bones on Hispaniola prior to Columbus.

electric stimulation. In 1665 a rumor that syphilis could ward off an approaching plague led men to storm the Paris brothels.

Beginning in the seventeenth century it was believed that disease could be transferred out of the body by intercourse with a healthy virgin of either sex, and many children were infected as a result.[1] The myth still survives today. On 22 May 2000 the *San Francisco Chronicle* reported: "Some of the growing number of child rapes [in South Africa] are attributed to an alarming urban myth that the government is doing very little to counteract—that a man can cure himself of HIV if he has sex with a virgin." Families buy expensive insurance for their children to pay for AIDS medications in case infection results from one of these encounters.

Mercurial remedies were developed by the alchemist Paracelsus (1493–1541) in an attempt to find the "Elixir Vitae," a substance that would purify the body of all disease. Gold, which neither rusts nor tarnishes and is the color of the sun, source of life and energy, was amalgamated with mercury derived from blood-red colored cinnabar ore. Mercury, which had for centuries been used by the Arabs to treat leprosy and yaws, was first used in Europe for the treatment of syphilis in 1497. Hawkers of remedies, or quacksalvers (those who quacked about their salves), promising speedy and complete cures, became known as "quacks," the pejorative aspect deriving in particular from those itinerant vendors who pushed toxic mercury salve, known as quicksilver or quacksilver, for the treatment of syphilis. Reputable physicians also used mercury as their main treatment; this chemotherapy was still found to be "the most potent weapon of attack on syphilis"[2] well into the twentieth century.

Mercury, a shiny element with the chemical symbol Hg, weighs 13.6 times as much as an equal volume of water. Iron, stone, and lead can float on its surface. Physicians who applied mercury-based ointments reported a lessening of their patients' pain and clearing of ulcers, but they tended to use such enormous quantities of the toxic metal that a price was paid in physical side

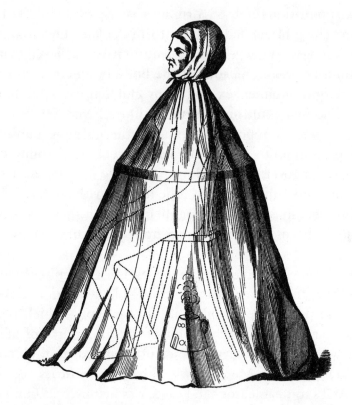

Figure 5.1 Woman seated over mercury pot.

effects, including new ulceration, dermatological eruptions, paralysis, shaking, anorexia, gastric distress, diarrhea, nausea, and rotting and loosening of teeth. The syphilitic overdosed with mercury would experience unquenchable thirst even while producing gushing saliva measured in pints and quarts, often while being encased in a steam box daily for a month. A hot iron applied to the skull to curtail salivation when absorbing vast quantities of mercury was one of the tortures these patients endured. Alchemists who distilled the quicksilver from heated cinnabar mixed the liquid metal with henna and herbs and heated it in a dry vessel over coals. The patient sat over a skillet under a cloak and inhaled the fumes. (See Figure 5.1.)

Today, when dentists debate whether people are wise to have mercury amalgam fillings removed to prevent trace amounts of mercury escaping into the system, mercury applied to the point of extreme salivation seems unconscionable and illustrates how desperate the early practitioners were to find a cure for the hideous malady. How to kill the spirochete without killing the patient or causing damage as serious as that of the original illness was the challenge facing the first doctors treating syphilis. Oncologists today face a similar challenge with chemotherapy.

Mercury added diagnostic confusion when it produced symptoms that also mimicked other diseases or even the syphilis itself. How, for example, could a doctor distinguish the neurological damage of tertiary syphilis from the neurological damage of mercury poisoning? Or mercury paralysis from that of tabes? It was thought that mercury could cause deafness, but so could syphilis.

When the "little blue pill," also known as the small-dose gray powder pill, took the place of salve as a way of dispensing mercury in the middle of the eighteenth century, syphilitics had a treatment that was easily administered and allowed them to keep their mortifying secret. They no longer gleamed with a blue sheen or smelled like a fried potato. Mercury pills contained rosewater, honey, licorice, and conserve of rose petals. During many years of practice, Jonathan Hutchinson found "warm advocates" of treatment with the gray powder pill when the dose was kept continuous, frequent, and small. He recommended one grain of powder every six, four, three, or even two hours according to circumstances, and found that one pill four times a day was sufficient to clear up a chancre or a secondary eruption. He forbade fresh fruits and vegetables and fresh air during treatment. He specifically advised against treatment to the point of salivation except in extreme cases.

Hutchinson believed that those who had kept to long regimens of mercury were less apt than others to develop tertiary symptoms. Irregular and excessive mercurial treatment would jeopardize health, but there would be no loss to general health, Hutchinson promised, if mercury were employed in the way suggested over a long enough time. In cases where there were premonitory symptoms of late syphilis, Hutchinson even advocated a lifelong course. In the early stages, mercury destroyed the parasite, Hutchinson maintained, while in later years it was useful against inflammatory damage. John Stokes also testified to an extraordinary factor of safety combined with therapeutic effectiveness after treating some ten thousand patients who had taken hundreds of thousands of mercury rubs in his clinic.

If some thought that only mercury in abundance cured, the founder of homeopathy, Samuel Hahnemann, proposed the opposite: to cure syphilis with infinitesimal doses. His student Hartmann wrote: "In that stage of the Syphilitic disease, where the Chancre or the Bubo is yet existing, one single dose of the best *mercurial* preparation is sufficient to effect a permanent cure of the internal disease, together with the Chancre in the space of a fortnight." As to the dose, "I was formerly in the habit of using successfully 1, 2 or 3 globules of the billionth degree, i.e., the 6th centesimal dilution, for the cure of Syphilis. The higher the degrees, however, even the decillionth (the 30th) acts more thoroughly, more speedily and more mildly. If more than one dose should be required, which is seldom the case, the lower degrees may be then employed."[3] Hahnemann claimed that he had never seen syphilis breaking out in the system when the chancre had been cured by homeopathy, unless there had been a previous overuse of mercury.

It is fitting that the remedies for early syphilis potent enough to kill spirochetes deep in the tissues were the heavy metals, mercury and bismuth, and a poison, arsenic. The other major syphilis medication, potassium iodide, used more for resolution of the gummy tumors of late syphilis and for advanced syphilis of the heart, was more benign, although patients complained of depression. Martin of Lubeck first administered an iodide for syphilis in 1821, using a burned sponge for the treatment of venereal ulcers of the throat. Wallace of Dublin used potassium salt in 1834.

Another popular treatment was the wood of the guaiac tree, imported from the Americas at great cost and thought to penetrate areas of the body mercury could not reach. Those who drank concoctions of warm sawdust hoped for a cure because the wood came from Hispaniola, the same place as the disease, and was therefore God's remedy. Arsenic in the form of a white powder was first used in the middle of the eighteenth century, primarily for lesions of the skin. King George II of England obtained a patent for "Greek water," an arsenic treatment. A cheap substitute called "Hot Hell Water" was often fatal.

The first blood test for detecting syphilis was developed in 1907 by a German bacteriologist, August von Wassermann. Although it proved remarkably effective in identifying early syphilis, it was grossly inefficient in later stages. Here the high percentage of false negatives resulted in many missed diagnoses that might have been found by physicians not lulled to complacency by a faulty laboratory finding. When the Wassermann test became routine for cases of suspected syphilis, wives were often told they were being tested for anemia and were treated for syphilis with no knowledge of having been infected by their husbands. One company manufactured chocolates laced with mercury so that the errant spouse could ply his wife with a cure disguised as a gift and keep his secret to himself: thus was family harmony maintained.

In 1909 Paul Erhlich, a Frankfurt scientist, discovered on his 606th modification of a certain molecule an organic arsenic compound named Salvarsan or arsphenamine (and later neo-arsphenamine) that supplemented mercury and the iodides as the treatment of choice in early cases. Ehrlich was searching for a "magic bullet," a toxin that would kill the parasite, visually identified by Fritz Schaudinn only four years before, without damaging the tissues of the host. For this discovery, Ehrlich is often called the originator of chemotherapy. Treatment with Salvarsan required weekly shots over a prolonged period, a difficult contract between patient and doctor, especially since Salvarsan had very unpleasant side effects. If at first Salvarsan seemed to cure, numerous relapses proved the opposite.

The various treatments available in the twentieth century were "complex beyond the dreams of a Fournier or a Jonathan Hutchinson," according to John Stokes, compared to when the goal of merely alleviating external lesions was "an affair of charming simplicity." He anticipated a future when "a turn of the wheel of inventive fortune may at any moment introduce us to the millennium of an infallibly preventative and curative pill."[4] Stokes's dream appeared to have come true when the wonder drug penicillin, discovered by British bacteriologist Alexander Fleming in 1928, was successfully used to treat syphilis in 1943 by John Mahoney and his colleagues at the U.S. Public Health Service. Liberating armies in World War II carried penicillin with them and found it such a valuable commodity that they retrieved it from their urine for reuse.[5]

Today penicillin is the recommended treatment for all stages of syphilis. It does not reverse damage done, and it does have a side effect, the Jarisch–Herxheimer reaction, marked by fever, chills, and headache. In cases of secondary syphilis, when the concentration of treponemes in the body is at the highest, 90 percent of patients have this response.[6] Although penicillin effectively kills spirochetes, it does not kill them all. A dark-field microscope can illuminate spirochetes found in "treponemal sanctuaries"—the brain, the aqueous humor of the eye, the lymph nodes, and temporal arteries—in patients given recommended penicillin treatment. Tissue from rabbits inoculated with syphilis and then "adequately" treated with penicillin will produce infection when injected into other rabbits.

Syphilis remains a public health concern today. In June 2002, the San Francisco Public Health Department, seeing syphilis on the rise, postered the city for Gay Pride Week with images of round, red cartoon chancres plotting against the Healthy Penis. Syphilis, a word previously only whispered, was for one weekend at least highly visible.

6

The Physician's Viewpoint

Know syphilis in all its manifestations and relations,
and all other things clinical will be added unto you.
—SIR WILLIAM OSLER, 1897

IN THE MIDDLE OF THE NINETEENTH CENTURY, PHILIPPE Ricord defined three stages of syphilis: primary (a chancre), secondary (lesions of the skin and mucous membranes), and tertiary (involvement of the inner structures of the body—the viscera, bones, and joints). When a few decades later Jonathan Hutchinson and Alfred Fournier showed that syphilis led to neurosyphilis—paresis, or general paralysis, and tabes dorsalis—in essence they added a fourth stage. But the terminology was already in place, and so "tertiary syphilis" came to mean all manifestations of disease after the initial infection. Nineteenth-century homeopaths, rightly emphasizing that the decades before tertiary syphilis deserved a discrete category, defined four stages. Finding three stages too simplistic, John Stokes identified *eight*, but there was so much overlap that he threw up his hands and concluded that with syphilis, "Almost anything may be expected at any time."[1]

Attempts to create neat categories that explain clinical manifestations (or their absence) in the decades between chancre and insanity have led to muddled and useless terminology, with phrases such as "early latent," "late latent," "early or late secondary," and "early benign tertiary" being used. Today *Harrison's Principles of Internal Medicine* simply calls the period after the early infection, when the clinical signs (chancre, fever, and rash) have disappeared, "latency" (from the Latin *latere*—to lie hidden, to lurk, present but invisible, concealed), and all manifestations of disease after that, very simply, "late syphilis."

When, then, does this "late syphilis" begin? According to *Harrison's,* the onset of slowly progressive inflammatory disease begins soon after the secondary infection resolves. For example, *Harrison's* lists iritis under "late lesions of the eyes," whereas according to Stokes, iritis usually appears between six months and two years after infection. Although this simplified categorizing is useful, the word "latent," or hidden, is now often associated only with its other meaning, "inactive." As a result, the painful manifestations of syphilis that Ricord originally described as the third stage involving the inner structures of the body and giving syphilis its nickname the "Great Imitator," have been underestimated.

Syphilitic infection begins when spirochetes enter the body at the point of infection. They quickly begin to reproduce by dividing. According to *Harrison's* text, before the appearance of a clinical lesion, the concentration of spirochetes reaches ten million organisms per gram of human tissue. The body's immune system wages war, and vast numbers of spirochetes die, but some remain clustered in tissues and periodically discharge showers of organisms from these reservoirs into the blood and lymph, thus starting lesions at numerous new sites. Syphilis is a chronic, inflammatory, relapsing disease.

Following is a brief summary of the course of syphilis, calling on the observations of physicians of the pre-penicillin era, when untreated syphilis, rarely seen in today's waiting rooms, was a common sight in its more chronic, florid, and late stages.

INFECTION: THE CHANCRE (PRIMARY SYPHILIS)

Spirochetes from one person wriggle through a break in the moist skin or a mucous membrane of another person. After an incubation period averaging three weeks, a sore or chancre appears at the point of infection. It may be so small that it goes unnoticed or it may enlarge to an unsightly ulcerating mass with a gristly base and callous edge, oozing a watery discharge teeming with infectious spirochetes. It is usually painless unless super-infected with another disease like gonorrhea. The body begins defensive action at the site of the chancre, and the highly infectious lesions disappear in two to six weeks. Spirochetes spread throughout the body via the blood and the lymph. Not finding the blood a congenial medium, they transfer to the tissues, where they establish colonies of infection. The spirochete reaches the brain in this early stage.

FEVER AND RASH (SECONDARY SYPHILIS)

A general systemic infection with fever, rash (see Figure 6.1), and extreme malaise follows five to twelve weeks after the appearance of the chancre. The fever may be slight or intense, continuous or remittent. The rash may be so subtle that it goes unnoticed or it may cover the body, including the palms of the hands and the soles of the feet, with a painless, copper-colored, non–itchy rash resembling measles. Mucous patches swarming with infectious spirochetes appear in the mouth and throat or on the lips. Patchy baldness (alopecia) may result when hair falls out in clumps.

At this time, the new syphilitic may experience aching in the bones and joints, loss of appetite, insomnia, sore throat, gastrointestinal distress, and headaches that appear at the same time every night and disappear in the morning. Inflammation of the iris (iritis) first in one eye and then the other is the beginning of ongoing vision problems. Jonathan Hutchinson noted that at the same time the skin is affected, the eye, the bones, the joints, and the nervous system—"indeed, all the tissues of the body—are liable to suffer."[2]

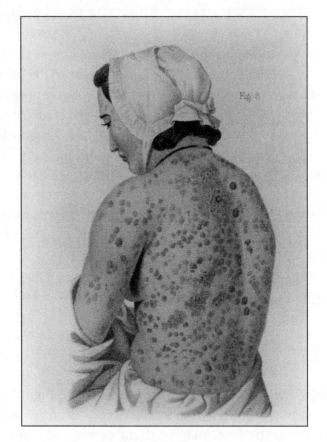

Figure 6.1   Clinical illustration of secondary syphilis,
M. A. Cullerier, *Atlas of Venereal Diseases*, 1868 (New
York Academy of Medicine Library)

This secondary infection may last a few weeks or as long as six
months. Early syphilitic infection imitates other fevers such as
malaria, typhus, or typhoid.

THE EARLY YEARS: HIDDEN SYPHILIS—INVOLVEMENT
OF THE INNER STRUCTURES OF THE BODY

In the years following the initial systemic infection, two
processes are unfolding beneath the placid surface. First, the host

becomes sensitized or allergic to the invading organisms. *Harrison's* text speaks of "an exaggerated delayed-hypersensitivity response to *T. pallidum*."[3] The body is no longer teeming with spirochetes; instead relatively few of them produce destructive tumors known as gummas, varying in size from the microscopic to several centimeters in length. They may be found anywhere in the body, except the hair, the teeth, and the nails. Second, a slowly progressive inflammation takes place in various sites where organisms are clustered, particularly in the nerves and the blood vessels.

It is during this time that syphilis is often missed entirely in a diagnosis. Apparent good health alternates with bouts of being bedridden or hospitalized as pain flares up and subsides in one part of the body after another. Severe headaches with vomiting, gastrointestinal pain, and joint and muscle aches are typical, as are iritis, deafness, episodes of paralysis, and numerous other manifestations. Syphilis in this inflammatory stage sometimes mimics several syndromes simultaneously. The patient, who often complains of feeling poisoned, travels from one specialist to another accumulating a laundry list of diagnoses as well as a reputation for neurasthenia or hypochondria. Syphilis is not suspected as the hidden cause of these complaints in every part of the anatomy. Of these early years, John Stokes wrote that syphilis was a disease with a low visibility but a wide dispersion of manifestations.

THE MIDDLE YEARS: WARNING SIGNS OF PROGRESSING DISEASE

Skin Lesions

Skin lesions occurring as rashes or as ulcerations are often the first signs of late syphilis. The late recurrent syphilitic rash consists of spots that are asymmetrical, grouped, localized, and sometimes itchy, as opposed to the generalized rash of the early secondary period.

Warning Signs of Paresis

General paresis (formerly known as general paralysis of the insane, or dementia paralytica) occurs anywhere from a few years to several decades after infection. Before its onset, prodromal or warning signs, often occurring over as much as a decade, may be obvious to family and friends, who are often shocked and confused when they observe long periods of extreme clarity and typical behavior alternating with episodes of bizarre, uninhibited, even criminal acts, and loss of previously held ethical values. William Osler described "a change in character . . . which may astonish the friends and relatives" and warned to watch for "important indications of moral perversions manifested in offenses against decency."[4]

In the final period close to the onset of paresis, mood shifts become more extreme as euphoria, electric excitement, bursts of creative energy, and grandiose self-reflections alternate with severe, often suicidal depression. Delusions of grandeur, paranoia, exaltation, irritability, rages, and irrational, antisocial behavior define the progression toward insanity. The patient may suddenly begin to gamble, go on absurd spending sprees, or imagine owning vast riches. A calm person becomes emotional, a neat person sloppy, a timid one aggressive. Here the condition is often misdiagnosed as paranoid persecutory psychosis or schizophrenia.

During this period, the syphilitic may be plagued by sensations of electric currents in the head, vertiginous attacks, humming and whistling in the ears, vertigo, and auditory hallucinations such as being serenaded by angels. This warning stage often has an explosive aspect, a sense of enormous contained energy, while the patient retains an ability to achieve the most rigorous control of expression. Syphilis is not suspected because of the extreme clarity of mind without dementia.

Physical signs and symptoms include episodic and progressive paralysis (especially of the limbs), headache, insomnia, weight loss, immense fatigue, tremor, and stumbling speech. Fleeting pains of a neuralgic or rheumatic character may be felt in various parts of the body. Exercise at this time causes exhaustion and the patient becomes inactive, often declining to walk even a short distance. The body becomes stooped and appears to be rapidly aging. There may be cerebral seizures or epileptiform fits and tremors. Handwriting shows tremor quite early, as well as characteristic changes: erasures, writing over, leaving out words and letters, piling up words at the end of a line, and change in the size of letters.

The patient is often misdiagnosed as having a manic depressive, or bipolar, disorder. Stokes wrote: "The possibilities of confusion of cerebral neurosyphilis with manic-depressive psychosis are numerous. . . . The depressive state appears to be the more difficult to differentiate, and no qualities seem to be wholly sufficient to distinguish the depression of general paresis from that of manic-depressive psychosis. . . . In the manic phase differentiation of the two types of disease may be equally difficult since identical delusions may occur in both."[5]

Warning Signs of Tabes Dorsalis

Tabes is the most painful syphilitic condition. Sudden intense "lightning pain" in the hands, feet, or eyes warns of its onset. Gastrointestinal agony, often experienced over many years, can be of such intensity that the patient is reduced to convulsive sobbing; uncontrollable vomiting leads to weakness and exhaustion.

Warning Signs of Cardiovascular Syphilis

Syphilis of the heart is one of the most dangerous manifestations of late syphilis. In the early months of infection, spirochetes exhibit a special affinity for the aorta. They launch a slow inflammatory process that may, decades later, close the vessels and weaken the walls with damaged tissue. Before penicillin, syphilis of the aorta accounted for almost all syphilitic heart disease. It was usually found only at autopsy because the tip-off sign found with a stethoscope—the clear, altered tonal quality of the aortic component of the second sound—was so often missed, or, if noticed, was attributed to simple hypertension. "Paradoxically speaking, of the warnings, the first may be sudden death."[6] Cardiovascular syphilis begins as early as five years after infection and may be experienced as pain in the chest and fear of heart failure, although the diseased heart may not become clinically obvious for thirty years.

THE LATE YEARS: TERTIARY

Paresis

Paresis often begins with a dramatic episode characterized by delusions; grandiosity; identification with religious, mythic, or royal figures; and sometimes rage and violent acts. In the following months and years, dementia alternates with periods of such clarity that there seems to have been a cure. Paralysis is progressive. Often the patient spends the last years in a mental institution. A mnemonic for "paresis" refers to personality disturbances, affect abnormalities, reflex hyperactivity, eye abnormality, sensorium changes, intellectual impairment, and slurred speech.

Tabes Dorsalis

Tabes is caused by damage to the nerve cells of the spinal cord, leading to loss of position sense and progressive inability to coordinate bodily movements. The sense of having unusual sensations haunts the tabetic. Stiffness of gait progresses to a wide-based, stumbling, zigzag pattern of walking, sometimes with the dragging of a foot. Symptoms include difficulty urinating, impotence, blurred vision, numbness in the hands or feet, and incorrect perception of temperature changes. Pupils that are small, irregular, and nonreactive to light but reactive to accommodation, known as Argyll-Robertson pupils, are often found in both tabes and paresis.

When tabes coexists with paresis, the condition is known as tabo-paresis. In these cases, especially with women, the paretic aspect is less severe than the tabetic.

Meningeal or Meningovascular Syphilis

Meningeal syphilis presents with headache, nausea, vomiting, cranial nerve palsies, and seizures, as well as personality changes.

Meningovascular syphilis begins with headaches, vertigo, insomnia, and psychological abnormalities. Strokes are common.

This abbreviated list of signs and symptoms illustrates the challenge to the clinical syphilologist at each stage of the disease.

Detective Zeal

The Fragile Art of Retrospective Diagnosis

> For the inquiring mind, no common disease
> is so exasperating and at the same time so fas-
> cinating as syphilis because of its ability to
> simulate so many other conditions even at
> post-mortem examination.
>
> —EVAN W. THOMAS

THE WORD "SYPHILIS" WAS TABOO IN NINETEENTH-
century society: rarely written, either in correspondence or in
print, and even more rarely spoken, and then only to a few intimate friends of the poor victim, with an implicit agreement that it
was never to be repeated. Doctors had to be trusted to maintain
confidentiality, often at the cost of great ethical conflict if there
was known risk of the disease being spread. A small-town doctor
in Upton Sinclair's novel *Damaged Goods* faces such a dilemma
when a young man comes to him with an early infection and an
intention to marry. Should the doctor warn the bride-to-be? He
does not, and she gives birth to an infected baby. The doctor again
experiences great conflict when the man wishes to engage a wet-
nurse for the dangerous infant.

In the rare biography that acknowledged syphilis, creative euphemisms pointed to the unspoken, as did medical substitutes

such as paralytica dementia or general paralysis of the insane, or paresis, or sometimes just "paralysis" for late-stage syphilis. Biographers have overlooked syphilis in their subjects for a variety of reasons. Often, having no reason to suspect it and seeing no whisper of it in the literary archive, they just miss it. Sometimes it has been covered up or discreetly ignored out of consideration for family members still alive. Some have found it irrelevant. Others have cited it parenthetically, or in a footnote, or at most in a paragraph, as if instead of being a life-changing and defining event, infection with syphilis was of no more importance than a passing head cold. And many have found mentioning it to be rude and inappropriate. The reluctance to attribute a shameful disease like syphilis to a great person, the danger that the work will in some way be linked to the disease, an oeuvre tainted and denigrated— all contribute to sparse references to syphilis.

Medical biographers have often fallen prey to the "Great Imitator," seeing only the diseases that syphilis mimics. A strong clue to syphilis is often in the number of posthumous diagnoses that specialists suggest, each in turn arguing against that of a predecessor, all ending with great head scratching and a pile of diagnostic loose ends that are adequately explained only by syphilis. Specialists focusing on one cluster of signs and symptoms when looking for evidence of their favored disease often do not step back to see the body, or the life, as a whole. If ever a disease required a holistic approach to detect and fathom, it is syphilis.

When Jonathan Hutchinson published *Syphilis* in 1887 (with several revised editions through 1909, after the spirochete had been viewed under Fritz Schaudinn's microscope), he provided his colleagues with an instruction manual for identifying and treating the hidden disease. Hutchinson was able to show how to link a variety of painful and inexplicable conditions to progressing syphilis. Using case studies gathered from his skilled observation of thousands of patients over his long lifetime, he counted himself fortunate to see youths he had treated with the "little blue mercury pills" become grandfathers.

For Hutchinson, syphilis posed a diagnostic dilemma: it both looked like other diseases and acted in concert with them. "There is scarcely a malady which has received a name which may not be simulated by it, and still fewer which it may not modify."[1] More vexing still, there was nothing that alone would prove syphilis: "Syphilis has no lesions or type-forms of disease which are peculiar to itself."[2] He looked to the patient's history and careful clinical observation to justify a diagnosis.

Stokes agreed with Hutchinson's two diagnostic challenges: that syphilis with extraordinary facility "apes every disease in any field of medicine,"[3] and that syphilis will never yield to one diagnostic key. He invited the syphilis detective to act like Sherlock Holmes, maintaining "an alert sense of nearness such as is experienced by the hunter stalking big and dangerous game."[4] The main obstacle to the identification of syphilis, he suggested, was a low index of suspicion among medical professionals toward a disease with a "Machiavellian facility in disguise, deceit and malevolence."[5] A disease of low visibility and wide dispersion of manifestations, syphilis requires from medical sleuths an alert suspiciousness, a "ferret-like instinct for a scent,"[6] and a constant vigilance to detect a pathologic process beneath a seemingly flawless surface.

Physicians suspecting syphilis often had to depend on what could be learned from a single clinical interview. If the initial sore had been small and the fever mild, the patient might not have noticed it, or would recall it only with encouragement. Return again and again to the patient's history, syphilologists advised. Be aware that a patient who has kept this secret for years knows only how to lie. Inquire of the patient's family to find hints of aberrant and even criminal behavior anticipating tertiary syphilis. Use a stethoscope to hear the clear, altered tonal quality of the second aortic sound that warns of syphilitic heart disease. If syphilis is suspected, look for pain that moves around in the body: joint pain, muscle pain, headaches, stomach aches. Look for euphoria and depression. Look for "nerves," nervous disorders, apparent hypochondriasis. Look for crises, attacks, time spent in the hospital. But most of all, look to the accumulation of clues and convergent indications to establish a pattern of disease over a lifetime that will lead to an overwhelming probability of syphilis.

If syphilologists had so much difficulty diagnosing living patients, how is it possible to establish a retrospective diagnosis with any certainty for a person who has been dead for a century or more? Sometimes the case is clear-cut, but what about cases where there is room for doubt? A biographer has certain advantages over a doctor who had to make the difficult choice whether to treat with toxic mercury on the basis of a few office visits: the perspective of a whole life, including the circumstances of death and autopsy, and an often vast literary estate—diaries, letters, journals and letters of friends, medical records, plus the aggregate work and cumulative insights of previous biographers and diagnosticians. The nineteenth-century custom of chronicling everything (except syphilis) while maintaining an extensive correspondence produced daunting archives: hundreds and even thousands of books and articles to be looked at according to each one's sources of information, weighing what was known about the disease at the time and factoring in the prejudices of the decade in which it was written.

The syphilologists left lists of questions to ask when interviewing a patient about a suspected syphilitic infection that can be modified for the retrospective biographer digging through a literary archive. First, was there a pattern of infection during youth? Look for indications of high-risk sexual behavior, especially with prostitutes; an admission of having syphilis, perhaps written circumspectly to a friend or close family member; or a diagnosis by a physician, even if revealed only posthumously. Was there at the possible time of infection a severe fever (typhus, typhoid, malaria) accompanied by extreme malaise? At any time were there indications of treatment with mercury or arsenic or, later, potassium iodide? Was there a sudden change from relatively good health to a lifetime of mysterious, painful ailments? Was there an unexpected vow of chastity? Social withdrawal? Sudden misanthropy, reworking of values, taking on (or casting off) of religion?

Next, over the following decades, was the person subject to a wide variety of illnesses, in one part of the body after another, that were suspicion arousers of a developing case of syphilis? Were there episodes of bizarre, uncharacteristic behavior? In the later stages, were there personality changes that warned of approaching neurosyphilis: grandiosity, euphoria, rages, violent or criminal behavior, extreme depression? Or were there sharp and mysterious pains, acute gastrointestinal distress, or an imbalanced gait that warned of tabes dorsalis?

Was the subject committed to a mental institution with a diagnosis of general paralysis of the insane, paresis, or dementia paralytica? Was there heart disease indicative of syphilis? Did an autopsy report yield useful information? And finally, was there great diagnostic confusion as the Great Imitator mimicked one illness or syndrome after another? Where Stokes, limited to a diagnostic interview, left three inches at the bottom of his patient record for comments, the biographical sleuth reserves megabytes on a hard drive and fills filing cabinets full of data.

The following pattern of revelation is often seen when researching a biographical history where syphilis is suspected:

1. *Keeping it secret.* Although statements are made privately by friends and doctors, syphilis is not publicly acknowledged during a person's lifetime.
2. *Diagnosing it.* The first medical biographies, often written by physicians with experience in long-term untreated syphilis, accept a diagnosis based on the mental and physical condition of the subject and on the statements of friends and doctors.
3. *Ignoring it.* Syphilis is then dropped by subsequent biographers, who for decades sideline the question of health in general as being rude or irrelevant.
4. *Missing it.* The file is reopened and a debate begins in the literature. Specialists not trained to identify syphilis, often harboring mistaken ideas about the disease, tend to look at

and reject each clue in turn without considering the larger pattern over the lifetime. Medical consensus runs against syphilis.

The zeal for accumulating clues must be balanced by caution against racing enthusiastically to a false diagnosis. Indications of syphilis must each be looked at and balanced with caution in the context of the life; retrospective diagnosis is a dangerous game. Witnesses can be unreliable. Not everyone who visited a prostitute got syphilis. Genital sores could be gonorrhea or chancroid. Not every fever was secondary syphilis. Gout, headache, arthritis, rheumatism, and iritis could be nothing more than they seem to be. Mercury, arsenic, and potassium iodide were used for other conditions. Toxic substances—especially mercury, lead, and the drink absinthe (now illegal)—could cause neurological and other problems that in turn imitate syphilis. Seizures could be epileptic. Mania, depression, and episodes of seemingly mad behavior could indicate a bipolar disorder, or schizophrenia, or paranoid delusions, or any number of psychological disturbances listed in the psychiatrists' diagnostic manual. And of course there is no reason why a syphilitic could not have more than one malady. Syphilologists repeated over and over that a lifetime of observation was necessary; a single clue was never enough.

A retrospective diagnosis of syphilis based on archival information cannot be affirmed with definitive scientific proof, any more than a diagnosis could have been in the days before laboratory testing or even now, when laboratory tests are error prone. A syphilologist's diagnosis approached, but never reached, certainty, and as often as not a diagnosis was only confirmed when the patient got better with (toxic) treatment, or infected a lover, or provided postmortem proof such as a syphilitic heart.

For his study of syphilitics, neurologist MacDonald Critchley chose "illustrious neuro-luetics" (lues being another word for syphilis) whose diagnosis seemed to be, in retrospect, as definite as any clinical evaluation could ever be. And indeed, few would challenge his choice of Guy de Maupassant, Jules de Goncourt, Alphonse Daudet, Heinrich Heine, or the jester, Dan Leno. But what about those for whom the diagnosis is less certain?

The secret, undiscovered, or casually dismissed cases are the most fascinating to study, as are the actively disputed ones. In biography, we can follow the footsteps of the early syphilologists who looked for the first few clues, were acutely suspicious, and then with great care and attention put together a reasonable hypothesis, either pro or con. Detective zeal tempered with constant wariness and well-developed skepticism is necessary for retrospective biographical diagnosis. Like a good private investigator tracking down dubious, even disreputable witnesses, the syphilis sleuth must be aware that the best information sometimes comes from surprising sources, while the usual peer-reviewed journals can be filled with faulty assumptions about a disease no longer familiar in clinical practice.

The diagnosis of syphilis, then, relies on the observation of a pattern of disease that leads to a compelling conclusion based on overwhelming circumstantial evidence (perhaps with a pinch of intuition?). That is where Sherlock Holmes aids his medical counterpart in the search for the always-elusive spirochete.

Absence of evidence is not evidence of absence

If a diagnosis of syphilis cannot be proved, it cannot be disproved either.

The arguments *against* syphilis are as relevant, if not as compelling, and must be looked at with as much attention as the arguments for it. Syphilis cannot be discounted on a single detail: a late negative Wassermann test, the lack of dementia, normal pupils. Nor can it be rejected because the subject never admitted having it, or was too lofty to have had such a disease, or because previous researchers did not consider it, or because the writer just wishes it not to be true. And yet many medical biographers reject syphilis for just such incorrect reasons. Those who try to prove the no-syphilis position are on just as shaky ground as those who try to prove syphilis. At most, they can temper and add balance to the probability of a diagnosis based on cumulative clues and a preponderance of circumstantial evidence.

Although medical aspects of syphilis have been well chronicled in the texts, the experience of having it has not. Very little has been written about any aspect of having syphilis: the terror of infection (the first moment of observing a fresh chancre, especially an elaborate one), the choice between chastity and risking infecting a lover, the decision to marry or not, the fear that at any time open lesions could reveal the secret disease to the world. Perhaps worst of all was the loneliness of living with the secret, the pain, the feeling of being poisoned, the intimations of insanity, and the inability to work for consistent periods.

Over the decades conventions in biography about how to handle sexual secrets and scandalous information have changed. In writing about rumors of Nietzsche's sexuality in 1880, Mazzino Montinari apologized: "I beg the reader's pardon for having once again concerned myself with a pseudo-problem, sickness, sexual relations, chastity, etc., which should no longer interest anyone."[7] And yet we are interested, indeed fascinated. How is it possible to look at a life through the lens of a biographer, with respect for the subject, while ignoring the influence of a disease that affected every aspect of that person's daily life, self-concept, social situation, career, decision to marry and have children, and even, with neurological changes, personality?

In the following chapters, the question of syphilis is looked at in the lives of a number of well-known men and women who have greatly influenced Western culture, both creatively and, in the last case, destructively. Before we look at what the experience or effects of having the disease might have been, we have to ask how secure the diagnosis is. Few if any who review the literature today would disagree that Schubert, Baudelaire, Flaubert, Maupassant, Blixen, and Schumann had syphilis. Most would agree about Nietzsche, although there is still some debate. There is hot debate over Beethoven, Wilde, and Joyce. The question has been discreetly avoided for the most part in respect to Mary and Abraham

Lincoln, and it has not been considered seriously at all in the van Gogh scholarship. Clues to syphilis in Hitler's life are scattered throughout the vast Hitler literature and, although plentiful, have never been gathered together or looked at through the selective filter of a diagnosis of syphilis.

The question of diagnosis must come first. Once syphilis is seriously considered, it becomes impossible not to wonder how it affected daily life. Only then can we ask the fascinating yet delicate question: what influence did syphilis have on the life's work? Here the danger lies in the *faux pas* of the pathographer: defining or reducing the work to being *nothing more than* the product of syphilis. If syphilis defined one as an outsider ("ghastly miserable and hated in society"[8]), how can knowledge of being infected not be reflected thematically in the work? If late-stage neurosyphilis resulted in creative euphoria, grandiose self-definitions, and freedom from moral restraint, then can we look at the last, and often most influential, work of someone who was on the verge of a final syphilitic breakdown and say that syphilis was irrelevant?

PART II
The Nineteenth Century

8

Ludwig van Beethoven
1770–1827

That green monster, my dreadful health.
—BEETHOVEN

O N 1 DECEMBER 1994 A SMALL BLACK LOCKET IN A DARK
wood oval frame containing a coil of Ludwig van Beethoven's brown, gray, and white hair (582 strands) pressed between
two pieces of glass was auctioned at Sotheby's for $7,300. The enthusiastic new owners were Alfredo "Che" Guevara, a Nogales,
Arizona, urologist, and Ira Brilliant of the Ira F. Brilliant Beethoven Center. Assuming that they were hoping to prove that Beethoven had syphilis or was poisoned by finding traces of mercury
and arsenic, the *New York Times Magazine* found the story of the
new owners' plan to test the hair sample worthy of a cover story,
"Beethoven's Hair Tells All."[1]

The *Times* published my fanciful letter to the editor: "Will
Beethoven's hair 'tell all'—or nothing? Mercury was used to block
hats in the nineteenth century—hence the phrase 'Mad Hatter'—
and arsenic was used to treat syphilis as early as 1498. If Beethoven's hair does contain mercury or arsenic, will it indicate that he
had syphilis? That he was poisoned? Or just that he may have
worn a hat!"[2] More to the point, since mercury grows out with

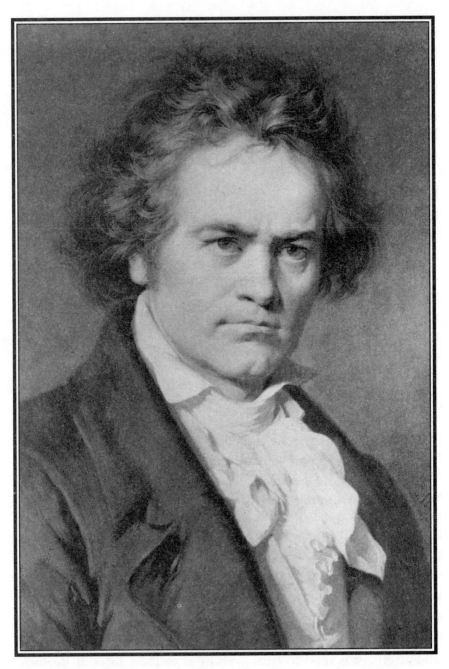

Figure 8.1   Ludwig van Beethoven (Library of Congress)

the hair, a deathbed sample would be of no use in determining treatment during youth. When the carefully guarded secret of the hair test results was finally revealed with great fanfare by Russell Martin in *Beethoven's Hair,* a charming book alternating stories of Beethoven's life with the picaresque saga of the hair sample, the mercury question was left ambiguous with this unfathomable logic-twister: "Beethoven's hair had evidenced levels of mercury so low they were undetectable."[3]

Guevara and Brilliant, who were serious about their science, had not enjoyed being called syphilis-obsessed by the nation's leading newspaper, according to Martin, and so they were pleased at what they did find: lead, and no small quantity—sixty parts per million. Lead poisoning, which the author speculated came from dishes, or wine plumbed (sealed) with lead, could have caused many of Beethoven's complaints, including his deafness. The popular media picked up the story and soon newspapers, radio, and television proclaimed the startling news: *Ludwig van Beethoven did not have syphilis after all.* But the syphilis question does not go away that easily.

Beethoven could have had lead poisoning *and* syphilis.

For over three decades, Martin pointed out, "Beethoven cognoscenti" have soundly discredited the idea that he had syphilis. The website of the Ira F. Brilliant Center for Beethoven Studies at San Jose State University tells us that for this reason no syphilis tests were even done on the hair. Interestingly, Guevara does not count himself one of the cognoscenti, since he appeared open-minded on the syphilis question when interviewed by Philip Weiss: "You have to remember that syphilis and gonorrhea were rampant in those days. Absolutely rampant. Case in point: We know for a fact that Beethoven hung out with prostitutes. It's documented by a cellist friend of his. Beethoven was a romantic, he wanted to be loved. . . . Remember, a syphilis infection manifests itself in many different ways. Deafness was one condition you could develop."[4]

The syphilis debate has raged in the Beethoven literature ever since George Grove of the prestigious *Grove's Dictionary of Music and Musicians* revealed the diagnosis in 1879. He concluded that a postmortem examination of Beethoven's auditory system showed that its abnormalities were "most probably the result of syphilitic affections at an early period of his life."[5] Since then, passionate proponents of this finding have been opposed by fervent deniers. George Marek wrote: "For every ten authorities who said that he had it, there are ten who said that he did not."[6] (And another ten, perhaps, couldn't care less.)

There was a great deal of agreement about the syphilis diagnosis among those of Beethoven's time, as well those who wrote in the pre-penicillin decades of the twentieth century, when interest in syphilis was at its height. Weighing in on the side of the pro-syphilis argument are Beethoven's own doctor and friend for ten years (1806–1816), Andreas Bertolini; his best-known biographer, the young lawyer from America, Alexander Wheelock Thayer; and the famous physician and syphilis expert Sir William Osler. Grove referred to two prescriptions in Beethoven's name for mercurial ointment given for lues, or syphilis, once in the possession of an otologist, Adam Politzer, author of the first *History of Otology*. His information came from Thayer, who had been told by Bertolini. As Beethoven's doctor, Bertolini had firsthand credibility, and Thayer was a reputable if fastidious biographer. Having written a life of Beethoven up to the year 1817, Thayer gave up in disgust, according to some sources, when he heard the news. When Bertolini thought he was terminally ill, he burned all of Beethoven's letters and notes, saying that a few were not of the nature to fall into careless hands. What medical knowledge could have been so damaging, scholars have wondered, except information about syphilis?

In 1910 (and again in 1927) Leo Jacobssohn, an otologist, argued in favor of syphilis as a cause of deafness from damage to the eighth cranial nerve and of liver disease. In 1912 Theodor von Frimmel, Beethoven scholar and physician, wrote that it was "practically impossible that there was not a contributory cause in the form of a previous infection. Beethoven's deafness was a symptom. The disease itself had another name."[7] Frimmel wrote of "something else about which I may not keep entirely silent since many years ago I received, thanks to the kindness of A. W. Thayer, definite written facts about this other illness of Beethoven."[8] Thayer had also said that Beethoven's disease, coyly unnamed, was well-known to many people.[9] In short: there was a great deal of agreement in the early biographical literature that Beethoven did have syphilis, and that it was well known.

Ludwig van Beethoven was born to a poor family in Bonn in 1770. He studied harpsichord, piano, viola, and organ, and while he was still quite young his ability to improvise on the piano gained him access to the musical drawing rooms of the city. There is a story that he once played for Mozart, who remarked that some day he would give the world something to talk about. Beethoven had brilliant eyes and blemished skin, some say from smallpox when he was young. He dressed elegantly, like a court musician, in a sea-green frock coat, green knee breeches with buckles, black silk stockings, an embroidered vest sewed with gold cord, and a crushed hat. His silver belt sported a sword. When he was twenty-two he received a stipend that allowed him to support his mother and two brothers—his father having just died of alcoholism—and to move to Vienna. He studied with Franz Joseph Haydn, among others. His brilliant improvisations on the piano gained him fame and patronage from the titled of Vienna, including Archduke Rudolph, the half-brother of the emperor, who was his pupil.

Other than some gastrointestinal complaints, Beethoven was relatively healthy as a youth, and his future was most promising. But a fever during his first year in Vienna marked a turning point. And one of his doctors, Alois Weissenbach, wrote of another severe fever in 1797: "He once had a terrible typhus, from this time on dated the ruin of his nervous system and probably the ruin of his hearing, so calamitous in his case."[10] Of note here is the identification of what might otherwise have been a temporary fever as a starting point of long-term health issues.

The information about Bertolini's diagnosis leads to the next question: could either of these severe fevers have been secondary syphilis? It could. In 1907 Sir William Osler postulated that Beethoven's typhoid infection was of syphilitic origin.[11] It is worth pausing to consider the value of the opinion of Osler, one of the most influential physicians in history and the best known in the English-speaking world at the turn of the century. His textbook, *The Principles and Practice of Medicine,* was widely used for decades, and his system of postgraduate training for physicians is still followed today. Osler was one of the great experts on syphilis.

Because there is no known sexual relationship in Beethoven's life, some biographers have asked whether Beethoven might have lived and died a virgin. Today most agree that Beethoven visited prostitutes frequently. Maynard Solomon decoded Beethoven's letters to his friend Zmeskall in which he referred to *Morsche Festungen,* literally rotten fortresses, in terms that indicate he was referring to brothels and prostitutes. In several letters he linked these "fortresses" to sex, disease, and danger, as well as wounding: "Enjoy life, but not voluptuously—Proprietor, Governor, Pasha of various rotten fortresses!!!!!" "I need not warn you any more to take care not to be wounded near certain fortresses." "Keep away from rotten fortresses, for an attack from them is more deadly than from well-preserved ones." "Be zealous in defending the fortresses of the empire, which, as you know, lost their virginity a long time ago, and have already received several assaults." "I thank you most heartily, my dear Z, for the information you have given me concerning the fortresses, for I thought you had the idea that I did not wish to stop in swampy places."[12] But he longed for something more: "Carnal pleasures without communion of the souls is always brutish; afterward, one enjoys no trace of noble feeling, but only of regret."[13]

A syphilologist reviewing Beethoven's medical record thus far would find high-risk sexual activity, a severe fever that marked a turning point in health, a medical doctor's diagnosis of syphilis, a number of other doctors agreeing with that diagnosis, and indications of treatment with mercury salve. The next step would be to look at the medical history for the next decades to see if there were indications of progressing syphilis: episodes of general ill health alternating with periods of apparent good health, with a long list of otherwise inexplicable maladies and no reasonable diagnosis. If Beethoven had been infected in 1797, as Osler suggested, then the disease would have been almost a decade old by the time Bertolini saw him professionally. That he found syphilis then indicates persistent illness. And if Beethoven did take mercury, there is no way of knowing for how long. Mercury could have been responsible for some of his complaints at that time.

Many scholars have asked if Beethoven's deafness may have had a syphilitic origin, but the long list of his other ailments has largely been ignored, opening the question of the extent to which the "Great Imitator" is lurking behind them. To summarize briefly, Beethoven's medical chart would include severe gastrointestinal distress ("truly dreadful colics"), terrible headaches (he had several teeth pulled hoping that would relieve his head pain), an infected fingernail that required an operation, surgery for an abscess of the jaw, a rheumatic attack with severe inflammation of the lungs (1815, after which he never regained full health), recurrent rheumatic pain with one "terrible rheumatic seizure," "gouty arthritis of the chest," jaundice, bleeding from the esophagus and nose, and a painful eye affliction for five months (with a recurrence) that required a darkened room and bandaged eyes. Doctors told him his heart was fatigued. He had frequent cardiac arrhythmias, which he set to music (piano sonata opus 81a, *Les adieux*). In his later years, he had facial spasms. Since this list is only a partial compilation of the miseries endured, Anton Neumayr seems especially ungenerous when he writes: "Beethoven was inclined to hypochondria in his later years."[14]

One of the most characteristic signs of the middle period of syphilis is a recurrent inflammation of the iris and the membranes lining the eyelids. When Beethoven was completing his *Missa solemnis* for a ceremony for Archduke Rudolph, he was hindered by such an eye condition. He wrote to Schindler: "Nights I have to cover my eyes and am supposed to take good care of them, otherwise, Smetana[15] writes me, I shall not write many notes more."[16] Anton Neumayr finds that the eye condition was "almost certainly a case of iridocyclitis, inflammation of the iris and the conjunctiva (the delicate membrane lining the eyelids and covering the eyeball)."[17]

Any number of Beethoven's complaints might argue routine poor health. However, a severe fever followed by chronic ill health including rheumatism, arthritis, gout, inflammation of the eyes, headaches, stomach ailments, and other complaints arouses strong suspicion of a syphilitic cause. He went from one doctor to another and tried any number of strange remedies. So little did he trust his corps of physicians that he labeled them (at least fifteen in all) "medical asses." His correspondence overflows with misery because of his physical complaints, and letter after letter describes his despair. To Franz Brentano (12 November 1821) he lamented: "Honored friend! Don't consider me a shabby or selfish genius— For the past year up to the present I have been continually ill; likewise during the summer I had an attack of jaundice, which lasted until the end of August."[18] To Zmeskall he confided that he wouldn't be in London the following year but in the grave; thank God, he said, that his role was about to be played out.

The loss of his hearing caused Beethoven distress above all else. In June 1801 he wrote to Franz Gerhard Wegeler: "That green-eyed monster, my dreadful health, has played a rotten trick on me, specifically: for the last three years, my hearing has become steadily worse."[19] At the theater he could not hear the higher tones of the instruments and singers. Treatment with oil of sweet almonds did not help, nor did Dr. Gerhard von Vering's remedy of a certain bark that caused painful blistering on both arms that supposedly would alleviate the buzzing in his ears (Vering "really has too little interest and patience for such a disease"), nor did Dr. H. Graff's suggestion that he grate fresh horseradish on a cotton cloth and insert it in his ear. On the advice of Dr. Johann Schmidt, he agreed to try galvanism, the direct application of electric current, for his hearing. Even seven months before Beethoven died he wrote hopefully of a new remedy for deafness, a few drops of green nut-rinds in lukewarm milk dropped in his ear.

To Wegeler he complained that his deafness followed him like a ghost; imagine how empty and sad a life he was living. But he experienced mood swings, and happiness alternated with the depression: "There is no greater joy for me than to apply and display my art. . . . I want to grab life by the throat; and this is certain, it shall never bring me down. —O, life, it is so beautiful, O to live a thousand lives."[21]

On 1 July 1801 Beethoven wrote to Karl Amenda: "Let me tell you that my most prized possession, *my hearing*, has greatly deteriorated. When you were still with me, I already felt the symptoms; but I said nothing about them. Now they have become very much worse. We must wait and see whether my hearing can be restored. . . . *I beg you to treat what I have told you about my hearing as a great secret to be entrusted to no one."*[22]

On 6 October 1802 Beethoven visited a village outside Vienna, where he wrote to his brothers (but never mailed) the suicidal declaration known as the Heiligenstadt Testament, blaming his loss of hearing for much of his despair:

Oh you men who think or say that I am malevolent, stubborn, or misanthropic, how greatly do you wrong me. You do not know the secret cause which makes me seem that way to you. From childhood on, my heart and soul have been full of the tender feeling of goodwill, and I was ever inclined to accomplish great things. But think that for six years now I have been hopelessly afflicted, made worse by senseless physicians, from year to year deceived with hopes of improvement, finally compelled to face the prospect of *a lasting malady* (whose cure will take years or, perhaps, be impossible). Though born with a fiery, active temperament, even susceptible to the diversions of society, I was soon compelled to withdraw myself, to live life alone. If at times I tried to forget all this, oh how harshly I was flung back by the doubly sad experience of my bad hearing. . . . But what a humiliation for me when someone standing next to me heard a flute in the distance and *I heard nothing*, or someone heard a *shepherd singing* and again I heard nothing. Such incidents drove me almost to despair; a little more of that and I would have ended my life—it was only *my art* that held me back. Ah, it seemed to me impossible to leave the world until I had brought forth all that I felt was within me. So I endured this wretched existence—truly wretched for so susceptible a body, which can be thrown by a sudden change from the best condition to the very worst. . . . How happy I shall be if I can still be helpful to you in my grave—so be it.—With joy I hasten to meet death.[23]

Four days later he wrote a letter to be read after his death, bidding sad farewell, abandoning hope of a cure, wishing for one day of *pure joy;* it had been so long since real joy echoed in his heart.

What is there in Beethoven's medical history and the details of his everyday life that points to a syphilitic cause of deafness? The syphilis texts tell us that deafness often manifests in the first year after the initial fever. It is caused by damage to the eighth cranial nerve. Tinnitus, a ringing, buzzing, or rushing sound, is almost always present. A loss of acuity for upper tones comes before loss of hearing of the range of sound including the spoken word. The onset of hearing loss is gradual, with periods of remission, and is often marked by a stressful event. Taking these indications of syphilitic deafness as a starting, point, it is possible to find illustrations in Beethoven's biography, enough at least to warrant a review of the first otologists' opinions. For example:

- The eighth cranial nerve. Neumayr wrote: "The most probable explanation of Beethoven's deafness is that it was a disorder of the auditory nerves of the labyrinth or inner ear."[24]

- Gradual onset. Again from Neumayr: "The insidious, almost imperceptible start was characteristic of a hearing loss associated with pathological change in structures within the inner ear or in the auditory nerve."[25] From Larkin: "Beethoven's deafness was progressive but with periods of standstill."[26]

- Tinnitus. In 1801 Beethoven wrote that Dr. Vering had given him pills for his stomach and tea for his ears, and so he felt stronger, but his ears "whistle[d] and buzz[ed] continually, day and night"; he wrote "I would be happy if the devil had not made his home in my ears."[27]

- A sudden incident marking a sharp decline in hearing. In 1810 Beethoven threw himself on the floor in a rage: "When I got back up," he wrote: "I found I was deaf and have remained so ever since; the doctors say the nerve is damaged."[28]

- Beethoven noted loss of higher tones from the outset of the hearing problem. He put cotton wool in his ears to muffle loud noises that were particularly painful.

Jonathan Hutchinson wrote: "I am not aware that any opportunities have occurred for dissecting the ears of those who have become deaf in the manner described."[29] He had no way of knowing that the most famous ears of all time had been autopsied. Beethoven's pathology report revealed that the auditory nerves were shriveled and lacking in the usual layer of myelin and that the left auditory nerve was much thinner than the right.[30] Doctors Johann Wagner and Karl Rokitansky performed the autopsy in Beethoven's house. To examine the ears more carefully, Wagner sawed out portions of the temporal bone on both sides of the head. The bones remained in a covered glass jar at the University of Vienna until they disappeared, rumored stolen by a departmental assistant and sold to a foreign doctor.

In 1863 Beethoven's body was disinterred and placed in a metal casket to be preserved. Several more bones were removed from the skull at this time. Gerhard von Breuning stored Beethoven's skull in his bedroom for nine days prior to reburial. Beethoven was dug up once more in 1888. This time the skull was too decayed to make a cast of the inner surface. The ungracious exhumation report read: "The skull of Beethoven did not correspond in the least to our ideas of beauty and harmonious proportions."[31]

Did the autopsy report point to syphilis? Otologist Sean Sellars suggests that it might have done so: "The postmortem finding of changes in the surround of the brain stem suggests a chronic localized meningeal reaction, thought to be syphilitic meningovasculitis. Syphilis was the cause that his contemporary medical attendants diagnosed and for which they treated him. His cirrhosis was at that time attributed to the same disease."[32]

In his last years Beethoven was often seen wildly stomping down the fashionable promenades of Vienna with wild hair flying, howling, humming off-key, and appearing as if he had been in mortal combat. On walks he bellowed so loudly that he stampeded cattle. The street children made fun of him, and once the police arrested him for staring in windows looking like a tramp. He had ceased to care for his appearance. At night his friends would steal into his room and leave clean clothes by his bed. He didn't seem to notice.

Word was spreading that the famous Beethoven might be more than merely eccentric. A German composer passed rumors on to Goethe that Beethoven was a lunatic. Charlotte Brunsvik wrote: "I learned yesterday that Beethoven had become crazy."[33] He had frequent outbursts of temper. Franz Lizst too had written of this imbalance: "The works for which I openly confess my admiration and predilection are for the most part amongst those which . . . are commonly described nowadays as belonging to Beethoven's *last style* (and which were, not long ago, with lack of reverence, explained by Beethoven's deafness and mental derangement)."[34]

Edward Larkin paints the following picture of Beethoven's last years: "persistent ill-health, of a prevailing mood of depression, a highly strung, suspicious, 'persecuted' man, unstable under stress, hypomanic at times, impulsive to the point of aggression, perfectionist, deaf, irritable."[35] Beethoven once heaved a stew at a waiter. Maynard Solomon summarized: "Signs of neurotic eccentricity— sudden rages, uncontrolled emotional states, an increasing obsession with money, feelings of persecution, ungrounded suspicions—persisted until Beethoven's death, reinforcing Vienna's belief that its greatest composer was a sublime madman."[36] All these symptoms are consistent with the stage of syphilis before the onset of paresis.

In 1827 Beethoven came down with pneumonia. When, after a long and difficult illness, it was clear the end was approaching, he signed a short will and testament naming his nephew Karl as sole heir. The handwriting in this document shows bunched letters, writing over, and curved lines that can indicate the beginning of paresis. When Dr. Wawruch warned his friend that he had little time left, Beethoven asked for a priest. With friends surrounding him, he said: "Plaudite, amici, comoedia finita est." *Applaud, friends, the play is over.*[37] When four bottles of wine arrived, Beethoven murmured his last words: "Pity, pity, too late."[38] He died on 26 March 1827.

Why in the past three decades has the tide turned so completely against a diagnosis of syphilis in Beethoven's case? The answer, which requires some tracking through the medical literature, is that a series of specialists, each one debunking a predecessor, has attempted to find an alternative diagnosis that would cover a large number of Beethoven's complaints, often suggesting one of the inflammatory syndromes that gave syphilis the name the "Great Imitator." Edward Larkin's 1970 essay "Beethoven's Medical History" marked the turning point in the history of Beethoven diagnosis when he came to this conclusion: "It is likely that Beethoven, like everybody else, caught gonorrhea but there is no evidence that either his lifelong illnesses or his deafness were syphilitic, and the substantial medical writers make other diagnoses."[39]

Larkin's malady of choice, systemic lupus erythematosus, was dismissed in a 1996 *Lancet* article as "an unlikely diagnosis" by Kubba and Young, who put various medical biographies "under the knife of a gastrointestinal surgeon,"[40] listing and disagreeing one by one with the other previous substantial medical writers. They considered, and gave medical reasons for rejecting, Paget's disease of bone, tuberculosis, sarcoidosis, inflammatory bone disease, and Whipple's disease. That done, the authors then proposed their own favorite, Crohn's disease (inflammation of the colon). This in turn was rejected in a *Lancet* letter to the editor listing all the reasons why Beethoven's autopsy report does not support a

Crohn's diagnosis. Although syphilis might well explain the wide range of Beethoven's illnesses, it is missing from the *Lancet* authors' list of candidates, being mentioned briefly at the end only as a possible cause of his deafness. Their conclusion: "His systemic illnesses remain largely unilluminated." And in *Beethoven's Hair*, Russell Martin underestimated the vast potential of syphilis to do mischief when he wrote: "Syphilis now clearly could not explain Beethoven's cruel concert of diseases."[41]

Larkin's 1970 essay contains information about Beethoven's diagnosis of lues (syphilis), his treatment with mercury, the opinions of the early biographers that he did have syphilis, and finally, a medical history that points clearly to a developing case of syphilis with increasing mental disorder. In short, his essay, while denying syphilis, gives us just what we need to reopen the question. Similarly, Neumayr's summary of Beethoven's health, while vehemently denying syphilis, gives us the very health history that points to it.

In his last months, Beethoven was showing signs that point to approaching paresis. In the stage that warns of the horrible end of the syphilitic path he would have experienced certain changes of personality and behavior. Dementia would not have been part of the picture, but elation and rage would. Because the warning period of general paralysis of the insane can last for years and can be characterized by the wildest euphoria, the most extreme and even seemingly mystical states, while maintaining *the most austere precision of form*, Beethoven's changes in behavior were not inconsistent with early tertiary syphilis. Because there is no proof that Beethoven did or did not have syphilis, the question and its implications have been put aside, dismissed casually in articles that look in a fragmented way at the circumstantial evidence, usually considering only a few of the clues and therefore finding them wanting. From the viewpoint of nineteenth-century medicine, however, Beethoven had many times the number of warning signs that would raise the index of suspicion of a sharp clinical syphilologist high enough to warrant treatment.

Why has syphilis been rejected? The arguments against it, in summary, are that although Beethoven regularly visited prostitutes, he may have avoided infection; the original diagnosis could have been gonorrhea instead of syphilis; the early information about infection was "gained in a manner comparable to Chinese whispers"[42]; lues may have meant another venereal disease; mercury salve may have been for another condition (according to Thomas G. Palferman, finding prescriptions for lues to be proof of syphilis is "ignorant and mischievous"[43]); the fever may have been typhoid after all; the string of illnesses after youth may have been unrelated; the character changes may have been just the crankiness of an aging, deaf composer; the shriveled auditory nerves and the inflamed meninges may have had other causes; and finally, because there was no dementia, there was no neurosyphilis.

The no dementia argument is worth an additional comment. Palferman found the most overwhelming argument against syphilis to be that Beethoven's history did not conform to the way the disease presents. It was not congenital, not meningovascular (discounting the condition of the meninges at autopsy), not tabes, and not gummatous. But he also claimed it was not general paralysis of the insane, because "GPI is usually fatal within about 3 years" and because Beethoven was not demented: "eccentric, wildly so at times, yes, but demented, no."[44] This common assumption, that GPI equals dementia, ignores the complex and long warning period of exquisite clarity in which dementia is but the next step. Once the corner is turned, GPI can be fatal within three years, although it often is not, but that is not relevant to Beethoven's case.

Did Beethoven think he had syphilis? If he was treated for lues with mercury, it is likely that he knew why. He lived when insanity and paralysis had not yet been linked to syphilis, but he would have known, as would Dr. Bertolini, that his chronic ill health began with his infection. In one of his conversation books of 1819 he noted the name of a book, *On the Art of Recognizing and Curing All Forms of Venereal Disease*, by L. V. Legumnan. Beethoven wrote

about a malady he could not change, one that brought him gradually to death.[45] Throughout his letters Beethoven refers to his "disease," which appears to refer to his deafness, but since deafness
would not cause death, here the deadly malady must be something
else.

Three trustworthy close observers—Bertolini, Thayer, and
Grove—were convinced that Beethoven had syphilis and was
treated with mercury, and several doctors agreed. Beethoven associated prostitutes with disease in his letters. As a young man he had a
fever after which he never fully recovered his health. Sir William
Osler linked that fever to syphilis. The Heiligenstadt Testament reveals suicidal depression and an expectation of imminent death. In
the last decades of his life, Beethoven had many physical complaints
that match with illnesses characteristic of secondary syphilis. Edward Larkin summarizes the various manifestations of disease during those years as "colitis, rheumatism, rheumatic fever, skin disorder, abscesses, endless infections, ophthalmia, and inflammatory
degeneration of arteries,"[46] all of which point to syphilis. Damage
to the eighth cranial nerve indicates syphilitic deterioration that
would cause deafness. At the end of his life there were rumors of
madness; contemporaries noted personality changes, rages, erratic
behavior, and paranoid thoughts, all suggestive of the period pre-
ceding the onset of paresis. At this time as well, Beethoven's compositions achieved their most exquisite form and expression.

The nineteenth-century medical consensus was that Beethoven had syphilis. Nonetheless, Beethoven cognoscenti of the past
three decades have denied that diagnosis. Anton Neumayr is one
of the most passionate opponents of the syphilis diagnosis. This
clinician, musician, and pathographer scolded Thayer in 1994 for
unleashing into the literature the "demon" of syphilis, which
"should be banished once and for all from serious medical discussions of Beethoven's illnesses."[47] He condemned Dr. Jacobssohn as
"a fanatic advocate of the syphilis thesis." What exotic blossoms
bloom in the garden of speculation by the medically untrained
and sometimes by reputable physicians as well, Neumayr complained, finding fault especially with Brunhold Springer (like

Thayer, a lawyer) for including Beethoven in his book, *The Brilliant Syphilitics*. Springer blames Beethoven's doctors for administering excessive mercury treatment. Neumayr thundered: "Confused, incompetent results are obtained when amateurs attempt to draw inferences about a venereal disease from methods of treatment and medical prescriptions."[48] He rejected syphilis so categorically because the autopsy did not show soft spots on the brain, changes in the membranes covering the brain, or gummas. (But would these signs have been present in a brain that had not yet reached the full flowering of the tertiary stage?) Neumayr does acknowledge, however, that the autopsy report described a swelling of the soft meninges at the base of the brain, which itself has led some to suggest syphilis.

Maynard Solomon does not mention syphilis in his Beethoven biography but notes parenthetically that "(it is thought that he may once have suffered from a minor venereal disease which responded successfully to treatment)."[49] The parentheses are significant; not only was the venereal disease both minor and successfully treated, but it was of mere parenthetical importance in Beethoven's life history. "If it was difficult then to diagnose living patients, it is impossible to diagnose a dead man after more than a century and after facts have been obfuscated, whether carelessly or willfully," wrote Marek, bemoaning lack of agreement among "a whole clinic of physicians" who had published retrospective diagnoses of Beethoven.[50]

Why have so many scholars who have considered syphilis in the life of Beethoven only discussed the initial stages of the disease without considering that so many of the other illnesses, as well as evidence of mental imbalance in his last days, might be clues? In Beethoven's case, no small part of the reason is the great reverence shown to the man who created the sublime compositions that so changed the course of music. Neumayr wrote: "His immortal works have such an aura of inviolability that, to the present day, not the slightest hint of disparaging criticisms has been cast in their direction. Beethoven's music fills us with the reverence we feel on entering a holy shrine."[51]

Richard Wagner's reverence toward the Master acknowledged serenity: "The deaf musician who listens to his inner harmonies undisturbed by the noise of life, who speaks from the depths to a world that has nothing more to say to him—now resembles a seer. . . . Never has an art offered the world anything so serene as these symphonies in A and F major, and all those works so intimately related to them which the master produced during the divine period of his total deafness."[52] Heinrich Heine (who had syphilis) found an ominous note at the end of Beethoven's life: "The sounds living in his mind were no more than memories, specters of dead sounds, and his later works had on their forehead a stamp of death that makes one shiver."[53]

As much as we might like proof for a diagnosis of syphilis, there is none. Sean Sellars concluded that without the contents of the missing Viennese specimen jar, no firm conclusion can be reached, but even then it is questionable whether the ear bones gone astray would provide definitive proof. The late music of Beethoven marked a turning point in the history of music with the Ninth Symphony, in particular the "Ode to Joy," a moment of surpassing perfection. When asked about the piano sonatas, Beethoven replied that they were not for the present but for a later age. What does it matter to us, in that later age, if Beethoven had syphilis or not? George Marek had this opinion: It goes without saying that it makes not the slightest difference, at least to the music, if Beethoven's complaints were due to spirochetes or to a hangnail.[54]

9

Franz Schubert
1797–1828

See, abased in dust and mire,
Scorched by agonizing fire,
I in torture go my way,
Nearing doom's destructive day.
— FRANZ SCHUBERT

THE SWATCH OF BEETHOVEN'S HAIR THAT WAS EVENTUALLY to land in the laboratories of Guevara and Brilliant was not the only sample taken, according to *Beethoven's Hair*. Another lock from the Master's head was supposedly snipped by Franz Schubert. Anton Schindler, Schubert's friend and first biographer, had taken sixty of Schubert's songs to Beethoven a few weeks before the master's death. Beethoven supposedly said that in Schubert there dwells a divine spark. Schubert, with a white lily pinned to his coat, was one of the torchbearers at Beethoven's funeral, attended by thousands of people in Vienna.

Schubert was mentioned in the famous conversation book that Beethoven used to communicate with friends once he was deaf. In August 1823 Beethoven's nephew Karl wrote that although Schubert was praised highly, he was hiding himself. Schubert was indeed hiding, since he was exhibiting the socially em-

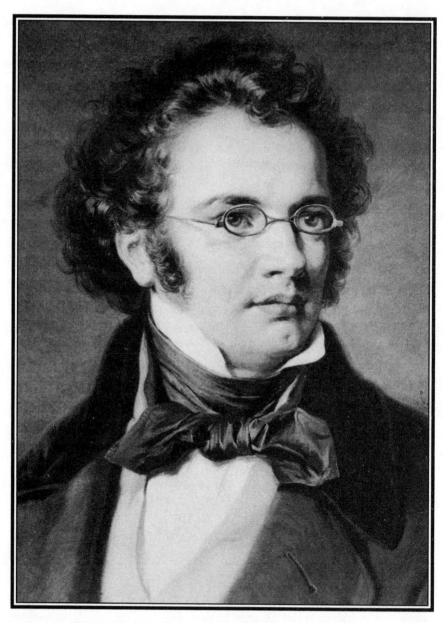

Figure 9.1   Franz Schubert (Bettmann/Corbis)

barrassing signs of relapsing syphilis. At first he kept his illness a secret, but it became common knowledge among his friends, shared
in their letters, although, of course, it was never named. The gossip
may have started with a comment Dr. Josef Bernhardt made to his
son-in-law. He was treating both Schubert and his friend Franz
von Schober, who appears to have had syphilis at the same time.
Friends thought Schober had a bad influence on Schubert. Schubert dedicated songs to Bernhardt, who became a close friend.

Three friends of Schubert eventually made guarded statements
about his syphilis, although not until several decades after his
death: Josef Kenner in 1858, Wilhelm von Chezy in 1863, and
Franz Schober in 1868. In the words of the first: "Anyone who
knew Schubert knows how he was made of two natures, foreign
to each other, how powerfully the craving for pleasure dragged his
soul down to the slough of moral degradation," ending with an al-
lusion to "an episode in Schubert's life which only too probably
caused his premature death and certainly hastened it."[1]

The syphilis diagnosis did not appear in print until 1907, and
then circumspectly, in an article by Otto Erich Deutsch. The case
presented was straightforward, and since then it has not been
questioned. Most medical authorities nonetheless assumed that
Schubert died of typhus, until Eric Sams published "Schubert's Illness Re-examined"[2] in 1980, summarizing the reasons to consider
syphilis as a cause of death instead. Schubert died at the age of
thirty-one after six years of illness.

Franz Peter Schubert was one of fourteen children in a Viennese
Catholic family. His father was a schoolteacher. He studied violin
and piano at home and learned the organ in church. His lovely
choirboy's voice gained him entry to the Royal Seminary, where
his teacher was Mozart's adversary, Antonio Salieri. He wrote his
first symphony when he was sixteen. By the time he died he had
produced one thousand compositions, including six hundred
poignant songs full of sorrow and yearning, the height of romantic
lyricism. Much of his music was heard for the first time during
private evenings known as Schubertiads. He received little recog-

nition in his lifetime outside his close circle of friends, and he lived in relative poverty.

Most scholars now assume that Schubert was infected during the last months of 1822, when he was twenty-five. From then on his excellent health was replaced by painful episodes and deep depressions, alternating with periods of apparent good health. No record exists of Schubert attending any social events in December 1822. On 7 January, "Schubert is almost entirely well and in the company all the time of Bernhardt."[3] At his birthday party on 31 January he was in high spirits. A two-week fast followed. In February Schwind told Schober that Schubert, no longer wearing his wig, was showing "the first signs of sweet little curls."[4] On 28 February 1823 he wrote to the publisher of his music saying that the "circumstances of my health still forbidding me to leave the house,"[5] which may have meant either that his syphilis was infectious or that it was conspicuous. That month he composed his Sonata in A Minor, a moody piece filled with sadness and regret.

In early March he was feeling better; "everything was different." He was living on a special diet proposed by Bernhardt—bread soup alternating with veal scallops, tea by the gallon—and a regimen of baths and fasts, typical treatments for early syphilis. But the improvement did not last. Schubert observed: "No one knows another's pain."[6] A few days later he expressed sheer despair over his condition in a letter to Leopold Kupelweiser:

In a word, I feel I'm the most unhappy, most wretched man in the world. Imagine a man whose health will never be sound again and who in despair only makes it worse and not better; imagine a man, I say, whose most shining hopes have come to naught, for whom the bliss of love and friendship offers nothing but the greatest pain, for whom the passion (at least something stimulating) for beauty threatens to die away, and ask yourself then if that isn't one wretched, unhappy man?—"My peace is gone, heavy is my heart, find it again shall I never, never again," this I can certainly sing now every day, for every night when I

go to bed I hope I'll never wake up, and every morning only reminds me of yesterday's grief.[7]

He ended the letter affectionately, kissing his friend one thousand
times. On 29 March he entered in his notebook: "Pain and not joy
sharpens the understanding and strengthens the mind."

In July Kupelweiser reported to Schober that he had heard
Schubert was ill; later reports said "seriously ill." By August Schubert was feeling better. He informed Schober: "I correspond
busily with Schäffer and am fairly well. Whether I shall ever quite
recover I'm inclined to doubt";[8] and on 12 November he reported himself "really quite ill at the time."[9] In October or November he spent several weeks in the Vienna General Hospital for
treatments. Deeply depressed, he threw himself into his work and
composed an entire cycle of songs. He wrote to Schober: "I hope
to regain my health, and this recovered treasure will let me forget
many a sorrow."[10]

On Christmas eve Schwind wrote to Schober: "Schubert is
better, and it won't be long now before he will have his own hair
again, which had to be cut off because of the rash. He is wearing a
very comfortable wig."[11] The first fever and rash of syphilis are often accompanied by alopecia, or patchy baldness, but Schubert's
condition in December suggests relapsing rash, since Schwind's
note mentions that his hair was cut, not that it fell out.

Next, his left arm was too painful to play the piano,[12] and he
complained of pains in his bones. Lesions of the mouth and throat
prevented him from singing. Schubertiads were no longer sched-
uled. He felt as if he had taken poison. But he could compose. To
his brother Ferdinand he wrote: "True, it is no longer that happy
time during which each object seems to us to be surrounded by a
youthful gloriole, but a period of fateful recognition of a miserable
reality, which I endeavour to beautify as far as possible by my
imagination (thank God).. . . A grand sonata and variations on a
theme of my own, both for 4 hands, which I have already written,
shall serve you as proof of this."[13] Schubert was referring here to
the *Grand Duo*, Sonata in C and the A-flat variations.

Again Schubert's health improved; in November 1824 he felt "newly rejuvenated." But time in the hospital followed. In the middle of the year he was well, but later too ill to attend a New Year's party. During a good period Schwind observed that Schubert was "carefree as a cloud and healthy," and Schober expressed joy that his friend was doing so well. Anton Ottenwalt wrote of one of the recoveries: "Schubert looks so healthy and energetic, is in such a cheerful mood, so friendly to talk to, that you have to take heartfelt pleasure in it."[14] To his parents he jubilated: "Am glad about everyone's good health, to which I—the Almighty be exalted—can add my own."[15] In a period of good health, Schubert composed songs from Scott's *Lady of the Lake*, including the *Ave Maria*. Robert Schumann observed that the sonatas of this period "can bring you to tears."

In the late summer of 1826, Schubert was again ill. His friend Bauernfeld recorded in his diary that "Schubert [is] half sick, he ought to have 'young peacocks' just like Benvenuto Cellini."[16] Cellini, the late Renaissance goldsmith, sculptor, and braggadocio, claimed to have cured his syphilis by eating peacocks, a coded reference, some suggest, to young men.

At this time Schubert was composing *Die Winterreise* (The Winter Journey), a song cycle of heart-rending beauty and profound sorrow. He was exhausted and depressed. His friend Spaun wrote: "For some time Schubert was in a gloomy mood and looked worn out. When I would ask him what was going on with him, he would only say: 'Come to Schrober's today and I will sing you a cycle of ghastly songs. I'm curious to see what you'll say. They have shaken me more than it ever was with any other lieder.' And he was right, for soon we were all enamored of these mournful songs . . . more beautiful German lieder than these do not exist."[17] With a voice full of emotion, Schubert sang the whole of *Die Winterreise* for his friends. They were dumbfounded by the gloomy mood of the songs. Various notes of friends indicate that from this time on, Schubert was consistently a very sick man.

On 26 March 1828, at the urging of his friends, Schubert gave his sole concert, which was greatly successful. This event marked the beginning of a remarkable period of creative production, including his own requiem, the grand mass in E-flat. At this time he was experiencing chronic headaches, dizziness, and rushes of blood to his head. He was also drinking heavily and subject to uncontrollable and aggressive rages. As Chèzy related: "As soon as the blood of the vine was glowing in him, he liked to withdraw into a corner and give in to a quiet, comfortable anger during which he would try to create some sort of havoc as quickly as possible, for example, with cups, glasses, and plates, and as he did so, he would grin and screw up his eyes tight."[18]

In September 1828 Schubert left the city and joined his brother in a new house in a suburb of Vienna. One night he went to dinner with Ferdinand, who recalled in his memoirs: "On the last evening in October, he was intending to eat some fish when, after taking the first bite, he suddenly threw down his knife and fork and declared that the food nauseated him and it was just as though he had taken poison. From this moment on, Schubert ate almost nothing more and merely took medicines."[19] He took a three-hour walk, thinking exercise would help, but on 12 November he wrote to Schober: "I am sick. For eleven days now I haven't had anything to eat or drink and I wander, lurching and exhausted from my chair to my bed and back again. Rinna is treating me. Even if I eat something it comes right back up again."[20] On 14 November Schubert was so weary he felt he was falling right through the bed. He continued to work in bed, making corrections to *Die Winterreise*. Two days before his death he complained of a burning in the head. On the evening of 17 November delirium set in, leading to manic singing. He was held in bed with difficulty. On the evening of 18 November he imagined himself under the ground. He asked Ferdinand not to leave him there. His dying words for his doctor were: "Here, here is my end."

The last music that Schubert heard was Beethoven's String Quartet in C-sharp Minor, Op. 131, a private bedside performance at his request. He was buried three graves away from Beethoven. With Beethoven, he was disinterred and reburied. His head was removed from his body and photographed.

The official cause of death was ambiguous: nervous fever. Eric Sams noted reasons why this term did not imply typhoid fever, as had been accepted for some time, suggesting instead that Schubert's last days were in no way different from his ongoing health complaints but were quite different from typhoid. In September Schubert had been treated for giddiness and rushes of blood to the head. He was well enough to amuse himself reading James Fenimore Cooper and correcting proofs. His friends noted that his condition did not look at all serious and he was planning future projects. Sams poses this question: "Could such comments conceivably have been made about, let alone by, a dying typhoid fever victim in the terminal stage of a manifestly serious illness with clearly marked and clinically familiar symptoms?"[21] He thinks not and suggests further that Schubert's feeling of being poisoned, and his giddiness, insomnia, and headache, might have been mercurial poison. Schubert's doctor of the last days was Josef von Vering, whose father had treated Beethoven in the summer of 1801 and who wrote two books on syphilis, one on the use of mercury, *Concerning the Treatment of Syphilis by Applying a Mercuric Liniment.* He found Schubert's case hopeless on first examination due to advanced decomposition of the blood.

Sams wonders that previous authorities have not suggested tertiary syphilis as a cause of Schubert's death. He notes that deteriorative anemia characterizes tertiary syphilis and cites a 1963 medical opinion by Dr. Kerner that the terminal event was an occlusion of a cerebral artery, "the direct and uncomplicated consequence of brain syphilis."[22] To our inquiry into the experience of having syphilis, Schubert adds one of the most poignant testimonials of a man with that self-knowledge, expressed in his correspondence and still more in his death-ridden, deeply brooding, romantic music. His work pace was that of a man fearing an early death. He did not live long enough to experience the exhilaration that sometimes marked tertiary syphilis right before the final stage. He knew only the initial misery: "Every morning only reminds me of yesterday's grief."

Robert Schumann
1810–1856

In 1831 I was syphilitic and treated with arsenic.

—ROBERT SCHUMANN

CELESTIAL ANGELS DICTATED (TO ROBERT SCHUMANN) AN entire work composed by the spirit of Franz Schubert—or so he thought in the week when he experienced his sudden turn to madness. On Friday night, 10 February 1854, Schumann suffered an acute attack of tinnitus, with strong and painful auditory disturbances that continued for a week, until they developed into musical tones and "wondrous" angelic voices consisting of a set of five variations on the angelic theme. Schubert as an angelic being had been anticipated in Schumann's diary in 1828. He had sobbed throughout the night when he heard of Schubert's death: "And you, heavenly Schubert, all too soon called home. . . . You are the over-arching celestial spirit that enshrouds its flowers of spring."[1]

Following this episode, Schumann was taken to an insane asylum near Bonn where his doctor, Franz Richarz, kept a journal about his famous patient, recording his meals, medications, rages, and fantasies. Some of the time Schumann was agitated and delusional, as when Richarz noted: "Was restless, violent, loud; hit the

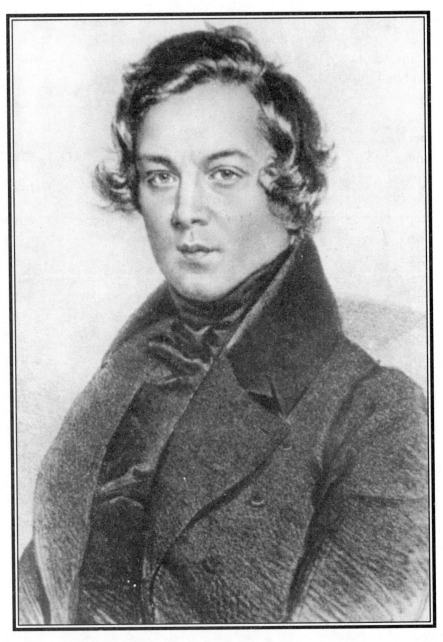

Figure 10.1   Robert Schumann (Library of Congress)

orderly, saying that 'everything was poisoned'; also during the night constantly excited, roaring, raging."[2] At other times he was calm and rational, playing the piano, composing, writing letters, and making entries in his diary. One of Richarz's entries is of particular interest: "12 September 1855. During rounds busy with calculating his financial circumstances and very calm. Recently has been writing down all kinds of brief jottings and reflections of melancholy content, e.g., 'In 1831 I was syphilitic and treated with arsenic.'" [3]

In the years after Schumann's death, the Richarz diary was kept secret, passing from the godson of Richarz's aunt to that godson's nephew, Aribert Reimann, who inherited it in 1973 and kept it at home, as his uncle had requested, in the interest of doctor-patient confidentiality. After sleepless nights of indecision, he finally handed it over to the Archive of the Academy of the Arts, Berlin, in 1991. Franz Hermann Franken, a medical historian and pathographer, commented on the report, pleased to put to rest rumors that had been printed "even in renowned journals" that Clara Schumann had shoved her husband into the asylum to carry on a love affair with Johannes Brahms, concluding that the legend of Robert and Clara as a "nightmare couple" is banal "and ignores the fact that Robert Schumann's fate is the greatest human tragedy of German Romanticism."[4] Comments in Richarz's records, such as "physically attacked the doctor," "spilled wine given to him at dinner into the stove because he thought it was urine," and "struck the orderlies" justified Clara's decision to turn her husband over to the care of Richarz's clinic.

Franken asks, "Does Richarz's progress report now clarify the diagnosis of Schumann's illness? The question is to be answered in the affirmative. Richarz described the characteristic development of a cerebral degeneration, in which the indications are convincing that it had to do with a progressive paralysis caused by syphilis."[5] Franken lists the various indications of progressive paralysis in Richarz's report, noting speech that became difficult and less understandable, convulsions, deterioration of his personality, and, most telling, differing dilation of his pupils. The autopsy report as well suggested syphilis: "the yellowish, gelatinous mass that he described at the base of the brain therefore corresponded, as we had already suspected in 1981, most likely to a syphilitic gumma."[6] Bone tumors found at the base of the skull are also suspicion-arousers, as is the condition of the heart, which Ostwald described as "big, flaccid, thick-walled, in all chambers symmetrically too large," commenting: "If Schumann had had syphilis affecting the valves or the aorta that might have caused cardiac enlargement."[7] Richarz diagnosed incomplete paralysis; Franken observed that what is self-evident today—the causal relationship between progressive paralysis preceded by decades of syphilitic infection—was not known to Dr. Richarz.

"In 1831 I was syphilitic and treated with arsenic." The specific date and remedy indicate that Schumann knew he was infected. He may have harbored the knowledge as a secret for more than twenty years. Was this secret kept from Clara? One of Clara's biographers, Nancy Reich, suggests that she did not know of her husband's infection and thought along with Schumann's doctors that he had a nervous condition aggravated by overwork. But perhaps it was a secret they shared to the end. Why would Schumann finally reveal a secret he had not previously even written in his private diaries? Approaching death, fearful of the episodes of madness, isolated from Clara due to Richarz's belief that visitors from the outside could excite a patient with Schumann's type of restless dementia—all this might have made Schumann feel that his secret was irrelevant. He may have jotted this note in a private moment, not realizing that Richarz was carefully copying the journal in his own doctor's log.

Robert Schumann's father broke with the family tradition of farming to be a bookseller and writer, and his mother, the daughter of a surgeon, was known for her operatic voice. Robert was an artistic child who composed music and poetry, sang, and played the flute and cello as well as the piano. When he went to Leipzig to study law, he was not following his own heart or abilities. "I shall never warm to bleak jurisprudence that shatters you from the very beginning with its ice-cold definitions,"[8] he complained to his mother. He was physically active, enjoying fencing, horseback riding, and gymnastics. His 30 July 1830 diary entry reads: "My whole life has been a twenty-year struggle between poetry and prose, or call it music and law. . . . Now I stand at the crossroads and I cringe at the question: whither?"[9] Music won out when Schumann persuaded the noted piano teacher Friedrich Wieck to take him on as a student.

Robert met Wieck's daughter Clara when she was nine. As a child prodigy she gave concerts that earned her a European reputation and even praise from Goethe in a private performance. Although Clara would be the love of Schumann's life and the mother of his children, his affections in 1831, the year he gave in the asylum as the time of his infection, were directed toward a woman named Christel, sometimes called Charitas in his diaries, who lived in the Wieck household, perhaps as a maid or a student.

References to Christel are clearly sexual: "Charitas came completely and was bleeding," "full of fire and flames," "Christel in one minute," "Christel didn't come either." In May 1831 his diary refers to a "wound" on his penis leading to a "biting and devouring pain," along with an aphorism: "Only guilt gives birth to Nemesis." Christel turned pale when she heard of the condition. The unhappy lovers separately consulted Schumann's cellist friend Christian Glock, who had just graduated from medical school. Glock suggested that Schumann bathe the sore in narcissus water, a herbal treatment in use since the time of Galen. Schumann wrote in his diary, "Foreskin stung from narcissus water."[10]

Soon after this episode Schumann complained to his mother of what he thought to be cholera or something similar. Unable to collect his thoughts, he stayed in his room for six days with pains in his stomach, heart, and head, along with memory loss and feelings of anger. Right after seeing Glock he wrote: "If only I could be a genius, so I could kill all the rotten people with it. I'd like to

load them all into a cannon and shoot something to death."[11] On
8 June, he turned twenty-one, took control of his inheritance, and
qualified for military duty.

Glock prescribed abstinence. On 15 June Schumann once
again had sex with Charitas, but this time "with fear and little enjoyment." He began drinking excessively and confided to his diary
about a terrible tendency to seek self-destruction. "I'm sinking
back into the old slime. Will no hand from the clouds come to
hold me?"[12] He referred to "evil days for which I hope God and
my heart may forgive me."[13] Schumann's mood did not improve
when the sickness passed. On September 21 he wrote to his
brother Julius: "I'm in a fatal state of restlessness and would like to
put a bullet through my head." That same day he instructed his
mother how to dispose of his belongings, including his piano, in
the event of his death.

Was the "wound" a syphilitic chancre? Was the cholera-like
fever, accompanied by such distress, secondary syphilis? Primary
chancres are usually painless, but they can be quite painful if they
are super-infected with another venereal disease. The diffuse body
pains, the loss of memory, the inability to concentrate accompanying the fever, and the subsequent depression all point to secondary
syphilis.

Although 1831 remains the most likely time of infection, it is
possible that Schumann only thought he was infected that year
when in fact the disease began either earlier or later. In 1825
Schumann's sister Emilie, suffering from "grief approaching dementia," committed suicide, whether by drowning or by throwing
herself from a window. She was twenty-nine, fourteen years older
than her brother. Emilie suffered from a chronic skin disease that
"threw its poisons onto the most precious parts of her body."[14]
The skin condition alone could have been psoriasis, but the genital involvement and the relentlessly progressive depression with
"occasional traces of quiet madness" point to syphilis. Peter Ostwald suggested: "But of course Emilie might have had a toxic-or-
ganic psychosis, even syphilis, given the skin disease."[15] If Emilie
did have syphilis, she may have infected Robert through the shar-

ing of a glass or a moist towel. According to John Stokes: "The family in which a syphilitic member has been discovered will include between twenty and forty per cent syphilitic individuals."[16]

Eric Sams has a third hypothesis, that Schumann was infected at the time that he was a student. He was treated by Franz Hartmann, a homeopath and student of the founder of homeopathy, Samuel Hahnemann. Sams tracked the records of Hartmann's clinic and found a patient who was being treated for a syphilitic finger chancre. Could that patient have been Schumann? Although this theory is tenuous at best, it does connect with a line from Schumann's journal. Before beginning studies in Leipzig, Schumann took a vacation and noted at various places: "Pretty girls—the cute innkeeper's wife—Rosen's endangered virginity—kiss-wild goings on—smiling maidens—finger-play under skirts."[17] It only takes a few spirochetes slipping through a small abrasion in the skin to cause the "physicians' chancre."

Schumann experienced lameness in the third and fourth fingers of his right hand and "the most pervasive pains in the arm."[18] Since at the time he was planning on a career as a piano virtuoso, the stiffness was of great concern, and he sought numerous medical opinions and remedies. In June 1832 he wrote to his mother that his brother would tell her of a strange misfortune that had befallen him. He was traveling to Dresden (with Wieck) for medical advice. In August he told her that his apartment looked like a pharmacy. For fear of the knife, he put off seeing a surgeon. He experimented with a mechanical device to strengthen his hand, which Wieck called a "finger-torturer." Though believing that the hand was incurable, Schumann still sought imaginative treatments. One such strange remedy was an "animal bath" cure recommended by Professor Karl August Kuhl. Schumann was to thrust his ailing hand into the belly of a large, freshly slaughtered animal and leave it there until the animal cooled, an experience he found to be, if not charming, at least strengthening, although he feared some of the cow nature might mingle with his own. Kuhl also had him bathe the hand all day in warm brandy and sleep with his aching arm encased in an herbal wrap.

Schumann also saw Dr. Otto, a practitioner of electrotherapy, who applied galvanic currents that deadened the sickly parts even further. In November 1832, he gave up on the piano, telling his mother that henceforth he would be a cellist since that instrument demanded functional fingers only on the left hand. In March 1833 he was treated by Karl J. Portius, who claimed to read psychic qualities with an electromagnetic device; this man is "no windbag or swindler,"[19] Schumann assured his mother. In 1838 Schumann wrote to Clara: "Sometimes I feel unhappy, especially since I have an ailing hand. And I'll let you in on a secret; it's getting worse. . . . I can only play in a pinch, since one finger stumbles over the other. . . . Now I have you as a right hand."[20] Schumann's friend Dr. Reuter, who passed letters between the lovers, Clara and Robert, when they were separated by her father, wrote two affidavits to get Schumann excused from military duty. He stated that since his index finger and the middle fingers of his right hand had been quasi-paralyzed for some time, he was incapable of using a rifle. Syphilis may have caused the hand problem, or it may have exacerbated a preexisting condition.

In the summer of 1833 Franz Hartmann, a Leipzig general practitioner and recognized authority on the homeopathic treatment of syphilis, told Schumann no allopath could cure him and promised to cure him himself within three months, whether of syphilis or the hand ailment is not clear. Although Schumann found the practice of homeopathy to be "flimsy," he was reassured by Hartmann's confidence. Hartmann insisted on a strict diet with no coffee or wine and just a little beer, and he prescribed a mysterious "tiny, tiny bit of powder"[21]—perhaps the arsenic that Schumann remembered in the asylum. Treatment for relapsing secondary symptoms two years later would be expected, and white arsenic, arsenic albicans, was frequently prescribed for syphilis by homeopaths.

When Schumann came down with another fever, Hartmann quarantined him for fourteen days, suggesting an infectious condition. Schumann wrote to Clara: "Today however I took all the bandages away from the wounds and almost laughed at the doctor

in his face when he tried to keep me from writing. I even threatened to attack him and infect him with my fever if he didn't let
me do as I like. Now he does."[22] If the bandages covered lesions of
relapsing secondary syphilis, Hartmann was wise to stay clear.

Biographers and medical writers alike have uncritically accepted the diagnosis of P. J. Möbius (the neurologist who first revealed Nietzsche's syphilis) that Schumann was suffering from
malaria. Peter Ostwald added the interesting twist that malaria is a
modern treatment for syphilis. However, Anton Neumayr argues
that Schumann's illness did not match malaria at all. Homeopaths
noted the similarity between the secondary infection of syphilis
and malaria: "It may be mild continuous or it may take on a remittent character, but the most remarkable form is the intermittent,
simulating Malaria, with a temperature running even up to 105
degrees persisting on for months."[23]

While he was feverish, Johanna urged her son to come home
to visit his brother Julius, who was dying of pulmonary tuberculosis. Schumann's response indicates how very sick he was: "You
seem to have no understanding of my tormenting disease. . . . Almost every breath of air produces an attack. . . . Were I to take the
mail coach I would have to go straight to bed and might never get
up again."[24] Julius died, as did Schumann's sister-in-law Rosalie.
Upon her death Schumann wrote:

> The most terrifying thought that a person can ever have sud-
> denly occurred to me, the most terrible with which heaven can
> punish you, that of 'losing my mind.' It overwhelmed me so vio-
> lently, that all consolation and every prayer became as ineffective
> as scorn and mockery. The anxiety drove me from place to
> place—my breathing was disrupted by the idea 'what would
> happen if you could no longer think?' . . . In my endlessly terri-
> ble excitement, I ran to a doctor, told him everything, that I of-
> ten seemed to lose my senses, that I didn't know where to turn
> because of the anxiety, yes, that I could not guarantee whether
> in such a condition of utter helplessness, I might not raise a
> hand against my own life.[25]

Later that year in a letter to his mother he wrote:

> I was hardly more than a statue, without coldness, without warmth. Only by forcing myself to work did life return, bit by bit. . . . Violent flushing, unspeakable dread, shortness of breath, and momentary lapses of consciousness fluctuate rapidly, although less now than in the days gone by. If you had an inkling how depression has totally shattered my peace of mind, you would surely forgive me for not writing.[26]

In 1834 Schumann pursued a possible engagement to a woman named Ernestine, although as she accepted his proposal he changed his mind: "In my tormented condition, I am afraid to accept the precious jewel into my accursed hand."[27] In 1840 Schumann married Clara after a terrible legal battle with her father, who opposed the marriage. Marriage to Clara was followed by several good years.[28] Schumann was many years past the infectious period when he married Clara.

"After a typical period of latency," Franken writes, "the neurasthenic pre-stage of progressive paralysis began in Schumann no later than 1850."[29] Here again, as we so often see in studies of those who had syphilis, the focus is on the initial infection and then the final stage of syphilis, leaping over decades as if during the "typical period of latency" nothing of medical interest were happening. And yet, if we look at Schumann's life during those years, we see one physical complaint after another, most, if not all, pointing to a progressing case of syphilis.

Schumann engaged Dr. Reuter to diagnose an apoplectic constitution: "dizziness brought about by blood-congestion to the brain, heart, and major vessels" involving the danger of an apoplectic stroke. He constantly complained of increasing poor health, "sad melancholia," and colic, and sought treatment for depression—hydrotherapy and cathartic salts—but the depression deepened. Clara observed that he could barely get across a room without great effort. He reported severe malaise after working. He had periods of sickness alternating with productivity. His journal is full of such comments as "sick in the evening—sleepless night," and "sick, half imaginary, half real." He complained of "nervous disease," "bad anxiety at noon," "sick, sick, and very sick," "anxiety and depression," "melancholy," "exhausted" and "weak." He described himself as "living in the country with some hypochondria," and spoke of "stupid hypochondriacal brooding." Schumann consulted with another member of Hahnemann's school of homeopathic medicine, Dr. Wolfgang Müller, who postulated that drug-induced toxicity was making many patients even more sick, and he consulted a phrenologist. He was often gloomy, nervous, and irritable, and he expressed fears of madness.

After a "violent nervous attack," Schumann had an appointment with Dr. Carl Gustav Carus. They discussed ongoing problems with his eyes, and Carus gave him some medication. A second doctor, Helbig, a hypnotist, concluded that Schumann had fallen into a diseased state while composing. He refused medication from Dr. Helbig but accepted his suggestions of cold plunge-baths. He began to have trouble with his ears, hearing a constant singing and rushing, with every noise turning into a tone. He had insomnia. He complained of "dreadful rheumatism" in his feet.

A severe nervous attack in March 1852 marked a turning point in Schumann's health. That summer he had another bad attack, lost his appetite, and experienced an overall weakening. On a vacation he fainted after a strenuous hike. Upon returning home he consulted Dr. Müller, who dismissed the event as the result of too much exertion and prescribed eighteen cold plunges in the Rhine. Schumann complied. In July he described being "still always very unwell"[30] and, after several experiences conducting, reported a "sad weakening of my strengths. Very exhausted."[31]

Clara spoke of her husband having a "nervous convulsion."[32] In August he complained of continual nervous agitation and in September of "a burning feeling in the back of the head" as well as "nervous dizziness." He felt pricking sensations in his fingertips and backbone. He was bled by leeches. He had an attack of dizziness and reported "strange afflictions of hearing." He experienced difficulty with speech and had a convulsive attack.

Schumann began holding séances to contact dead composers. His table thumped out the opening to Beethoven's Fifth Symphony on command. On a trip to Bonn he suffered a severe attack of rheumatism and consulted Dr. Domenicus Galt (or Kalt). Slater suggests that a cerebral vascular stroke at this time may have been linked to syphilis: "congestive attacks, with the clinical features of very temporary strokes, are common in the early stages of general paresis."[33] He experienced a "strange weakness of the speech organ"[34] and his handwriting became less legible, although his musical manuscripts remained orderly. When Schumann began to drop his baton while conducting, he tied it to his wrist with a string. He responded to being told that he could no longer conduct anything but his own music with: "Impertinent effronteries."[35] Clara agreed: "Vulgarity is in charge."[36] In November the couple left for a month of concerts in Holland. Schumann was experiencing more auditory problems.

The angels who dictated to Schumann on the Friday evening at the beginning of his first mad episode had turned into devils by morning. Schumann was a sinner headed for hell fire. Hyenas and tigers circled him. On Sunday, 24 February 1853, he worked himself into a "joyous exaltation" and, bathed in sweat and fearing that he might harm Clara, insisted on being taken to an asylum. He laid out all the things he would take with him. The next day he wandered out of the house in a rainstorm, walked toward the Rhine, and having no money with him, gave his silk scarf to the toll collector at the bridge. He leaped into the water but was rescued by a fisherman.

On 4 March, he was finally taken to the asylum. Clara lamented: "Oh what agony it is for me! . . . My heart breaks completely when I don't even know how he lives, what he does, whether he still hears the voices. . . . How does he sleep, what does he do during the day, and does he ask for me or not?"[37] The delirious symptoms passed, leaving Schumann placid, but in the subsequent weeks he was agitated and had another acute psy-

chotic phase with hallucinations and confused talk. The doctors
had very little of his medical history, in part because Clara was not
consulted. Brahms wrote to Clara that Schumann asked if she
were dead, it had been so long since he had heard from her. Her
letters had been withheld.

When Julius Grimm visited, he reported that his friend spoke
softly, seemed gentle and friendly, and looked well and strong, having put on some weight. But at dinner he had poured his wine on
the floor, declaring it was poisoned. He thought he was being fed
the feces of other patients. Brahms visited as well, reporting that
Robert was well and strong, clear and sensitive. A doctor told
Brahms that there were alternating periods of confusion and clarity. Schumann wrote, but illegibly, and often had no memory of
what he had done an hour before.

Schumann declined in his third year in the hospital, and when
Brahms visited he babbled incoherently. Clara, who was support-
ing the family and paying for the asylum, interrupted a concert
tour to go to him when she heard of his worsening condition. She
recalled his greeting: "He smiled at me and embraced me with
great effort, because he could no longer control his limbs. Never
will I forget it. For all the world's treasures I wouldn't exchange
this embrace."[38] The next day when she went to see him his limbs
twitched and his speech was violent. He drank a little wine she
gave him, and she thought he knew her. He died at 4:00 P.M. the
following day, 29 July 1856, while Clara had gone to the train de-
pot with Brahms. Her diary entry when she returned read: "I
stood by his corpse, my ardently beloved husband, and was quiet;
all my thoughts went up to God with thanks that he is finally free.
And as I knelt at this bed . . . it seems as if a magnificent spirit was
hovering over me—ah, if only he had taken me along."[39] Brahms
eulogized: "The remembrance of Schumann is sacred to me. I will
always take this noble, pure artist as my model."[40]

Opinion is divided about the value of the fifty compositions
Schumann produced in the last four years of sanity. Eric Sams
thought them substandard: "The songs of 1849 are a decline; the
later ones a descent, first steep and then precipitous."[41] John

Davario disagreed, saying that anyone who heard signs of decay in Schumann's later music did not know it well. Clara destroyed some of his last songs as unworthy.

Schumann's body is buried in Bonn. His head, like Schubert's, was removed from his body for scientific study. Like the parts of Beethoven's ears removed at autopsy, it has been misplaced.

Psychiatrists might have been content to attribute Schumann's psychological problems to syphilis if Richarz's diaries of his incarceration had been revealed earlier. Instead, they have gone to such great lengths to find an adequate diagnostic category that the resulting list of hypotheses reads like the table of contents of the American Psychiatric Association diagnostic standards manual. At various times Schumann's mental condition has been described as psychotic, schizophrenic, manic-depressive, borderline, narcissistic, catatonic, paranoid, depressive, and obsessive-compulsive.

The diagnostic literature split early between those who thought that Schumann was schizophrenic and those who favored a diagnosis of a bipolar disorder. P. J. Möbius opted for schizophrenia, whereas the younger Professor Hans Gruhle argued against Möbius that Schumann's illness was "a cyclothymic form of manic-depressive madness." Möbius countered that daementia praecox, as schizophrenia was then called, and manic-depressive disorder were often difficult to distinguish, but insisted that Schumann's condition was not caused by an outside invader, such as a spirochete.

Peter Ostwald (who left the syphilis question open) maintained that Schumann was psychotic, dismissing both schizophrenia and manic-depressive disorder. Anton Neumayr politely took exception to his colleague Ostwald with an elaborate diagnosis touching most of the bases: composite psychosis or periodic catatonic schizophrenia, "one in which the symptoms of schizophrenia are also evident amid signs of cyclic depression."[42]

Ostwald wrote: "Genius and madness have often been thought to be related in some way. In the life of Robert Schumann it is particularly difficult to draw a line between the two. The problem of distinguishing between his creative and psychotic behavior has confounded many biographers, musicologists, and psychiatrists. Thus far no single diagnosis has done justice to the facts."[43] Does syphilis do justice to all the facts? Is there anything in Schumann's condition that does not fit under the umbrella of a diagnosis of syphilis?

Eric Sams neatly summarized these signs of syphilis in Schumann: continuous general malaise, tinnitus, vertigo, insomnia, headache, depression, premonition of insanity, numbness, cramp, difficulty writing, speech disturbance, loss of memory, a stroke, pains in bones and joints, florid psychosis, and postmortem signs.

Although there is still some controversy, the weight of scholarly opinion now opts for a diagnosis of syphilis. Anton Neumayr states: "As for the organic process affecting Schumann's brain that became evident from 1850 on, there are now incontestable indications for the presence of progressive paralysis resulting from syphilis."[44] John Davario adds: "Although there has long been a strong suspicion that Schumann had earlier contracted syphilis, we can now be reasonably sure this was indeed the case. Other pieces of the puzzle fall into place."[45]

Schumann continued his productive and creative career despite the many illnesses he experienced over the years. Paresis has been called a Faustian bargain because of the periodic euphoric joy that offsets the misery in the months before its onset. Schumann appears to have missed that reward, except perhaps for the brief episode during his breakdown when an angelic chorus blessed him with Schubert's celestial concert. On the other hand, his happy marriage to Clara and his children provided a stability missing in the lives of many syphilitics.

Charles Baudelaire
1821–1867

> We all have the republican spirit in our veins,
> just as we have the pox in our bones. We are
> democratized and syphilised.
> —CHARLES BAUDELAIRE

CHARLES BAUDELAIRE'S VOLUME OF POETRY, LES FLEURS *du mal* (Flowers of Evil) so scandalized his contemporaries with its theme of beauty and corruption that he was charged with obscenity, and six of the poems having to do with lesbians and vampires were suppressed by the French Public Safety Section of the Ministry of the Interior. Gustave Flaubert wrote a deeply indignant letter of sympathy to the young man, asking against what had he offended: religion? public morals? It was something new, Flaubert wrote, to prosecute a book of verse. To his mother Baudelaire explained that *Les fleurs du mal* was a witness to his disgust and hatred of everything. The poet Paul Verlaine called him *le poète maudit* (the cursed poet).

How much of this disgust and hatred was related to Baudelaire's knowledge of being syphilitic? (*Mal* means both evil and malady.) Baudelaire never made any public statements about his disease, although he did speak of it in letters to his family. He con-

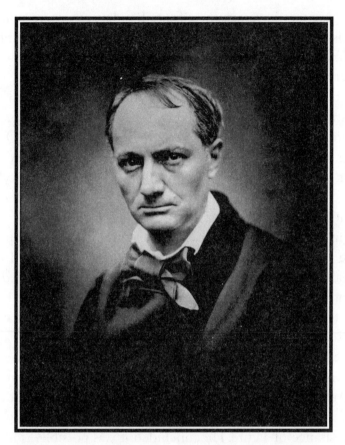

Figure 11.1   Charles Baudelaire (Spencer Museum of Art, University of Kansas)

fessed to his mother on 6 May 1861: "You know that when very young I caught a venereal infection, which I later supposed to be totally cured. In Dijon after 1848 it erupted again. It was made to subside once more. Now it is returned in a novel form, marks on the skin, and extraordinary stiffness in all the joints. You may believe me; *I know about it*. Perhaps in the state of sadness in which I am plunged, my terror makes it worse."[1] This sadness contrasts with Baudelaire's famous statement of bravado: "On the day that the writer corrects his first proof, he is as proud as a schoolboy who has just caught his first pox."[2]

Biographers have assumed from Baudelaire's correspondence with his brother that the date of his infection was November or December 1839, when he was eighteen and living in the Latin Quarter in Paris. He had just been expelled from a military boarding school for refusing to relinquish a note he had written to another student; he had swallowed it instead. He prepared privately for exams and passed. For two years he lived in the Latin Quarter, writing, until he set out for India in 1841 on a trip planned by his mother, who hoped he would give up his bohemian lifestyle. He returned early to Paris, where he lived lavishly when he received a substantial inheritance. After he had squandered nearly half of it by 1844, his family obtained a court order to have a lawyer appointed to dole out an allowance to him for the rest of his life. In Paris Baudelaire wrote reviews, essays, and poetry, and he achieved some recognition for his art criticism of Courbet and Delacroix. He also completed an autobiographical novel, *La fanfarlo*. He translated his "twin soul," Edgar Allan Poe (another syphilis suspect), and he published poetry in journals.

Twenty years later Baudelaire cautioned his friend and publisher Auguste Poulet-Malassis to be careful with his pox, because of his own experience of relapse, warning him to be wary about the appearance of a cure. He concluded it was possible, as he himself had been so fortunate: "You have just given me the exact description of the symptoms I once had. Be assured, however, that no one is more hale and hearty than one who has had the pox and has been quite cured."[3] But hale and hearty was not to be his future; there was no cure for syphilis.

Baudelaire's love life remains a mystery. Some biographers think that his relationship with Jeanne Duval was voyeuristic only and that he remained a virgin, a difficult hypothesis to reconcile with his venereal infection, and perhaps with the addresses of prostitutes found in his notebooks. Nadar subtitled his study of Baudelaire *le poète vierge* (the virgin poet). André Gide recorded in his journal (1921) that Proust was convinced Baudelaire was gay: Gide: "'You don't believe that he ever practiced'... Proust: 'What!

He cries. I am convinced of the opposite; how can you doubt that he practiced? He, Baudelaire!'"4

Baudelaire lived with Jeanne on and off for nineteen years. She was his inspiration for the "Black Venus" section of *Les fleurs du mal*. Little is known about her. She spoke infrequently and has left no literary trail. Baudelaire was a rich man when she met him but reduced to poverty later, although he managed to continue to support her off and on over the years whether they were together or not. When she left him, he confided to his mother that she had been his sole distraction, sole pleasure, sole comrade. For ten days he did not sleep, he vomited frequently, and he cried.

Biographers have not been as fond of her as he was. Roger Williams described her as "a vicious and insatiable prostitute, a lecherous animal, experienced in all manner of sexual indulgence. She had neither mind nor heart, and if not a prostitute in title, she had the appropriate professional skills and instincts. She easily would have recognized his perversions and known how to cope with them."5 Others have called her stupid and obscene, a gutter-snipe, a dishonest, drugged, and alcoholic woman. Baudelaire himself described her as "an impassive, cold goddess, cruel, hard, and deceitful, so sensual yet so remote that one can only worship the image of her indifferent and destructive sexuality."6 Jeanne was last seen in 1870 dragging herself along the streets of Paris on crutches.

When he was twenty-four, Baudelaire stabbed himself (inef-fectually) in the chest after leaving a will and suicide note with Jeanne. "The fatigue of going to sleep and the fatigue of waking up have become insupportable. I kill myself, because I am useless to others and *dangerous to myself*."7 However, death was not to come for many painful years.

In later years, Baudelaire experienced many physical and mental complaints indicative of progressing syphilis. "Is it illness which saps the intelligence and the will, or is it spiritual cowardice which tires the body? I don't know. But what I feel is an immense sense of discouragement, a feeling of intolerable isolation, constant fear of some vague disaster, complete lack of faith in my powers, total lack of desire."[8] He complained of digestive and nervous trouble, culminating in a mild bout of paralysis, which he did not connect with the old syphilitic infection. Early in 1858, he complained to his mother: "I believe I am sick, and a sick man, even if the sickness is imagined, is a sick man. What else could be these perpetual fears, these palpitations, and this breathlessness, especially during sleep?"[9]

Baudelaire left one of the most poetic descriptions of an intimation of insanity: "I have cultivated my hysteria with enjoyment and terror. I always have vertigo now, and today, 23 January 1862, I have experienced an unusual warning: I felt pass over me *the wind of the wing of madness*."[10]

In February 1865 he described his seizures:

I am writing to you in the respite allowed by one of my attacks. They are sometimes so violent, that this morning it took me more than an hour to decipher your letter. . . . You congratulate me on my good health. For the past week, I have suffered diabolically. I have had both eyes blocked up, in turn, by a cold, neuralgia or rheumatism. I had begun, as you know, with four months of troubles with my stomach and intestines. In August and September, there was just a little light and warmth here. And then I was well. But for the last two months I have generally been seized by a fever at midnight. The long hours pass in continual shuddering and cold; finally, when morning comes, I go to sleep exhausted, having been unable to take advantage of my insomnia to write, and I wake up later in a dreadful sweat, quite exhausted by my sleep. For the past week, especially, there has been an increase of pain. And you know that there is no possible courage, except passive courage, in pain. It is an absolute abdication of willpower. . . . I am suffering and I am bored. . . . I do not stir from my room.[11]

He added: "Several times I have thought that I was free of it, and then, without apparent reason, there was a recurrence the next morning."[12] He wrote to his legal guardian, Ancelle: "I have been seized by neuralgia in the head, which has lasted for more than a fortnight. You know that this drives one stupid and mad; and, in order to write to you, Lemer, and my mother today, I have been obliged to swaddle my head in a pad which I soak every hour in cooling water. The attacks are not as violent as they were last year, but the pain lasts very much longer."[13] They left him feeling vague. He was taking opium, digitalis, belladonna, and quinine, doubling and quadrupling the doses of opium because the doctor did not know of his past familiarity with the drug. Later he took laudanum, and for vertigo, ether and valerian.

In January 1866, after waiting in the rain and cold for four hours for a package at the post office, Baudelaire developed a severe migraine. The next day he collapsed and rolled on the floor vomiting. Probably not knowing about the syphilis, his doctor diagnosed hysteria. One of his doctors warned him not to read or study, a curious medicine, Baudelaire observed. That doctor was a brute, worse than the "bloody cruel" one who forced him to give up wine. He complained: "I have been ill again, very ill. Vertigos and repeated vomiting for three days. I was obliged to lie on my back for three days; for, even when I crouched on the floor, I fell. . . . A moment ago, I was obliged to throw myself on my bed, and that's a great problem, because I'm always afraid of dragging down the furniture I cling to."[14] Baudelaire provided the "brutal" Dr. Marcq with details of his illness: "I think that food and fasting have no effect on it at all. But I am never hungry; I can go for several days without wanting to eat. Order of sensations. Vagueness in the mind. Suffocating fits. Horrible headaches. Heaviness; congestion; complete dizziness. If I'm standing, I fall. If I'm sitting, I fall. This is all very rapid. When I come round again I want to be sick. Extreme heat in the head. Cold sweats."[15]

In February 1866 Baudelaire wrote to his friend Charles Asselineau that to be honest he had been ill for almost all of the previous twenty months. He described violent neuralgia in the head, acute twinges of rheumatism, falling down, and vomiting bile. He would feel quite well, and then without apparent cause, he would have a sensation of vagueness, followed by an atrocious pain in the head, then a cold sweat, vomiting, and stupor. He did not associate his condition with syphilis, asking: "Do you know this kind of illness? Have you seen it before?"[16] In March Victor Hugo heard from his wife that she often saw Baudelaire, a rare and noble spirit, but "his mind has gone a little odd, and he has a nervous illness—the combination makes him a hypochondriac."[17]

In his last months spent in Belgium, Baudelaire drank large quantities of brandy and wondered if he had been poisoned by digitalis and belladonna. In March 1866 he had an onset of paralysis that was rumored in literary circles to be due to alcoholism and drug abuse. When he dined with the photographer Neyt, he was gloomy, confused, and spoke with difficulty. Pierre Dufay recorded: "He was preoccupied, seized by fits of shuddering, his eyes sometimes wild, and as if lit up by a flash of terror."[18] After dinner Baudelaire went to a tavern and got drunk on brandy. Neyt found him there and assisted him back to his hotel; in the morning he discovered Baudelaire partially paralyzed. The exact date of that event is not known, but it was probably near 20 March when Baudelaire wrote the last letter in his own hand. ("My dear mother, I am neither ill nor well."[19]) Two days later he had to stay in bed with a paralysis that affected his right side. He had a second attack, but recovered enough to call on Madame Hugo, who told her husband the next day: "Baudelaire is finished. . . . The illness has almost entirely destroyed his brain, they despair of the invalid. . . . It is very sad, for Baudelaire was a rare spirit."[20] In April, Poulet-Malassis observed that although it was unclear even if Baudelaire could still think, he had the sense of intelligence in his friend's face, as if ideas were somehow flashing through *like lightning.*

Baudelaire was sent, paralyzed and mute, to a nursing home run by the Sisters of Charity. They tried unsuccessfully to get the sign of the cross from him. When he managed to utter one phrase, a curse, they notified his mother, who removed her blasphemous son to the Hôtel du Grand Miroir while making plans to return to France. At first she planned to place him in the famous asylum of Dr. Ésprit Blanche in Passy; Dr. Blanche had met Baudelaire when he visited the poet Gérard de Nerval there. However, she placed him in another nursing home instead in July 1866. On 31 August 1867 he died in his mother's arms, with a smile on his face. The cause of death was cerebral hemorrhage or stroke.

Roger Williams, assuming Baudelaire was in the "latency" stage and therefore would have no symptoms, wrote: "In any case, when Baudelaire related ailments in 1848 and 1861 to his venereal infection of late 1839, we must deduce that those later maladies had nothing to do with syphilis."[21] And so Williams concludes that Baudelaire's protestations of illness have a theatrical ring. Williams supposed that when Baudelaire had seizures in the streets of Paris they were caused by worry over money.

Although there is general agreement that Baudelaire had syphilis, and a graphologist analyzing handwriting from 1858 on found clear anticipatory signs of mental disorder consistent with approaching paresis, the lack of other anticipatory signs (like megalomania) argues that he died early in the paretic progression.

For decades Baudelaire suffered from daily complaints consistent with syphilis: fever, palpitations of the heart, nervous stomach, diarrhea, fatigue, rheumatism, neuralgia, piercing gastrointestinal pain, migraine, shortness of breath, intestinal complaints, vertigo, seizures, paralysis, severe depression, and fear of madness. In his poetry he knew himself to be the vampire of his own heart, forsaken, condemned to eternal laughter. If he expressed doom in his poetry ("And step by step, toward Hell we wend our way/Blithely, through stinking vapours black as pitch"), he could also write that a multitude of small delights constitutes happiness. And if he saw elegance in rotting flesh, he observed this carrion while dressed as a dandy, immaculate, carrying a slim gold-tipped cane, and wearing pink gloves, a fine white shirt, a long waistcoat, and corkscrew trousers.

12

Mary Todd and Abraham Lincoln
(1818–1882) and (1809–1865)

> I am now the most miserable man living. If
> what I feel were equally distributed to the
> whole human family, there would not be one
> cheerful face on the earth.
>
> —ABRAHAM LINCOLN

MARY TODD'S FAMILY WAS SOCIALLY PROMINENT IN Kentucky. In 1839 she met Abraham Lincoln, a self-educated lawyer and state legislator, and after a long courtship and one broken engagement they were married in 1842. Of their four sons, only Robert survived to adulthood. Mary became first lady when her husband was elected the sixteenth president of the United States in 1860, a term of office that began with eleven southern states declaring their independence.

The ensuing Civil War lasted five years and resulted in an estimated 629,000 deaths, over half, by some reports, from disease. Lincoln was reelected president in 1864. Mary Todd became a widow when her husband was shot at Ford's Theater by John Wilkes Booth on 14 April 1865 and died the following day. After his death, Mary Todd traveled in Europe and eventually moved to Chicago.

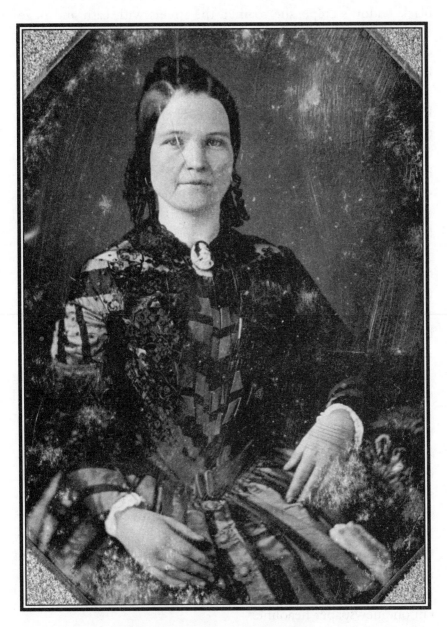

Figure 12.1   Mary Todd Lincoln (Library of Congress)

The people of Chicago found her to be quite odd. Dressed in black widow's crepe, she roamed the streets with cash and negotiable bonds pinned in her undergarments. She went on elaborate shopping sprees, buying trunkloads of drapes when she had no home to furnish. David Davis, the executor of Abraham Lincoln's estate, thought it insane that she had bought eighty-four pairs of kid gloves in less than a month. In 1875, when she was staying at the Grand Pacific Hotel with her son Robert, she wandered half-dressed into the elevator, mistaking it for the bathroom. When a hotel employee tried to help Robert return her to her room, she screamed that her son was trying to murder her. Hotel employees reported that she was nervous and excitable. A waiter overheard her repeating: "I am afraid. I am afraid."

A despairing Robert finally swore out a warrant for her arrest, to assure her safety and that of the community. At her trial, it only took ten minutes for the all-male jury to find her fit to be in a state hospital for the insane, another way of saying she was unfit to be elsewhere. A homeopathic surgeon from Chicago, Dr. Willis Danforth, had testified that Mary had "nervous derangement" and "fever in her head." She imagined that an Indian spirit was trying to pull wires out of her eyes, bones out of her cheeks, and steel springs from her jaw bones, while lifting her scalp and placing it back again.

Dr. Samuel Blake had added that she had degeneration of the brain tissue, or dementia, that would become worse. She thought she was being followed by nefarious men—not entirely a delusion, since Robert hired Pinkerton detectives to follow her. Robert's words ensured her committal: "I have no doubt that my mother is insane. She has long been a source of great anxiety to me." *Oh Robert,* lamented Mary, *to think that my son would do this to me.* "Another Sad Chapter in the Life of the Demented Widow," ran one newspaper headline.

Mary was sent to Bellevue Place, a private asylum where Dr. Robert Patterson tended twenty-five genteel ladies. (He refused known syphilitics.) His inventive diagnosis: Mary Todd was suffering from "moral insanity," a compulsion that overrode the moral

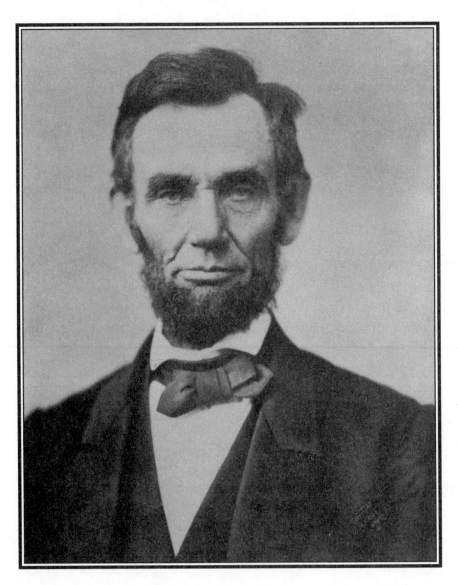

Figure 12.2   Abraham Lincoln (Library of Congress)

instincts "so critical for women,"[1] brought on in spiritualists when séances caused too much blood to go to the brain. Mary said she kept in touch with her dead husband and three dead sons that way. The end result, said Dr. Patterson, was lunacy. Mary spent less than four months in Bellevue. Later the court determined that her reason had been restored.

On 1 January 1882 four doctors rendered a medical opinion to request an increase in Mary Todd's widow's pension. They reported to Congress that she was suffering from a number of complaints, including "disorder of the spinal cord and reflex paralysis of the iris."[2] The spinal condition was progressive and would end in paralysis of the lower extremities. She was unable to walk safely without assistance, and her sight was reduced to one-tenth of normal.

One of the physicians, Lewis A. Sayre, gave a statement to the *New York Times* that Mrs. Lincoln's condition had resulted from a serious injury to her spine sustained when she fell from a chair while she was in France. Adequate sympathy was aroused in Congress to increase her widow's pension from $3,000 to $5,000 and award her $15,000 in back payments. Before she was able to collect a penny, she died of a stroke on 15 July 1882.

Syphilis was suggested in Mary Todd's medical history when Norbert Hirschhorn and Robert Feldman published an article in 1999 reviewing the work of the four doctors who had diagnosed her progressive spinal trouble.[3] Finding a clear case of tabes dorsalis, Hirschhorn and Feldman argue convincingly that the doctors would have known very well by then that tabes was caused by syphilis in the majority of cases and would have opted to save her reputation (and to assure a benefit that might have been withheld by a censorious Congress) by stating that her tabes dorsalis was caused by an injury to her spine when she fell from the French chair. "Given the widespread medical knowledge about tabes dorsalis at the close of 1881 and what then was considered its most likely cause [syphilis], it was inevitable that the four physicians chose the least pejorative diagnosis, however marginally acceptable it was to progressive medical opinion."[4] Jonathan Hutchinson concluded that it was generally accepted that tabes occurs "almost solely" in those who have previously suffered from syphilis. P. J. Möbius went one step further: "The longer I reflect upon it, the more firmly I believe that tabes never originates without syphilis."[5] Hirschhorn and Feldman note that tabes can also be caused by diabetes, something the doctors of the time did not know. Since Mary Todd was probably diabetic, they chose that as the most parsimonious diagnosis, while not, however, eliminating syphilis from consideration.[6]

The tabes diagnosis gives a fresh interpretation to the reasons for Mary Todd's incarceration: "Symptoms imputed to insanity at her trial clearly had their origin in the organic disease of tabes dorsalis."[7] The authors point out that the lightning pains of tabes were often described with vivid images appropriate to such extreme agony, such as having wires taken out of the eyes or, as Mary also complained, of being hacked to pieces by knives, of having a sharp, burning *agony* in the back, or feeling as if one were on fire.

But tabes only explains those aspects of her alleged insanity that have to do with physical pain. What about the "moral insanity" described by Dr. Patterson, and the other odd, uncharacteristic behavior so lacking in judgment, described by Robert? And what about the behavior, summarized by Hirschhorn and Feldman, that seems at first glance more criminal than like a first lady: "Mary Lincoln had already been publicly denounced for bribery, spying, extortion, profligacy, and stealing, so the only possible accusation left was adultery."[8]

Hirschhorn and Feldman point out numerous allusions to that possibility: "Contemporary gossip about her unfaithfulness was plentiful,"[9] citing Illinois Republican Senator Richard Yates, for one, who had circumspectly told the Senate: "a woman should be true to her husband. . . . I shall not go into details. Mr. Lincoln's memory is sweet to me. God Almighty bless the name and fame of Abraham Lincoln." Herndon, who did not like Mary Lincoln, wrote to Weik: "You know that Mrs. Lincoln is charged with unchastity and the like."[10]

Mary Todd was certainly sharp and witty to the end, with no slurring of speech or other signs of paresis, an argument against full-blown paresis, but not against the anticipatory stage, which can last many years and is characterized by bizarre and even criminal behavior, the "moral lapses" described in the old texts. A shopping compulsion too was a frequent warning sign.[11] Mary Todd's handwriting showed definite degeneration from her previous neat script. A letter written in 1882 to Noyes W. Miner shows warning signs of neurosyphilis when the inability to concentrate to the end of the line results in large, bunched up letters and blotches at the right side of the sheet.

That Mary Lincoln may have had the warning signs of taboparesis, a common manifestation of late-stage syphilis, accommodates both the physical and the mental symptoms.[12] Since the paretic aspect is atypical in women and usually takes a longer and milder course than in men, and psychotic features are not as characteristic, Mary Todd's behavioral changes over many years, along with her gradual paralysis, fixed pupils, and sharp pain, argue that she may have been exhibiting the warning signs of that manifestation of syphilis when she died in 1882.

According to Lincoln's biographer, friend, and law partner for eighteen years, William Herndon, Lincoln told him that he had been infected with syphilis in Beardstown in 1835 or 1836. Herndon wrote to his co-author "Friend Weik" in January 1891, wishing that he had not put the confidence in writing:

> When I was in Greencastle in 1887 I said to you that Lincoln had, *when a mere boy*, the syphilis, and now let me explain the matter in full, which I have never done before. About the year 1835–36 Mr. Lincoln went to Beardstown and during a devilish passion had connection with a girl and caught the disease. Lincoln told me this and in a moment of folly I made a note of it in my mind and afterwards I transferred it, as it were, to a little memorandum book which I loaned to Lamon, not, as I should have done, erasing that note. About the year 1836–37 Lincoln moved to Springfield and took up quarters with [Joshua] Speed; they became very intimate. At this time I suppose that the dis-

ease hung to him and, not wishing to trust our physicians, wrote a note to Doctor Drake, the latter part of which he would not let Speed see, not wishing Speed to know it. Speed said to me that Lincoln would not let him see a part of the note. Speed wrote to me a letter saying that he supposed L's letter to Doctor Drake had reference to his, L's crazy spell about the Ann Rutledge love affair, etc., and her death. You will find Speed's letter to me in our *Life of Lincoln*. The note to Doctor Drake in part had reference to his disease and not to his crazy spell as Speed supposes. The note spoken of in the memorandum book was a loose affair, and I never intended that the world should see or hear of it. I now wish and for years have wished that the note was blotted out or burned to ashes. I write this to you, fearing that at some future time the note—a loose thing as to date, place, and circumstances—will come to light and be misunderstood. Lincoln was a man of terribly strong passion, but was true as steel to his wife during his whole married life, as Judge Davis has said, saved many a woman, and it is most emphatically true, as I know. I write this to you to explain the whole matter for the future if it should become necessary to do so. I deeply regret my part of the affair in every particular.[13]

In a postscript, Herndon adds that Mrs. Dale saw the book and took note of its contents, and so he fears that the contents might come to light from that source.

Herndon tells us that Lincoln moved in with Speed in 1836–1837 and, to repeat from the letter, "*at this time I suppose that the disease hung to him* [emphasis added] and, not wishing to trust our physicians, [he] wrote a note to Doctor Drake." But there is an odd discrepancy in the Speed letter to Herndon published in the *Life of Lincoln*. Here Speed puts the date of the letter to Drake several years later:

Lincoln wrote a letter—a long one which he read to me—to Dr. Drake of Cincinnati, descriptive of his case. Its date would be in December 1840, or early in January 1841. I think that he must have informed Dr. Drake of his early love Miss Rutledge, as there was a part of the letter which he would not read. . . . I remember Dr. Drake's reply, which was, that he would not undertake to prescribe for him without a personal interview.[14]

The first reference to a contact with Dr. Drake, in 1836–1837, would have been within one or two years of the initial infection in Beardstown, thus in the highly infectious stage. The second reference, December 1840–January 1841, would have been four to five years after Beardstown, or well into the middle stage of the disease. Hirschhorn, Feldman, and Greaves assign the Drake contact to the later date.[15]

Was anything unusual happening in Lincoln's life around December 1840–January 1841 that might be linked to a doctor's appointment for treatment for an ongoing syphilitic infection? Lincoln refers to "that fatal first of Jany '41" when he broke his engagement to Mary Todd. According to Herndon, he left her at the altar on New Year's Day: "The bride, bedecked in veil and silken gown, and nervously toying with the flowers in her hair, sat in the adjoining room."[16] That story has been disputed. Lincoln had such a severe case of what he called "hypochondriaism" around then that he missed all but a week's attendance in the legislature. He sank into so deep a depression that friends kept his razors from him. Were these events connected to a confidential visit to Dr. Drake for syphilis?

Herndon's letter shows deep regret for inadvertently letting the Beardstown story slip. Gore Vidal suggests that a "Mount Rushmore" Lincoln image has kept people from accepting this statement by Herndon, whom he finds a most reliable source. "Since there is no reason for Herndon to lie about this, I suppose we should all agree upon it as a fact. But since no saint has ever had syphilis, Herndon is a liar and so the consensus falls against him."[17]

Herndon, believing both Mary Todd and Abraham had syphilis, suspected it in the premature deaths of three Lincoln children. "Poor boys, they are dead now and gone! I should like to *know* one thing and that is: What caused the death of these children? I have an opinion which I shall never state to anyone."[18] Since syphilis was thought to be hereditary then, it is not surprising that Herndon held this opinion.

Lincoln fans were angered when Gore Vidal suggested on *NBC's Today* show, and again on the Larry King program, that Mary Todd Lincoln had tertiary syphilis, or paresis. They were further enraged when he speculated that she had been infected by her husband. Vidal based his idea about Mary Todd's mental condition on something a doctor friend had told him in Chicago years before: "that an autopsy had been performed on Mrs. Lincoln (but only on the head, an odd procedure even then) and that the brain was found to have physically deteriorated, ruling out mere neurosis, the usual explanation for her behavior."[19] Vidal knew of no such autopsy existing and wondered if Robert Lincoln might have destroyed it or whether it might exist today somewhere in the depths of Walter Reed's extensive presidential collection along with Abraham Lincoln's autopsy report and seven bones of his body. (The autopsy story originated with a mistake in W. E. Barton's *The Life of Abraham Lincoln*.[20])

Lincoln historian Richard N. Current responded hotly that if Gore Vidal had "the slightest concern for truth" he could have learned from *The Merck Manual of Diagnosis and Therapy* that Mrs. Lincoln's symptoms did not correspond at all to those of a paretic. Vidal defended himself against the attack in an article in the *New York Review of Books* by quoting the Merck manual back at Current, whom he dubbed the Mr. Magoo of the History Department leaping bravely in the dark and falling on his face. Paresis is insidious in origin and identified by behavior changes, defective judgment, headache, insomnia, and so forth, all matching Mrs. Lincoln's behavior as seen by contemporaries: "I am in Current's debt for handing me this smoking gun."[21] They could both be correct: Mary Todd did not have paresis—yet. The Merck manual describes its *insidious* origin.

Hirschhorn and Feldman, with a third author, Ian A. Greaves,[22] followed their article on Mary Todd's tabes with another find from a letter written by Herndon: "Mr. Lincoln had an evacuation, a passage, about once a week, ate blue mass."[23] They found elemental mercury to be the active ingredient in blue mass, or blue pills, a medication Lincoln took over an extended period. They even had the blue pills recreated in the laboratory using a recipe from 1879 consisting of licorice root, rosewater, honey, and sugar, plus mercury and dead rose petals. Each pill contained approximately 65 grams of elemental mercury. The authors suggest that Lincoln may have been treated with the blue pills for melancholia, or hypochondriasis. Since syphilis sufferers were both depressed and had so many mysterious ailments that they often thought themselves to be hypochondriacs, the blue pills could have been prescribed for the "syphilis that hung to him" and melancholia and hypochondriasis at the same time.

In the "Blue Pills" article, Hirschhorn, Feldman, and Greaves find Lincoln's secrecy about the medication explained by the "opprobrium that would have been attached to the diagnosis of hypochondriasis in a person who aimed for high office."[24] Syphilis would have been very much more of a reason for circumspection, and a good reason to consult an out-of-town doctor. They suggest that Lincoln suffered from the neurobehavioral consequences of mercury intoxication—rage, for example. Herndon recalled that Lincoln looked like Lucifer when he was in an uncontrollable temper; he once shook a man until his teeth chattered.[25] Prone to moody silences, he was also observed talking "wild and incoherent nonsense" to himself. He had insomnia and headaches and worried about a tremor in his signature. An observer noted in 1863 that Lincoln "certainly is growing feeble. He wrote a note while I was present, and his hand trembled as I never saw it before, and he looked worn and haggard."[26] Lincoln had premonitions that he did not have long to live, and he feared madness. He took the little blue pills at least until 1861, a few months after his inauguration, and may have started them much earlier. Mary Todd tried them in

December 1869. She had a quick and severe reaction and supposedly discontinued them immediately.

Abraham Lincoln has been voted the most popular of all the American presidents, and there is lasting affection for Mary Todd and her sad condition. In *A Foreigner's Quest*, Jan Morris observed that "the American people as a whole were almost deranged in their obsession with their sixteenth President."[27] Still, it is odd that Lincoln's own statement to Herndon about contracting syphilis has been so ignored. Hirschhorn and Feldman's article puts a diagnosis of tabes dorsalis on firm ground in Mary Todd's case. Their later article with Greaves about Lincoln's taking little blue mercury pills when he consulted Drake about a syphilis that "hung to him" increases the probability that both Lincolns were suffering from syphilis. If so, Abraham Lincoln's "hypochondriasis" and melancholia and Mary Todd's erratic behavior in her last years can be seen in a fresh light.

The National Museum of Health and Medicine in Washington, D.C., part of the Armed Forces Institute of Pathology, has on display fragments of bones from Lincoln's skull, as well as strands of hair taken after his death and bloodstains from the cuffs of a shirt worn by one of the physicians attending him after his assassination. In the 1990s, when the question was raised of DNA testing of the Lincoln biological material for Marfan's syndrome, a genetic condition characterized by long, bony fingers, large feet, and a gaunt face, a committee convened to discuss the ethics of such testing. Victor A. McKusick of the Johns Hopkins University School of Medicine, spokesman for the panel, reported approval on legal and moral grounds but concern that testing might damage the delicate samples. Perhaps someday the Armed Forces Institute of Pathology will be able to announce that bone tests have put the question to rest one way or another. Abraham Lincoln described himself as the most miserable man living. He certainly had reason in his life for despair aside from syphilis, but if we believe Herndon's statement that he thought he was infected as a youth, then we can't discount that the diagnosis, if not the disease itself, was a part of his experience in subsequent years. In their two articles, Norbert Hirschhorn and his colleagues have summarized well the historical and medical information about syphilis in regard to both Abe Lincoln and Mary Todd. Unlike Gore Vidal, they do not conclude that either had syphilis, but they cautiously open the question, its relevance, even its appropriateness, to debate in a new and more serious way.

13

Gustave Flaubert
1821–1880

> Scarcely have you been born before you begin rotting.
>
> —GUSTAVE FLAUBERT

FLAUBERT KNEW ABOUT THE POX BEFORE HE CAUGHT IT. IN 1836 at age fifteen, the year of his sexual initiation with one of his mother's maids, he wrote: "Happiness is like the pox. Catch it too soon, and it wrecks your constitution."[1] He did catch it, probably while he was a student in Paris, and it did wreck his constitution. There he dressed in black, with white tie and gloves, even for early morning classes. His long flowing blond hair, sea-green eyes, and impressive stature commanded attention. But if his dress was gallant, his behavior was not; he told a friend he spent New Year's Eve in a brothel, having sex with the ugliest prostitute there while being observed by friends—with a cigar in his mouth to show his contempt. One prostitute may have had her revenge. In 1842 he went from having a very active sex life to taking a vow of abstinence. According to several sources, including the Goncourt *Journal*, he maintained that he was chaste for several years, although letters of 1843 reveal that he was once again visiting prostitutes.

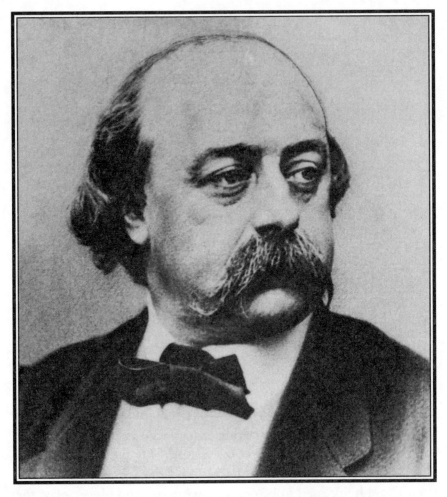

Figure 13.1   Gustave Flaubert (Hulton-Deutsch Collection/Corbis)

A long-censored passage of a letter of 1849 to his friend Ernest Chevalier indicates that he knew that he had contracted syphilis years before, and that it was recurrent. The initial infection was apparently mild, since he recalled: "You must know that your friend is, apparently, undermined by kind of a pox, the origins of which are lost in the mists of time. Although the symptoms get cured, it reappears again from time to time. My nervous complaint, from which I still suffer intermittently, and which cannot be cured in the circumstance in which I live, may well have no other cause."[2]

The "nervous complaint" began on 1 January 1844 when Flaubert experienced his first nervous seizure, falling to the floor of a two-horse carriage he was driving. For about ten minutes he appeared to be dead. His brother bled him immediately. Their father, who was the chief surgeon in the town of Rouen, took over his care and bled him frequently, since at the time such attacks were attributed to an excess of blood in the system. Flaubert experienced four more attacks in the next two weeks. In February he complained: "I am purged and bled, they treat me with leeches, and good food and wine are kept away from me. I am a dead man."[3]

The syphilis was no secret from Maxime du Camp, who had witnessed and described several of Flaubert's seizures. He inquired: "And your nervous condition? And your pox, that lovely pox of which you were so proud?"[4] Flaubert used his father's library to read about nervous diseases and told Ernest Chevalier that he had experienced a cerebral congestion, which he called an apoplectic attack in miniature. His nerves, he said, vibrated like violin strings while his stomach, shoulders, and knees fluttered like leaves. The fits began with a feeling of having a flame in the left eye, then a flame in the right eye. He threw himself on the bed convulsing, then slept. To his lover Louise Colet he later wrote that he had felt himself carried away in a flood of flame. A hundred thousand images would leap up at once, like fireworks. It was as if his soul were being wrenched from his body in those "hemorrhages of the nervous system."

Maxime du Camp "implied that Flaubert knew the truth of his malady and tried to conceal it out of shame,"[5] though whether du Camp meant syphilis, epilepsy, or both is unclear. Flaubert's comment that the nervous attacks may have been connected with syphilis implies that he thought them one and the same. He may have been right, since syphilitic epilepsy is a serious complication after the first year of syphilis. According to Robert Howland Chase: "One of the most serious forms of congestion is the epileptiform attack. There is a sudden loss of consciousness with the typical warning cry, pallor followed by flushing, foaming at the mouth and convulsions."[6] Du Camp noted Dr. Flaubert's "humiliation, despair, and a kind of resignation in the presence of an act of God that he could not dominate."[7] He was disinclined to talk about his son's illness and he never diagnosed it.

In the early months of 1844 Flaubert gave himself mercury rubs. He had dermatological outbreaks that made him speculate that they were caused by syphilis. Although the seizures became less severe in the summer, when he went back to Paris to register for law school they recurred almost daily, so he gave up and returned home. Carefully tracking his friend's crisis, du Camp noted that this condition marked the turning point in his life. Flaubert was later to tell Louise Colet that his youth had been terminated by a nervous complaint that lasted two years. Dr. Flaubert bought a house near his own just outside of Rouen and his son retired there to become a writer, "the Hermit of Croisset." The theme of illness and the reclusive life would frequently appear in Flaubert's future works.

The secrecy, the vow of chastity, the mercury rubs, the skin rash that Flaubert connected with syphilis, and especially du Camp's statement about "the lovely pox of which you were so proud," establish that Flaubert had syphilis by then. There has been considerable confusion in the medical literature about the attacks, with numerous hypotheses being proposed, including temporal lobe epilepsy, hysteria, apoplexy, and even hostility toward legal studies. In May 1849 Flaubert consulted a Parisian doctor who diagnosed a "chronic syphilis of long standing" as the cause of his nervous disorders. Later writers, believing that Flaubert had epilepsy, have criticized this doctor for misdiagnosing the nervous complaint.

Roger L. Williams suggests that Flaubert's attacks were not grand mal seizures but may have been partial, or epileptiform, seizures of the type to be described in 1863 as Jacksonian epilepsy, named after Dr. Hughlings Jackson.[8] This does not preclude syphilis. In his chapter "Pathology and Clinical Symptomatology of Early Neurosyphilis," John Stokes describes syphilitic epilepsy, identified by epileptiform convulsions, noting under clinical signs: "May present Jacksonian or other localizing signs of areas involved. No residual paralysis."[9] He also points out that "Jacksonian epilepsies present no features distinctive of syphilis and must be identified as such on serologic and collateral clinical evidence. True epilepsy and generalized syphilitic epileptiform convulsions are likewise clinically indistinguishable in some cases."[10]

Maybe Flaubert left Paris to become a writer instead of a lawyer, the "Hermit of Croisset" who produced *Madame Bovary* instead of legal briefs, because of syphilis. He has been credited with the development of realism, the death of romanticism. The grand novel *Madame Bovary*, the story of the love affairs of a romantic young woman married to a somewhat boring small-town doctor, triumphed against censorship in a court of law (and was praised for doing so by Baudelaire).

In the fall of 1849 Flaubert came out of hiding and embarked on a year-and-a-half journey to Egypt, Syria, Turkey, Greece, and Italy with Maxime du Camp, his mother having consented on the assumption that the trip would be good for his health. Gustave and Maxime spent two months in Cairo, then sailed up the Nile on a blue vessel with two crossed sails.

On 13 March 1850, Flaubert told Louis Bouilhet of his night with the famous courtesan Kuchuk Hanem: "I sucked her furiously, her body was covered with sweat, she was tired after dancing, she was cold. I covered her with my fur pelisse, and she fell asleep, her fingers in mine. As for me, I scarcely shut my eyes. My night was one long, infinitely intense reverie. . . . As for the *coups*, they were good—the third especially was ferocious, and the last tender."[11] He wondered (romantically) whether she might remember him. If not, many others surely did. The letters home were good tourists' reports, but to Louis Bouilhet went a sexual travelogue and an account of the spread of venereal disease. From Constantinople on 14 November 1850 Flaubert wrote to Bouilhet:

I want you to know, dear Sir, that in Beirut I picked up (I first noticed them at Rhodes, land of the dragon) VII chancres, which eventually merged into two, then one. In that condition I rode my horse from Marmaris to Smyrna. Every night and morning I dressed my wretched prick. Finally it cured itself, in two or three days the scar will be closed. I'm being desperately careful about it. I suspect a Maronite woman of making me this gift, or perhaps it was a little Turkish lady. The Turk or the Christian? Which? Problem![12]

He continued: "Last night Maxime discovered, even though it's six weeks since he did any fucking, a double abrasion that looks to me very much like a two-headed chancre. If it is, that makes the third time he's caught the pox since we set out. There's nothing like travel for the health"[13]—one's own or others!

Three months later he told Bouilhet (10 February 1851, from Patras): "As for me, my frightful chancres have finally closed. The induration is still very hard, but seems to be disappearing. Something else that is disappearing, and faster, is my hair."[14] Throughout the trip Flaubert was weak and debilitated, with a constant fever accompanied by small red spots on his lower belly. When he reached Rome he was in the sixth month of illness. One testicle was troublesome and he had a painful facial neuralgia.

Since syphilis does not manifest chancre or rash upon reinfection, Flaubert's venereal troubles in Egypt were probably another infection like chancroid. Philippe Ricord's dictum was: You cannot catch a double dose of the Pox. However, now it is known that because subsequent exposures do not produce the usual early lesions, this "silent reinfection" can go undiagnosed. According to the Merck manual: "A treated infection does not confer immunity against subsequent reinfection." The small red spots on Flaubert's lower belly were localized, not generalized like the rash of secondary infection.

Flaubert and his friend heard of widely available male prostitutes in Egypt. Since they were traveling for education and charged with a mission by the government, they considered it their duty to test this "mode d'éjaculation." He had succeeded, Flaubert told him, with a pockmarked young man wearing a turban in a Turkish bath. The experiment must be repeated to be well done, he promised. In Cairo they visited a hospital, where slaves suffering from syphilis dropped their pants and held open their buttocks to show their chancres. On their way home, they went to Italy and Greece. Whether for syphilis or for other newly acquired sexual diseases, Flaubert was having mercury massages and his hair was rapidly falling out. According to Benjamin Bart, Flaubert continued to dose himself with "mercury and ever more mercury"[15] over the years.

In Beirut the two friends visited a French colony, where Flaubert claimed to have availed himself of three young women before lunch and one after dessert; they were shocked when he washed his genitals in front of them. Du Camp had sex once at that luncheon even though he had a chancre from Egypt. In Constantinople both had venereal infections, the third for du Camp. Twice a day Flaubert used mercury dressings on a chancre he thought dated from the lunchtime adventure in Beirut. He visited a district of male brothels but, given his painful condition, only to look.

In *Flaubert's Parrot*, Julian Barnes wrote that his subject was a sweet man "unless you count the occasion in Egypt when he tried to go to bed with a prostitute while suffering from the pox. That was a little deceitful I admit."[16] She found a sore and booted him out. And Lottman observes, "The modern reader will note lack of prophylactics—even less concern for infecting others."[17]

During the following years Flaubert reflected often on his many illnesses, never being sure what was wrong with him. To George Sand he wrote: "Abnormal things are going on inside me. My depression must have some hidden cause. I feel old, worn out, disgusted with everything. . . . It may be the work that is making me ill, for this book is an insane enterprise."[18] In a letter to Mme. Roger des Genettes he worried: "As for me, I am *worse*. What is wrong with me I have no idea, and neither does anyone else, the term 'neurosis' expressing both a number of different phenomena and the ignorance of the physicians. . . . Judging from the way I sleep—ten or twelve hours a night—I have probably done some damage to my brain. Is it beginning to soften, I wonder?"[19] He continued: "My mood would make ebony look pink." Vaguely, he wondered: "Especially for the last six months, I don't know what's wrong with me, but I have been feeling profoundly sick, although I can't be more specific than that."[20] Before a trip to Switzerland, he declared himself to be deeply weary, exhausted, and stupid, in the last stage of decline. His nerves were taut as brass wire, his pen a heavy oar.

Flaubert's list of complaints included stomach cramps, intestinal discomfort, extreme nervousness, rheumatism (potassium bromide prescribed), a skin reaction that made him look like a leper, numerous rashes and boils as big as hens' eggs all over his body, a recurrent cough, severe pains in the back of his head, insomnia, chronic headaches, and lumbago.

In August 1854 Flaubert told Louis Bouilhet that he planned to consult the famous Philippe Ricord, although he apparently never did. He was receiving treatment with mercury and iodide for a syphilitic tumor, or gumma. His notation "terrific mercurial salivation" refers to an aggressive treatment with mercury; three pints of saliva was considered a good amount to gush forth with such a regimen. Flaubert's description of his treatment is one of the most graphic:

Laxatives, purges, derivations, leeches, fever, colic, three sleepless nights—gigantic nuisance—such has been my week, cher monsieur. I have eaten nothing since Saturday night, and only now am I beginning to be able to speak. To put it briefly, Saturday night my tongue suddenly began to swell until I thought it was transmuting itself into that of an ox. It protruded from my mouth: I had to hold my jaws open. I suffered, I can tell you. But since yesterday I am better, thanks to leeches and ice. . . . For a week I was hideously sick. Terrific mercurial salivation, mon cher monsieur; it was impossible for me to talk or eat—atrocious fever, etc. Finally I am rid of it, thanks to purges, leeches, enemas (!!!), and my 'strong constitution.' I wouldn't be surprised if my tumor were to disappear, following this inflammation; it has already diminished by half. Anyway . . . I won't go to consult the great Ricord for another six weeks. Meanwhile I'll keep stuffing myself with iodide. [21]

On 8 May 1880, with his trunks packed for a trip to Paris, Flaubert experienced faintness after a hot bath. He summoned his maid to call the doctor, who arrived to find him stretched out on a Turkish divan. His heart was still beating. On the fireplace mantel his pipe was still warm and full of tobacco. A "black collar" was visible on the surface of his skin. Guy de Maupassant rushed to Croisset. He recalled: "I saw in the failing light, stretched out on a wide divan, a great body with a swollen neck and red throat, as terrifying as a colossus who had been struck down."[22] He spent three days by the body and helped the doctors wrap Flaubert in a shroud. He wrote to Turgenev about the "black collar." There have been numerous theories over the years as to the cause of Flaubert's death, in addition to syphilis of the heart,[23] including apoplexy and epilepsy. One of the wilder ones was Edmond Ledoux's proposal that Flaubert hanged himself in his bath. Julian Barnes found this as plausible as that he electrocuted himself with sleeping pills.

Three hundred people attended Flaubert's funeral and burial in Rouen. The grave was too short and the gravediggers were unable to stuff the coffin in. The omnipresent Edmund de Goncourt recorded the event in his journal: "Ah! my poor Flaubert, here round your corpse are human documents with which you could have made a provincial novel."[24]

14

Guy de Maupassant
1850–1893

I've got the Pox! At last! The real thing!
—GUY DE MAUPASSANT

EMILE ZOLA MET GUY DE MAUPASSANT AT A LUNCHEON
at Flaubert's house. He described him as "a man of middle
height, strong-backed with iron muscles and a ruddy complexion.
He was a terrible [impressive?] oarsman in those days and used for
his pleasure to row fifty miles on one day on the Seine."[1] Shy at
first, the young man later amazed the assembled group by bragging about his love life in a way that sent Flaubert into enormous
fits of laughter. Maupassant claimed that he could climax twenty
times in rapid succession. It was said that he once had sex before
witnesses with six prostitutes in an hour. He was reputed to collect
lovers as others collect birds' eggs or stamps, although his biographer Robert Sherard maintained that stories of his fickleness were
false; alas, poor Guy was the victim of pursuing women.

That Maupassant had syphilis was known to many of his com-
panions. Sherard described its effects on his life and his work, even
though he never used the word syphilis itself. Instead he devised
poetic euphemisms, such as "the Monster of infinitesimal size but
Himalayan mischief,"[2] the "Neapolitan evil," and the "cruelest haz-

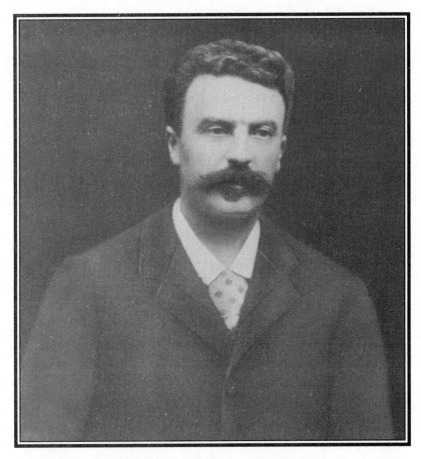

Figure 14.1   Guy de Maupassant (Bettmann/Corbis)

ard that awaits the passer through life which, since the days of
Columbus, has attacked the brightest and fairest intellects of the
world" while pursuing a "clandestine career in atrocity." His favorite synonym was the "Great Distress." There is no doubt that he
did mean syphilis because he noted in his preface that Maupassant's
disease began to be understood with the discovery of the spirochete in 1905 and the subsequent linking of this "pallid spirochaet"
to general paralysis of the insane. (Sherard's biographies of Oscar
Wilde also refer to syphilis euphemistically.)

Maupassant said that he had been infected with syphilis at age
twenty by a ravishing boating companion but did not learn the di-

agnosis, and the reason for his subsequent illnesses, until years later. To Robert Pinchon, the municipal librarian of Rouen, he wrote on 2 March 1877: "You will never guess the astonishing discovery which my doctor has just made about me. . . . Because my body hair had all fallen out and not grown back, because my father was fussing over me, and because my mother's lamentations could be heard all the way from Étretat, I took my doctor by the collar and said to him 'Find out what's wrong with me, you blighter, or you'll get what for.'" Maupassant's threat yielded the truth: "The pox," he replied. Maupassant thereupon provided the most straightforward acknowledgment of infection by the Pox in the literature of the nineteenth century, and a stunning show of dangerous bravado:

> I hadn't been expecting that, I can tell you; I was very upset, but at length I said "What's the remedy?" "Mercury and potassium iodide," he replied. I went to see another Sawbones, who made the same diagnosis, adding that it was an "old syphilis, dating back six or seven years." . . . In short, for five weeks I have been taking four centigrammes of mercury and thirty-five centigrammes of potassium iodide a day, and I felt very well on it. Soon mercury will be my staple diet. My hair is beginning to grow again . . . the hair on my arse is sprouting. . . . I've got the pox! at last! the real thing! not the contemptible clap, not the ecclesiastical crystalline, not the bourgeois coxcombs or the leguminous cauliflowers—no—no, the great pox, the one which Francis I died of. The majestic pox, pure and simple; the elegant syphilis. . . . I've got the pox . . . and I am proud of it, by thunder, and to hell with the bourgeoisie. Allelujah, I've got the pox, so I don't have to worry about catching it any more, and I screw the street whores and trollops, and afterwards I say to them "I've got the pox." They are afraid and I just laugh.[3]

If the infection went back six or seven years, then Maupassant had been infected in 1869 or 1870, when he was about twenty.

Not noticing or attaching importance to a slight initial lesion, he died of severe paresis many years later, confirming the lore that a gentle first infection often led to a particularly nasty demise.

His theme of cavalierly infecting others found its way into one of his later stories. In "Bed Number 29," Maupassant makes light fun of Captain Epivent, a handsome, strutting ladies' man, superb of leg, figure, and mustache (a glorified self-portrait?), proudly having an affair in Rouen with beautiful Irma. When he is called back to the Franco-Prussian War, the lovers spend a passionate night of good-byes, leaving furniture overturned and clothes mingled in distress on the carpet. After the war he returns, decorated, to find his Irma wasting away in Bed 29 of the syphilis ward. She asks him to kiss her. Overcoming his disgust, he places his lips on her wan forehead. "He believed he detected an odor of putrefaction, of contaminated flesh, in this corridor full of girls tainted with this ignoble, terrible malady."[4] She explains that she was infected by the invading Prussians, but she got her revenge by passing her disease on to as many soldiers as possible. When Epivent accuses her of consorting with the enemy, she boasts that her score of deaths is greater than his; she poisoned as many of them as she could. She died the next day.

An entry in the Goncourt *Journal* of 1 February 1891 tells another story about Maupassant's theme of infecting others. According to this tale, he painted a chancre on his penis, paraded it in front of a woman, and then forced his frightened companion to have sex.

Guy de Maupassant was born in Dieppe, France, in 1850. He grew up in Normandy, the location of many of his stories. His parents separated when he was eleven. He left the study of law in Paris to volunteer in the Franco-Prussian War. When he returned, he joined the literary circle including Zola, Turgenev, Henry James, and Gustave Flaubert, who was his friend and mentor. (There were rumors for a time that Flaubert had been Maupassant's mother's lover and was also his father.) On 15 July 1878 Flaubert sent his younger friend a letter of advice to an artist: "You *must*—

do you hear me, young man?—you MUST work more than you are doing. I am beginning to suspect you of being slightly idle." Do less boating, get less exercise; the civilized man does not require "so much locomotion as Messrs. the medical men would have us believe. You were born to write poetry."[5]

Sherard tells us that the "Great Distress," syphilis, began to give Maupassant reason for sorrow and despair around 1876, although to the world he wore a mask of gaiety, letting no one see "the snake gnawing at his heart." Here Sherard was quoting Heine, probably without knowing that Heine had syphilis as well. On this topic Maupassant practiced to excess the principle, "Hide thy life." He kept no diary and had minimal correspondence. Yet the word seems to have gotten out about his disease, perhaps because in the early days, as is indicated by his letter to Robert Pinchon, he was not very discreet.

Maupassant's passion was the Seine. He rushed from work to get to the water. In the introduction to the story "Mouche," he wrote: "Ah! The beautiful, the calm, the varied and the stinking river, full of mirages of filth. I loved it so much, I think because it gave me, as it seems to me, a sense of life."[6] A colleague in the government clerk's office where he worked recalled that Maupassant dreamed of nothing but open-air races and boating on Sundays. Every morning he would get up at daybreak and wash his boat, row, and sail, waiting until the last minute to catch a train to go to his labor, his official prison. He drank hard, slept well, and ate like four men.

Eight years of employment with the Ministry of Public Instruction was deadly boring, although Maupassant often found time to write while at work. When his health became "bad, really bad" as Sherard put it, he had reason to be absent as much as three days a week from a routine that would normally require him to be there from nine in the morning until six-thirty in the evening, six days a week. He finally applied for a three-month leave of absence (with pay) "to recover from nervous ills" in the spas of Switzerland. When he achieved some literary success, he left the civil service to pursue writing full-time, although for years he was officially still on a leave of absence arranged as a safety net in case the literary career did not work out or his health declined. In fact he had no need to return to the shackles of daily employment; his career as a writer progressed splendidly, and Flaubert could relax his concern about his young friend being lazy, as he turned out more than twenty-seven volumes—three hundred stories, six novels, three plays, travel books, and poetry—in the ten years before insanity set in.

Maupassant's chief physical concern was with his eyes; he feared losing his sight and reported early in 1880 that his right eye was almost blind. An ophthalmologist, Dr. Abadie, found paralysis in the accommodation of the right eye. The Goncourt journal records that Maupassant consulted an oculist, Dr. Edmund Landolt, who found that "the mischief lay behind the eyes." Sherard noted that the disease that causes general paralysis of the insane atrophies the optic nerve "behind the eyes."[7] Maupassant's pupil was dilated, and Landolt recalled later: "This disorder, apparently insignificant, caused me nevertheless to foresee, on account of the function troubles which accompanied it, the lamentable end which awaited (ten years later) the young writer formerly so vigorous and so valiant."[8] Dr. Gratz described Maupassant in 1891 as a "candidate for general paralysis."[9] He would have been warned by the many doctors he saw, Sherard explains, to be wary of the slightest spot on the skin, fatigue of the eyes, transitory failure of hearing, or trifling headache as a premonition of the "fatal mischief."

Sherard expressed his knowledge of syphilis in a flowery style. One of the hideous features of this evil, he wrote, is that destruction goes on relentlessly beneath the surface, ghastly ruin being done by "myriads of spiral-shaped germs darting to and fro in marrow, cell, and brain." He ponders whether the curious fact of Maupassant's literary leap from mediocrity in 1876 to the supreme mastery of the short story seen in "Boule-de-Suif," which made him the most talked of writer in Paris in 1880, might have been the result of a tremendous stimulation of the brain cells from this disease. Here he expresses the idea that the syphilitic's brain is for a time at the late stage of syphilis "capable of extraordinary production of far higher merit than they would ever have been capable of without this inoculation."[10] Sherard was repeating the idea that although syphilis led directly to decadence in most cases, it could take a genius to new heights.

Although Madame de Maupassant thought she saw the first signs of her son's madness in passages of the story "Sur l'eau" in 1888, many of his friends noticed changes during the following year, reporting that he had begun to talk rather wildly. Goncourt observed him on a train and noted that his face was brick-colored and had a fixed expression: "He does not seem to me fated to get old bones."[11] Goncourt saw Maupassant emaciated and shivering on a rainy Sunday as a monument to Flaubert was being inaugurated at Rouen: "As long as I live, I shall see that face, shriveled up with pain, those big eyes at bay, which a protestation against an iniquitous fatality lit up with dying lights."[12] Maupassant himself felt the approaching signs of madness. When he visited Juliette Adam, the editor of La Nouvelle Revue, he was agitated; she told him he was talking like a madman, and he responded: "My brother, you know, is already mad; yes, mad. Didn't you know that he is no longer at Antibes, but in a private asylum? When will my turn come?"[13] Goncourt wrote in his journal in June that Maupassant was haunted by fear of death and moved constantly on land and sea to escape from this fixed idea.

Maupassant consulted the popular Paris doctor David Gruby, who had gone into general practice after years of research (including on syphilis), and who counted among his patients Vincent and Theo van Gogh, Alphonse Daudet, Heinrich Heine, Chopin, and Georges Sand. Gruby put Maupassant on a special diet: boiled potatoes three times a day, as many eggs as he could swallow, two quarts of milk a day, saltwater fish at every meal, and abundant meat and fowl. He was forbidden green vegetables, wild game, and wine. Sherard speculated that Maupassant was anemic and overly sensitive to cold from having taken great quantities of what the famous Dr. Fournier described as "barometer syrup," or mercury. He had extreme feelings of coldness, neuralgia, sensitivity to noise, insomnia, and pain in the limbs. He tried vapor baths but feared an apoplectic stroke; in July he went to the health spa at Aix-les-Bains.

Creatively, Maupassant was in excellent form. He often thought of a story over time and then wrote it in a single sitting. In July he wrote a story that had not been carried around in this way but which "was there, complete, erect within my mind."[14] He wrote it in four days, about 14,000 words, without a single correction. He had the manuscript copied so that he could save the pristine original.

Maupassant's last sane year, 1891, was a restless one. He moved from place to place, avoiding the air and noise of Paris, which he said caused him horrendous headaches. "The dreadful pain racks in a way no torture could equal, shatters the head, drives one crazy, bewilders the ideas, and scatters the memory like dust before the wind. A sick headache had laid hold of me, and I was perforce obliged to lie down in my bunk with a bottle of ether under my nostrils."[15] Discounting syphilis, Roger Williams suggests that the headaches were an expression of repressed hostility, a vegetative neurosis originating in a repressed hostility to his family.[16]

Maupassant identified with dogs who howl: "Their howling—is a lamentable complaint addressed to nobody, going nowhere, telling you nothing."[17] At the same time he felt at the top of his form, planning a book, *L'angélus*, which he thought was to be his best: "I feel admirably fit to write this book. I have it all perfectly in my head. It was all thought out with an astonishing facility. It will be the crowning of my literary career."[18] But he feared madness and spoke often of suicide. Frank Harris wrote:

> Three or four years before the end, Maupassant knew that the path of self-indulgence for him led directly to madness and untimely death. . . . First an orgy brought on fits of partial blindness, then acute neuralgic pains and periods of sleeplessness, while his writing showed terrible fears. . . . Then came desperate long-continued depression broken by occasional exaltations and excitements. . . . and always, always, the indescribable mental agony he spoke of as *indicible malaise*.[19]

While riding a bicycle, Maupassant fainted and bruised his ribs. He wrote to his mother that his bruises were painful but announced that his health was suddenly admirable; he planned three weeks of fashionable life in Paris to prepare for more work. Once there, though, he suffered depression. In November 1892 he reported from Cannes: "There are whole days on which I feel I am done for, finished, blind, my brain used up and yet still alive. . . . I have not a single idea that is consecutive to the one before it. I forget words, names of everything, and my hallucinations and my pains tear me to pieces."[20] He imagined that the salt baths he had been giving his nostrils had started a salty fermentation in his brain, and that the dissolved brain was flowing back through his nose. In Paris he announced that he had been made a count and insisted on being so addressed. Goncourt's *Journal* recorded that in literary circles it was agreed that Maupassant had lost his mind.

At Christmas time Maupassant took two women sailing and seemed to be all right, but then he complained that he had just seen a ghost. New Year's Day marked the turning point. At a quarter past two in the morning his servant found him with his throat gashed. "You see, François, what I have done. I have cut my throat. It's a case of sheer madness."[21] He had also tried to shoot himself, but the wound was not serious. A doctor sewed him up and put him in a straitjacket. After being comatose for the day, he woke to announce that he must go to the frontier; war had been declared. His friends took him to see his boat, hoping that would orient him. On 6 January 1893 Maupassant was taken to Paris, still in restraints, and placed in the celebrated asylum of Dr. Ésprit Blanche in Passy.

Over the next months he was at times rational, delighting his visitors with hilarious stories; at other times he hallucinated, was violent, and had to be restrained. From April on, the decline was rapid. A doctor kept a daily record. Maupassant's last letters speak of vast fortunes of gold nuggets and buried treasure. He imagined he was the wealthy younger son of the Virgin Mary. He planted twigs around the gardens expecting them to sprout into baby Maupassants. He licked the walls of his cell, and retained his urine, thinking it was made of diamonds and jewels. He howled like a dog, recalling his fantasy of envying the dog its expression of anguish. When his thoughts seemed to escape from his head, he anxiously asked around after them ("You haven't seen my thoughts anywhere, have you?"), and he glowed with happiness when he thought he had found them in the form of butterflies colored by mood: black sadness, pink merriment, and purple adulteries. He tried to catch the imaginary butterflies as they flitted by.

At the end he was violent and had to be kept in mechanical restraints. When he died on 7 July 1893, his attendant said he went out like a lamp that has no more oil. His last words were reported to be "des ténèbres, des ténèbres"—*darkness, darkness.*

Maupassant's syphilis was not publicly known during his life, but there was gossip. Sherard tells us that at the end of November 1892, Oscar Wilde wrote to Lady Dorothy Nevill that he feared poor Maupassant was dying, having just heard so from "a friend" of Maupassant's who had just met his doctor on the boulevards. This friend turns out to be Sherard himself, as he revealed, probably unwittingly, in a later biography of Wilde.

After criticizing Frank Harris for never inquiring about his supposed friend Maupassant's condition during the entire time Maupassant was in "my friend Dr. Blanche's madhouse," Sherard added: "He knew very well what Maupassant's condition was, for I told Wilde about it after I had an interview with Dr. Blanche and Wilde had immediately sent the news to Lady Dorothy Nevill, who would of course pass it on to Harris."[22] Maupassant's condition was, of course, general paralysis of the insane, but no one on the grapevine would ever name it.

Vincent van Gogh
1853–1890

A human charged with electricity.

—VAN GOGH

WHEN THE HOLLAND HERALD ASSIGNED JOURNALIST KEN Wilkie to write a feature article on Vincent van Gogh, he began tracing van Gogh's steps in the previous century, interviewing descendants of relatives and friends. After the article was published, Wilkie was still bothered by unanswered questions. Why did Vincent's letters from Antwerp to his brother Theo, beginning in November 1885, express fears of going mad and dying? Why had death suddenly become a theme in his art? The grim *Skull with Cigarette* was a clear departure from previous themes, as was *Skeleton Hanging in a Closet*, in which a black cat contemplates a disintegrating skeleton. Wilkie wondered: Did Vincent's increasingly poor health then have anything to do with this change in his art?

Looking for a place to start, Wilkie recalled that biographer Dr. Marc Edo Tralbaut had told him about finding the name "Cavenaile" written on the back of one of Vincent's sketchbooks along with a notation of a consultation hour. He began there. First, he checked the Antwerp phone book and was surprised to find the name Cavenaille. (Tralbaut claims to have confirmed that

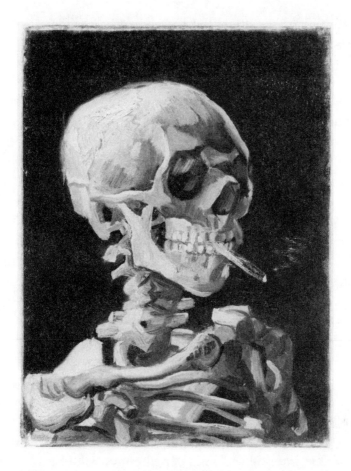

Figure 15.1   Skull with a Cigarette. Antwerp, early January 1886. (Vincent van Gogh Foundation, Amsterdam)

the correct family spelling has two *ls*). He was even more surprised when Dr. Amadeus Cavenaille, the grandson of Dr. Hubertus Amadeus Cavenaille, answered his call. When they met, the doctor seated Wilkie in the chair his grandfather had used when interviewing patients; presumably Vincent had occupied the same seat. "My grandfather treated van Gogh several times in 1885," Cavenaille told Wilkie.

"And did your grandfather ever tell you," Wilkie asked, "what van Gogh's complaint was?" Cavenaille shocked him with this answer: "He said he treated van Gogh for syphilis. He prescribed a treatment with mercury and sent him to the Stuyvenberg hospital for hip-baths."[1] When Vincent had pressed him for details, the doctor had told him the disease could affect his brain and be fatal. This consultation, held only a few years after Alfred Fournier's findings that syphilis led to paresis, shows that by then syphilitic insanity was widely accepted and the information routinely passed on to patients. From that moment on, Vincent would have had reason to fear and anticipate tertiary syphilitic insanity. Vincent paid for the consultation with a portrait, which has been lost.

Wilkie returned to Tralbaut's biography and found that his predecessor knew about this as well: "Moreover, Vincent had caught syphilis," Tralbaut reported as fact, "probably at Antwerp, and this certainly contributed to his physical and mental condition."[2] Vincent's Antwerp letters reveal numerous complaints of poor health, periods of fever and faintness, and gastrointestinal problems. He developed a chronic cough accompanied by grayish phlegm.[3] In Wilkie's copy of Tralbaut's book, the word "syphilis" was circled and a big "No!" penned in the margin, signed W.V. v G: Vincent Willem van Gogh, the painter's nephew. This nephew, when Wilkie interviewed him, vehemently denied the possibility of syphilis.

Scholars have had a tough time agreeing on a diagnosis for Vincent van Gogh. the *New York Times* (November 1990) counted a remarkable 152 posthumous diagnoses, which would be a new record for syphilis imitating other diseases. As one of these posthumous diagnoses, syphilis cannot be dismissed casually, given Vincent's noting of the doctor's name and the appointment time in his sketchbook, Cavanaille's diagnosis, Wilkie's observation of his sudden preoccupation with death, and the statement of Cavenaille's grandson, a reputable doctor himself. A good syphilologist armed with this information about a previous colleague's diagnosis would ask the basic questions: Was there a severe fever following a high-risk sexual experience? Was there a sudden change from relative good health to a lifetime of illnesses consistent with syphilis? And finally, were there indications of changes in character warning of approaching paresis? Since the answer to all of these questions is yes, the probability of syphilis in Vincent's case is very high, certainly more than sufficient to continue the inquiry.

Only Nietzsche's massive correspondence rivals the letters between Vincent and his brother Theo as a profound philosophical reflection on illness as it relates to a life's work. In these letters—874 of them or nearly 850,000 words—syphilis is not given as a cause of their mutual suffering, but Theo had syphilis and his brother knew it, and if Vincent was diagnosed with it by Dr. Cavenaille and he shared this information with his brother, then the letters may be read looking for a subtextual conversation of mutual acknowledgment. To make everything more complex, Paul Gauguin corresponded with the van Gogh brothers, and he had an undisputed case of syphilis. When the letters refer to Gauguin's illness, is it with knowledge of his diagnosis?

Vincent van Gogh was born in Holland on 30 March 1853, the son of a pastor of the Dutch Reformed Church. His mother commented that this blue-eyed, red-haired, freckled son was the strongest of her six surviving children. When he was in his twenties, Vincent attempted numerous careers: as art dealer at Goupil's in Paris and London, teacher at Ramsgate, and clerk in a bookstore. He considered the ministry but found himself unsuited for the academic part of training, so he arranged with the church to be an evangelist for the coal miners of the Borinage district of Belgium. Living in poverty with the miners, he began to sketch the harsh conditions of life there. In 1880 he decided to dedicate his life to art, a passion that he pursued until his death by suicide only ten years later. His art did not sell; sadly, he never expected to be recognized.

In 1881 Vincent fell in love with his widowed cousin Kee Vos, but to his advances she replied: "No, never, never." To his brother

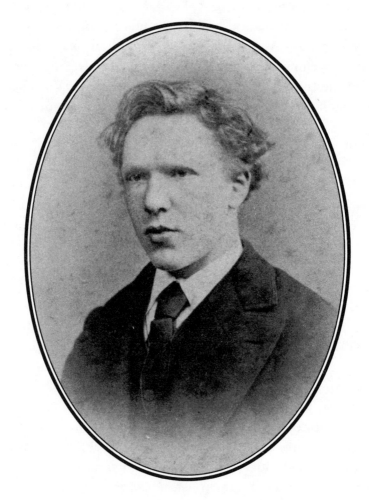

Figure 15.2   Vincent van Gogh as a young man. (Vincent van Gogh Foundation, Amsterdam)

he wrote: "Theo, I love her—her, and no other—her, forever."[4] Although it was against logic to desire another woman after he had pledged eternal love to Kee, in fact if she was not to be his, living without love was not something he wished to do forever: "I need a woman, I cannot, I may not, I will not live without one. I am a man, and a man with passions; I must go to a woman, otherwise I shall freeze or turn to stone—or, in short, shall be stunned.

. . . I think a life without love a sinful and immoral condition."[5] His post-Kee agenda was successful. The woman, a prostitute, was not young or beautiful, but her slight fadedness had a charm for him. He was not a baby in the cradle; it was not the first time that he was unable to resist affection (and love) for women who are damned by the clergymen in the pulpit.

With the voice of an older brother, Vincent lectured that one should not hesitate to go to a prostitute occasionally, to a woman you could trust and feel something for—something necessary, absolutely necessary, to keep sanity and wellness. Insanity and chronic illness were the result, however, if this prostitute gave him syphilis. Tralbaut assumed that Vincent was infected in Antwerp in 1885 because of the meetings with Dr. Cavenaille, but it is more likely that the doctor was treating syphilis of several years' duration. In January 1882 Vincent developed a severe fever. He wrote to his brother: "Now this morning I felt so miserable that I went to bed; I had a headache and was feverish from worry because I dread this week so much, and do not know how to get through it. And then I got up, but went back to bed again; now I feel a little better."[6] In the next letter he wrote:

> But I am so angry with myself now because I cannot do what I should like to do, and at such a moment one feels as if one were lying bound hand and foot at the bottom of a deep, dark well, utterly helpless. Now I have recovered enough so that I got up again last night and rummaged around, straightening things. When the model came of her own accord this morning, though I only half expected her, I put her into the right pose with Mauve's help, and tried to draw a little; but I could not do it, and I felt miserable and weak the whole evening."[7]

Vincent complained that he had always been healthy and had never had to spend a day in bed; now there always seemed to be something wrong with his health. "During the last fortnight I have been weak, not feeling well at all; I haven't given in to it and have gone on with my work. But, for instance, I have not been able to sleep for several nights, and have been feverish and nervous. But I forced myself to keep going and working, for this is no time to get sick. I must go on."[8] Since Vincent's health declined from this time forward, the December prostitute may have been the source of a syphilitic infection, and the subsequent fever and malaise secondary syphilis.

At about the same time that he had the fever, Vincent wrote to Theo that he had found a family to model for him: a woman, her mother, and her daughter. "The younger woman is not handsome as she is marked by smallpox, but the figure is very graceful and has some charm for me. Also, they have the right clothes, black merino and a nice style of bonnets and beautiful shawls, etc."[9] Clasina Hoornik, or Sien, was also willing to model nude.

Vincent's letters create an intimate portrait of Sien, revealing much about the hard life of a nineteenth-century prostitute. These women would often quickly become infected, spread the infection during its active period and the relapses of the following years, and then struggle with ongoing illnesses throughout their lives. The timing of the fever, and the likelihood that Sien would no longer have been infectious, points to the December prostitute rather than to Sien as the source of Vincent's infection. Although each worked as a washerwoman and had a young daughter, the description of the December woman as "strong and healthy," unlike poor Sien, also makes her the likelier carrier of a fresh dose.

Deserted when she was pregnant by a man of a higher class, Sien was not on the street long before she fell ill and was hospitalized. When she met Vincent she was pregnant again. He took her in with her daughter. In a letter to fellow artist Anton van Rappard, Vincent wrote: "I have to do with a woman who had one foot in the grave when I met her, and whose mind and nervous system were also upset and unbalanced."[10]

A year of illness and poverty in 1882 was also one of love and affection for Vincent and Sien. He planned to marry her, even though it would mean lowering himself socially. He told Theo that his lost love for Kee contrasted with his newly found love for

Sien: "Last year I wrote you a great many letters full of reflection on love. Now I no longer do so because I am too busy putting those same things into practice."[11] He insisted that he must not break his vow of marriage, which was not all altruism: "We both long for home life, close together; we need each other daily in our work and we are together daily."[12]

In June 1882 Vincent checked into the municipal hospital in The Hague with a new complaint. He admitted to Theo that he had been suffering for the past three weeks from painful urination, in short, gonorrhea—"but only a mild case."[13] Lecturing his younger brother that one should not aggravate these things by ignoring them, he also requested discretion. He was treated with quinine, his urethra being washed with a solution of alum and then painfully stretched: "Gradually the bougies they use get bigger, and every time one is introduced things are stretched a little more."[14] His bladder was catheterized and he complained of weakness. Drawing made him too feverish, so he read. "If only I were well again!"[15] On 22 June, Vincent wrote that he had not recovered as quickly as the doctors had expected and was extending his stay for two more weeks. Was there a complication, he asked the doctors? They assured him there was not.

"Vincent had to go into hospital to be treated for gonorrhea which he had caught from Sien,"[16] one biographer wrote, although this is also unlikely; she was a few weeks from delivering a baby, and was supposedly happily retired from a life on the streets. She assumed he had taken another woman,[17] which disappointed and puzzled him. In a letter to Theo he wrote that in every love there are many loves. "The principle thing is to continue and to persevere. He who wants variety must remain faithful. And he who wants to know many women must stick to one and the same."[18] Kee was still on his mind: "I had not forgotten another woman for whom my heart was beating, but she was far away and refused to see me; and this one walked the streets in winter, sick, pregnant, hungry—I couldn't do otherwise."[19]

While Vincent was in the hospital, Sien gave birth to a withered and jaundiced boy. During her confinement she found a doctor who hoped that in a few years she might regain her health and become strong once again. That health would depend on a stable and simple life; was this man she was living with to be trusted to stay with her? He was, she assured the doctor. Vincent wrote to Theo that he felt at home with Sien; they had developed a real need for each other. What Theo would see when he visited was a true home, with a baby and a cradle.

Vincent was released from the hospital but was soon readmitted; on the evening before he checked back in, he wrote Theo of his affection for Sien:

> It is a heartfelt, deep feeling, serious and not without a dark shadow of her gloomy past and mine, a shadow which I have already written you about—as if something evil were threatening us which we would have to struggle against continuously all our lives. . . . A woman changes when she is in love; when nobody cares for her, she loses her spirits. . . . what a woman wants is to be with one man, and with him forever. . . . So she now has quite another expression than last winter, and her eyes look different; her glance is calm and quiet, and there is an expression of happiness on her face.[20]

If anyone tried to separate them, they would leave the country together. "The chances of certain death are ten to one if one has no money and is not strong, but we would prefer that to being separated. . . . I will not leave Sien; I should be a broken man without her, and then I should also be ruined in my work and everything, . . . Sien loves me and I love Sien, . . . *There is love between her and me, and there are promises of mutual faithfulness.* . . Now I have recovered or am recovering in body and soul, and so is Sien, but it might be fatal if we were knocked on the head again, so to speak." Vincent and Sien both held hope for health: "The feeling of recovery thrills her, as I am thrilled by the urge to work again and to become absorbed in it. . . . I long for her complete recovery and for mine, for peace and quiet, and especially for some sympathy from you."[21]

Sien was exhausted after the difficult birth of her son. Vincent wrote to Theo: "I found her looking as though she had *withered*— literally like a tree which had been blasted by a cold, dry wind, its young shoots withering; and to make things complete, the baby was sick, too, and looked shriveled. . . . I had assured her as emphatically as I could that I should never leave her—less by words, however, than by doing whatever I could for her, but nevertheless in words too. Notwithstanding this, doubt and restlessness arose in her mind—but they disappeared as soon as I did my best to reassure her again."[22] He added: "I do not want her to fall back into that terrible state of illness and misery in which I found her, and from which she is saved for the present. This I undertook, this I must continue. I do not want her ever to feel again that she is deserted and alone."[23]

But poor Sien was right to be wary of Vincent's commitment. On 11 September 1883, he left for the fenlands of southern Drenthe, ending his period in The Hague having produced well over three hundred drawings, watercolors, lithographs, and oil paintings. Sien and her two children waved good-bye to him at the station. He saw her only one more time, when he returned to pick up some of his things. She did not go back to prostitution, as Vincent had feared she would, but worked as a washerwoman. Unable to support her children, she was forced to board them with her family. In 1901 she married a man in Rotterdam and three years later she committed suicide by drowning, as she had often threatened to do.

Although Vincent spoke of Sien tenderly, wished to marry her, and said that he would be a broken man without her, biographers have been singularly mean-spirited toward her. She has been called slovenly, crude and scheming, sad, ugly, despised, prematurely old, and a vicious drunkard. David Sweetman got right to the point in his biography of van Gogh: "She had fallen and he would save her, though, as the drawing of her smoking a cigar showed, her capacity for self-absorption and indifference must have made it hard to retain the illusion that she was anything other than a slut."[24] Although both Sien's doctor and Vincent were sure that life on the street would kill her, Sweetman refers to that option as "the easy life of prostitution." One drawing of Sien, "Sorrow," was one of Vincent's favorite pieces and the first in a line of drawings of pitiful, burdened women that one biographer called the ugliest, least appealing women in the history of art.

After two months in Drenthe, Vincent moved back in with his parents. The somber *Potato Eaters* was a painting of this time. He then moved for a few months to Antwerp (where he saw Dr. Cavanaille) and painted sailors and prostitutes around the docks. From there he moved to Paris for two years, living part of that time with Theo. The situation was strained; Theo later said his own illness made him less tolerant of his brother. Vincent learned about Impressionism and met fellow artists: Monet, Renoir, Degas, Seurat, Toulouse-Lautrec, and Paul Gauguin, who became a close friend. In February 1888, Vincent moved south to Arles on the advice of Toulouse-Lautrec, who inspired him to seek the intense colors there and also introduced him to absinthe. Vincent invited Gauguin to stay with him in his Yellow House. The two artists cooked and painted together and "talked a lot about Delacroix, Rembrandt, etc. Our arguments are terribly *electric*, sometimes we come out of them with our heads as exhausted as a used electric battery."[25] But on 23 December 1888 Vincent attacked Gauguin with a razor, then sliced off part of his own ear lobe and delivered it to a prostitute in the local brothel—at least that's the story that has usually been told, although a new hypothesis suggests that Gauguin did the hacking. Theo rushed from Paris to take care of his brother.

Vincent was hospitalized and released. On the advice of a doctor, he requested to be admitted to a mental hospital in Saint-Rémy, where he spent a year painting outdoor scenes and working from reproductions. In May 1890 he moved north of Paris to be near Theo, his wife Jo, and their new son, his namesake, Vincent. Dr. Paul-Ferdinand Gachet, a homeopath and amateur painter, cared for him. On 23 July 1890, he wrote: "This misery will never end." On 27 July he wandered out into the fields with an easel and his paints and a revolver and shot himself in the heart.

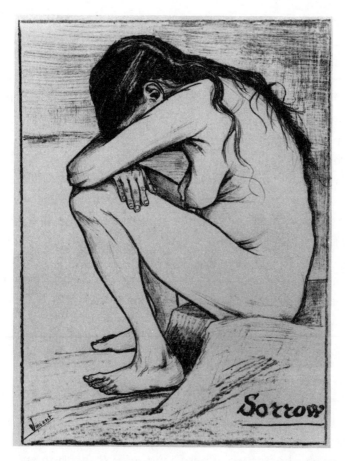

Figure 15.3   Sorrow: Drawing of Sien Hoornik. (Vincent van Gogh Foundation, Amsterdam)

The bullet was deflected to the diaphragm. He managed to stagger home. Gachet was called; he summoned Theo, who rushed to his brother's side, talked with him as he smoked a pipe, and climbed in bed with him and held him. Vincent's last words were: "I wish I could pass away like this." He died on 29 July at 1:30 A.M. The Catholic Church refused to bury him, but a nearby township accepted him. His coffin was covered with the yellow flowers he loved: sunflowers and dahlias.

In *Vincent van Gogh: Chemicals, Crises, and Creativity*, Wilfred Niels Arnold fell short of the *New York Times*'s 152 posthumous diagnoses; he gave up at 101. Of the dozen hypotheses worth considering, he found the key ones to be epilepsy, manic-depressive disorder, schizophrenia, Ménière's disease, and lead and absinthe poisoning. Others have suggested turpentine poisoning, sunstroke, and hypertrophy of the creative force. Dr. Urpar, director of the Arles hospital, chose "acute mania with generalized delirium."[26] Arnold's own disease of choice was acute intermittent porphyria, a hereditary disorder that can affect the nervous system and cause hallucinations, seizures, and paranoia. Epilepsy remained the diagnosis of choice until the 100th anniversary of Vincent's death, when the *Journal of the American Medical Association* announced Ménière's disease as a definite diagnosis, throwing out epilepsy. Arnold argued that they were wrong on both counts. There was no case for Ménière's, and epilepsy was no longer a diagnosis of merit. Kay Redfield Jamison countered in the *British Medical Journal* (1992) that Arnold's own selection, porphyria, was unlikely; she thought manic depressive disorder more likely for both Vincent and Theo. And, of course, manic depressive disorder is one of the most difficult conditions to distinguish from syphilis.

Arnold dismissed syphilis from consideration for two reasons: the relatively short interval between the first infection and insanity and the lengthy remissions from illness, a reason occasionally given against Theo's syphilis as well. Neither of these reasons holds up: John Stokes has described cases of syphilis with "extraordinarily long and extremely short courses, with and without remission."[27] Arnold argues further that there is no mention of syphilis in the letters, but the convention of the times would not allow mentioning syphilis in writing, and a careful reading reveals numerous references suggesting that Vincent and his brother were well aware of each other's disease and wrote of it in safe, veiled language.

Philosopher and psychiatrist Karl Jaspers, author of one of the most profound studies of the relationship between van Gogh's late mental state and his painting of that time (a parallel to his study of Nietzsche), saw no justification for the epilepsy diagnosis, given the absence of epileptic seizures. He concluded that "the only discussible possibility is that of a schizophrenic or a paralytic process,"[28] paralytic here meaning syphilitic. He opted for schizophrenia as the more likely of the two because van Gogh sustained the violent psychotic attacks for two years while keeping command of critical faculties, although because of a certain insecurity of hand, by van Gogh's own accounting, and a certain "dissoluteness," Jaspers did not discount a paralytic process completely. If he had known of Cavenaille's diagnosis, he might have been more inclined to favor syphilis. Wilhelm Lange Eichbaum, who wrote about genius related to madness (he too wrote a study of Nietzsche), rendered a diagnosis that accommodated both of Jaspers's hypotheses, with epilepsy thrown in for good measure: he suggested van Gogh had "an active luetic [syphilitic] schizoid and epileptoid disposition."[29] Once again, the astounding diversity of medical diagnoses in itself points to the possibility of the Great Imitator, syphilis.

Both Theo and Paul Gauguin progressed to tertiary syphilis. A brief look at their last days provides a context for looking at the correspondence of three men who had a diagnosis of syphilis and may well have shared this dismal secret with each other in their private conversations.

The month after Vincent's funeral, Theo collapsed. According to his painter friend Émile Bernard, he was temporarily paralyzed. On 10 October 1890, Theo's father-in-law Andries Bonger wrote asking Dr. Gachet to come to see Theo, who was in an unmanageable state of over-excitement and anger. According to a letter from Camille Pissarro to his son, Theo had gone suddenly mad, violently attacking his wife and child. At the same time, he had sent a grandiose telegram to Gauguin in Brittany, assuring him that funds for travel to the tropics would be available. Poor Gauguin, believing the offer, waited for the money. Theo was hospitalized two days after his violent outburst, and two days after that he was admitted to the celebrated asylum of Dr. Ésprit Blanche in Passy, where Guy de Maupassant had spent his last insane days. Gachet was unable to communicate with Theo when he visited. Dr. Louis Rivet, who had treated both brothers, concluded that Theo's case was "much worse" than Vincent's and there was not a spark of hope.[30] Because Theo died of syphilis, this statement implies that Dr. Rivet knew that Vincent had the same disease.

Gauguin probably picked up the disease in the days of his first sexual encounters in Rio de Janeiro, according to his biographer, David Sweetman. When he was forty-three (in 1891), Gauguin began to cough blood, a quarter of a liter a day, and he had pains as if his heart was giving out. His mind drifted lethargically. In 1892 he was admitted to a military hospital in Papeete, where he was treated for syphilis of the heart and was given a homeopathic specific, digitalis, according to Sweetman, although he provides no further details. Gauguin never acknowledged syphilis, "as if he simply could not face the truth of what was happening to him."[31]

He spent his last days in the Marquesas. Dirty bandages covered weeping sores on both shins and buzzing green flies followed him as he hobbled around leaning on a walking stick with a carved erect penis as a handle. At the end he was addicted to morphine for the pain, which he complained was everywhere, and laudanum, and he drank quantities of absinthe. His mood swings became progressively manic. With the arsenic he had for the lesions on his legs, he attempted suicide on a mountaintop, expecting ants to eat his body, but the poison was insufficient and he only vomited. He complained that his strength was gone and he was utterly exhausted from sleepless nights. He had an eye infection, probably conjunctivitis. "Ravages of syphilis were not confined to his suppurating body alone," Sweetman wrote, "but were also taking their toll on his sanity."[32] When he died in 1903, his friend Tioka bit into his scalp, a traditional island way of calling the dead back to life, but he was beyond recall.

The correspondence of Vincent and Theo is filled with philosophical comments on art and health, with opinions about their doctors. No diagnosis is given (other than epilepsy at the end), but the frequent references to a mysterious disease indicate that they were sharing information about syphilis. Although Rivet was their main physician, Vincent and Theo both consulted David Gruby, a Hungarian doctor living in Paris who was well-known for his treatment of syphilis.[33] The correspondence reveals that they were being treated by Gruby for something long-term; Vincent mentioned a year's trial. A letter of 4 May 1888 discussed his treatment.

In this letter Vincent expressed a wish to have a home of his own in which to regain his health. After comparing himself to a man he knew who became paralyzed, he mentioned that in Paris he was headed for a stroke, and then he told Theo of a cure that "would be very painful. Whereas one does not feel the disease itself." He said that Gruby was right about such cases with his advice "to eat well, to live well, to see little of women, in short to arrange one's life in advance exactly *as if one were already suffering from a disease of the brain and the spine* [emphasis added]. . . . Certainly that is taking the bull by the horns, which is never a bad policy."[34] Vincent continued: "And after all, doesn't it do one all the good in the world to listen to the wise advice of Rivet and Pangloss, those excellent optimists of the pure and jovial Gallic race, who leave you your self-respect."

Why would he link Rivet with Pangloss? In Voltaire's *Candide*, Pangloss, the castle tutor, ends up a beggar in the street ravaged by syphilis that eats away his eye and ear. Syphilis, says Pangloss, came from the New World with a man who traveled with Columbus; but in the end, it was necessary—after all, if Columbus had not made that trip, Europe would not have found chocolate! Vincent followed the Pangloss remark with this advice: "If we want to live and work, we must be very sensible and look after ourselves. Cold water, fresh air, simple good food, decent clothes, a decent bed, and no women."[35]

Two weeks later (17 May 1888), Vincent wrote a second letter, mentioning Rivet's reference to "the disease one has got":

What you write about your visits to Gruby has distressed me, but all the same I am relieved that you went. Has it occurred to you that the dazedness—the feeling of extreme lassitude—may have been caused by this weakness of the heart, and that in this case the iodide of potassium would have nothing to do with the feeling of collapse? Remember how last winter I was stupefied to the point of being absolutely incapable of doing anything at all, except a little painting, although I was not taking any iodide of potassium. So if I were you, I would have it out with Rivet if Gruby tells you not to take any. . . . I often think of Gruby *here* and *now*, and I am completely well. . . . Rivet takes things as they are . . . he hardens one against illness, and keeps up one's morale, I do believe, by making light of the disease one has got. If only you could have one year of life in the country and with nature just now, it would make Gruby's cure much easier. I expect he will make you promise to have nothing to do with women, except in case of necessity, but anyhow as little as possible. . . . I believe iodide of potassium purifies the blood and the whole system, or doesn't it? . . . Did you notice Gruby's face when he shuts his mouth tight and says—"No women!" It would make a fine Degas, that. . . . It doesn't matter if you don't shake it off all once. Gruby will give you a strengthening diet. . . . I shall not believe you if in your next letter you tell me there's nothing wrong with you.[36]

Gruby's diet was not easy: Alphonse Daudet tried it for his syphilis (as did Maupassant)—and decided that death was preferable. Potassium iodide was a standard treatment for syphilis then. Vincent suggested that it was affecting the state of his mind for the better: "The unbearable hallucinations have ceased, and are now getting reduced to a simple nightmare, in consequence of my taking bromide of potassium, I think."[37]

Another indication that Vincent considered that syphilis was causing his illnesses comes from this thought: "So I don't ask you to tell people that there is nothing wrong with me, or that there never will be. It is just that the explanation for all this is probably not Ricord's but Raspail's."[38] In mentioning Ricord, he is clearly thinking of syphilis, since Ricord was the foremost syphilologist of the time, but in favoring Raspail's "explanation," was he voting for Raspail's theory of syphilis over Ricord's? Or was he suggesting that Raspail had an explanation other than syphilis? Raspail was known for hypothesizing that a parasite caused alopecia, or patchy baldness. Alopecia often occurred with the fever and rash of secondary syphilis, but it was also found without syphilis. Vincent incorporated a picture of the cover of Raspail's annual book on health in *Still Life: Drawing Board with Onion, etc.*

When Vincent began to have his attacks, he did not connect them with syphilis, thinking instead that they were caused by epilepsy. From the asylum in Arles, he wrote to his brother: "Most epileptics bite their tongue and injure themselves. Dr. Felix Rey told me that he had seen a case where someone had mutilated his own ear, as I did."[39] Rey also told him that auditory and visual hallucinations were usual in the beginning with epilepsy. "Everyone here is suffering from fever, hallucinations, or madness." Vincent observed that their madness was no more frightful than if they had been stricken with something else: syphilis, for instance. But how much of Cavenaille's warning that syphilis would affect his brain haunted him as well? Was he thinking of Cavenaille when he said; "I am either a madman or an epileptic"?[40]

In the intense periods of long hours of work in the last months of his life, Vincent described himself as a human charged with electricity. Crazy religious ideas took hold of him. In these states, he wrote that his mind in a state of excitement always concerned itself with infinity and everlasting life. "I struggle with all my might to master my work," he wrote, "and I say to myself that if I win, it is the best lightning rod for my illness; I shall come out on top."[41] The brushes glide in his fingertips fast as a bow over a violin. Fired up with energy, he is able to bring out a rich blue background that assumes a mystical effect. In the intense colors of the coffeehouse, he paints a place where one could go insane, commit crimes. Religious images are too exciting; he fails with a picture

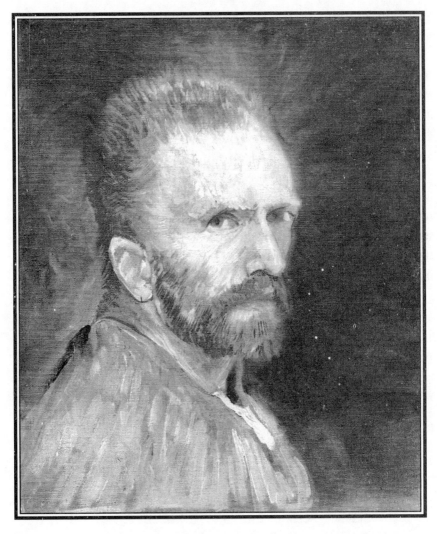

Figure 15.4   Vincent van Gogh, self-portrait. (Wadsworth Atheneum)

of Christ with an angel. He begins to work with larger canvases, thinking of his part in the art of the future. Theo calls him a great genius who will someday be compared with Beethoven. Vincent writes that it is necessary to get really fired up to bring the shades of gold he is achieving out in a painting; not just anyone can achieve those colors. He feels life only when flinging out the work. His brain is taut to the breaking point; he thinks a thousand things within a half an hour. He is engulfed in the work with the clearheadedness of a lover. He becomes unconscious of himself; the painting progresses like a dream. As he becomes more sick and fragile, he feels he grows in artistic stature.

Jaspers calls Vincent's last period one of vehement and ecstatic turbulence, but always disciplined. The imagery of restless energy, electric excitement, and almost mystical fervor, along with repeated statements of fear of madness and fear that he did not have long to live, raise a question that cannot be answered with certainty: Was Vincent experiencing the ecstasy and the misery of the stage that precedes paresis when he painted with such intensity in the last months of his life? Because he committed suicide, we will never know.

16

Friedrich Nietzsche

1844–1900

> The life I am living is really dangerous be-
> cause I am one of those machines that could
> explode.
>
> —FRIEDRICH NIETZSCHE

IN THE TOWN SQUARE IN TURIN, ITALY, ON 3 JANUARY 1889, Friedrich Nietzsche threw his arms around the neck of a horse being beaten, lost consciousness, and turned the bend to madness.[1] His landlord, Davide Fino, found the fallen philosopher in the square and took him home. That night Nietzsche kept everyone awake, singing, shouting, and banging on the piano. He composed a series of mad postcards, most of which were confiscated by the Turin post office. Of those that got through, one was to the Vatican signed "the Crucified," and one was to his old friend Franz Overbeck, a professor of church history at Basel: "I am just having all anti-Semites shot,"[2] Nietzsche wrote, and signed the letter Dionysos. When his former colleague, Jacob Burckhardt, received a four-page, clearly unstable letter from Nietzsche written in tiny, almost illegible script, he immediately consulted Overbeck, who set out that day for Turin in time to keep a frightened Fino from having Nietzsche arrested. Nietzsche's experience in the town

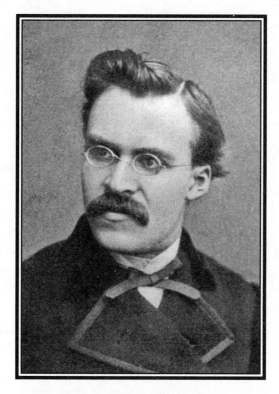

Figure 16.1 Friedrich Nietzsche (Hulton Archive/Getty Images)

square of Turin recalls similar sudden transformations from seeming sanity to syphilitic madness experienced by Schumann, Baudelaire, Hugo Wolf, and Maupassant.

Overbeck reported the details of his rescue mission in Turin to Nietzsche's friend Peter Gast, saying he must be silent about a few matters to "any soul who was the sick man's friend"—at least for now. Nietzsche had broken into tears and embraced Overbeck. Then he sang loudly, raving, uttering "bits and pieces from the world of ideas in which he has been living, and also in short sentences, in an indescribably muffled tone, sublime, wonderfully clairvoyant. Unspeakably horrible things would be audible, about himself as the successor of the dead God, the whole thing punctuated, as it were, on the piano, whereupon more convulsions and outbursts would follow."[3] Nietzsche, the clown of the new eternities: the breakdown was so complete that Overbeck wondered if it would have been a genuine act of friendship to have taken his life.

The next day Overbeck persuaded Nietzsche to accompany him to Basel, pretending that there was to be a great festival in his honor. Overbeck described a "quietly terrifying" train trip. They were helped and accompanied by a dentist who said he was used to dealing with madmen. As it happened, the French novelist André Malraux's grandfather's brother Walter was on the train as well. He told a young Malraux this eyewitness account.

Short of money, they had to travel third class. A peasant woman with a hen in a basket was in their compartment with them. Walter feared a violent incident. As they were going through the St. Gotthard tunnel, a thirty-five minute trip in complete darkness, Nietzsche began to chant a poem, his last, "Venice," accompanied by the sound of the hen pecking at the basket. Walter thought some of Nietzsche's poetry was mediocre, but this one— "well, by God, it was sublime."[4] In Basel Nietzsche was admitted to the nerve clinic of Dr. Wille, an expert on general paralysis of the insane. The sign-in sheet recorded: "Friedrich Nietzsche, Professor at Basel at age of 23. 1866. *Syphilit. Infect.*"

Scholars who find Nietzsche's last works to be the most mature expression of his philosophy oppose suggestions that there were signs of impending madness. The story of Nietzsche's sudden plummet from the most advanced thought of his time to raving dementia is often told as if there were a razor's edge demarcation between sanity and tertiary syphilis, as if on 3 January armies of spirochetes woke suddenly from decades of slumber and attacked the brain, instead of the biological reality that paresis is a gradual process presaged over many years. There were times before the well-known episode with the horse when Nietzsche was showing clear anticipatory signs of paresis, and times in the asylum when he seemed so normal that his friends wondered if it might all be a ruse. Gast observed: "The question of whether one would be doing Nietzsche a favor if one reawakened him to life must be left aside. . . . I have seen Nietzsche in certain conditions where it seemed to me—a terrible thought!—that he was *faking* madness, as if he were glad that it had ended *thus*. It is highly probable that he could write his philosophy of Dionysus only as a madman."[5] Overbeck agreed: "I could not help having the horrifying thought, at least momentarily—though this happened during several of the periods in which I witnessed Nietzsche's mental illness—that his madness was simulated."[6]

Many, perhaps most, Nietzsche scholars believe that Nietzsche's exquisite writing in his last months (and years) prove that he could not have been influenced by syphilis then. Scholar Claudia Crawford represents this approach well in an essay on Nietzsche's final production. She argues that his excesses in the last year, especially in the last quarter of 1888, in *Twilight of the Idols, The Antichrist, Ecce Homo, The Case of Wagner,* and in his notes and letters, were not "symptoms of megalomania and impending madness" or "signs of degenerative madness,"[7] but rather the conscious wielding of a grand style of prophecy and apocalypse. Nietzsche's language was appropriate to carry out his plan to assassinate two millennia of anti-nature, to play out "the psychological aim of becoming a redeemer on a par with Jesus and Socrates."[8] Here Nietzsche was confronting humanity with the most difficult demand ever made of it: "the attempt to raise humanity higher, including the relentless destruction of everything that was degenerating and parasitical." He possessed and expressed the "will to power" as no one had ever done.

However, since the syphilis texts tell us that the last expressions of sanity before paretic dementia sets in can be characterized by mystical vision, messianic prophecy, grandiose self-definition, clarity of expression, and extreme disinhibition, *while all the time maintaining exquisite precision of form,* then this remarkable final late work of Nietzsche's was not incompatible with or contrary to what we would expect from the paresis that was about to annihilate him. Over and over in those last works are images of tightly controlled energy and immanent detonation. The final chapter of *Ecce Homo,* "Why I Am Destiny," proclaims a crisis, decades of worldwide conflagration, with wars such as have never been seen before on this earth, and the certainty that the name Friedrich Nietzsche will be associated with it all: "I am not a philosopher. I am dynamite!" His brilliance seemed boundless. On 18 December 1888 Nietzsche wrote to his friend Carl Fuchs: "Never before have I known anything remotely like these months from the beginning of September until now. The most amazing tasks as easy as a game; my health, like the weather, coming up every day with boundless brilliance and certainty. I cannot tell you how much has been finished—*everything*. The world will be standing on its head for the next few years: since the old God has abdicated, *I* shall rule the world from now on."[9] On Christmas Day he promised in two months to be the best-known name on earth. He saw himself as a machine about to blow apart. Thomas Mann characterized Nietzsche's soaring intellect at that time as "blasted with ecstasy."[10] Karl Jaspers describes a mystical light, a dangerous shuddering at the boundary in this last work.[11] Since Nietzsche never sold more than a few hundred copies of any of his books during his lifetime,[12] his final proclamations seem grandiose. And yet his influence on every aspect of Western culture has been so profound that we have to ask if his most extreme self-aggrandizement has not proven understated.

Sigmund Freud acknowledged the influence of paresis when he praised Nietzsche's last achievements. On 28 October 1908 the Vienna Psychoanalytic Society devoted the evening to Nietzsche's *Ecce Homo*, just published posthumously. Freud said (and Otto Rank recorded in the *Minutes*):

> Nietzsche was a paretic. The euphoria is beautifully developed, and so on, and so on. However, this would oversimplify the problem. It is very doubtful whether paresis can be held responsible for the contents of *Ecce Homo*. In cases in which paresis struck at men of great genius, extraordinary accomplishments were achieved until a short time before the outbreak of illness (Maupassant). The indication that this work of Nietzsche is fully

valid and to be taken seriously is in the preservation of mastery of form.[13]

Illness became his fate, Freud said. (Thomas Mann went one step further: "His destiny was his genius. But there is another name for this genius: disease."[14]) Freud continued: "The degree of introspection achieved by Nietzsche had never been achieved by anyone, nor is it likely ever to be reached again. . . . The most essential factor must still be added: the role that paresis played in Nietzsche's life. It is the loosening process resulting from paresis that gave him the capacity for the quite extraordinary achievement of seeing through all layers and recognizing the instincts at the very base. In that way, he placed his paretic disposition at the service of science."[15] Alfred Adler agreed; in paresis one can find extraordinary accomplishments.

At the asylum Nietzsche was able to recognize his mother Franziska, who with Overbeck arranged to have him transferred from Wille's clinic to the psychiatric clinic of Jena University closer to her. There the head of staff, Dr. Stutz, concluded that "the data confirm progressive paralysis as being the correct diagnosis. There can hardly be any doubt on the subject."[16] The initial exam was conducted by Dr. Ziehen, the chief house physician. The examination at Jena revealed a scar on the penis, a possible indicator of a prior syphilic chancre. John Stokes wrote that the chancre resolves with "at most only the most superficial and minute scar,"[17] whereas an elaborate scar would indicate another venereal infection, chancroid. Nietzsche's handwriting showed tremor when he was upset. He gesticulated and grimaced continually while speaking. For the first five months he continued to be agitated and frequently incoherent. He smeared his feces and drank his urine. He screamed. At other times, he would seem perfectly normal. He received mercury rubs. According to the belief of the time that family would only further agitate a paretic, Nietzsche's mother was not allowed to visit for six months, just as Clara Schumann had not been allowed to visit Robert in the asylum.

Nietzsche was admitted to the Jena clinic with this entry: "type of Illness: Paralytic mental illness." Otto Binswanger, the head of the clinic at Jena, was an expert in general paralysis of the insane. His publications included "Contributions to the Pathogenesis and Differential Diagnosis of Progressive Paralysis" and "Brain Syphilis and Dementia Paralytica, Clinical and Statistical Studies." Professor Binswanger once presented Nietzsche to his class as a case study of paresis. Binswanger kept Overbeck informed of his patient's condition. Nietzsche, he wrote, spoke more coherently, with fewer outbreaks of screaming, and some delusions and auditory hallucinations. The outlook for recovery was small.

In March of the following year, Nietzsche was released from the clinic into the care of his mother, who watched over him until she died in 1897. Then his sister, Elisabeth, with the help of her mother's maidservant, Alwine, took over until the end. From early 1894 Nietzsche was house-bound. In 1895 he began showing signs of increasing physical paralysis. Overbeck recalled his last visit to Nietzsche. His friend was half-crouching in the corner, wanting only to be left in peace. Previously, he had been dreadfully excited, roaring and shouting.

One of the arguments against Nietzsche's having had neurosyphilis has been that he existed in the twilight zone of insanity for eleven years after the onset of paresis. However, syphilis texts tell us that the course of paretic neurosyphilis can range from three to six months in extreme cases to as many as thirty years or more in slowly deteriorative types.[18] This slow-moving or "stationary paresis" is different from the type known picturesquely as "galloping paresis." Relevant to the episode with the horse, John Stokes wrote that trauma can incite paretic manifestations in a case that otherwise would have remained quiescent.[19]

Nietzsche died of a stroke on 25 August 1900. He was buried in a traditional Lutheran funeral, a mockery of his philosophy. No autopsy was performed. Elisabeth confessed that at the time of her brother's death she never thought of permitting a dissection, and in fact no physician had suggested it. Besides, she added, at that time the "disgusting suspicion" of syphilis had not yet emerged. Of course, syphilis was part of the medical record, although it is quite possible that the diagnosis had not been shared with the family, and the doctors saw no reason to make it public.

No archivist has had more mixed reviews than Elisabeth Nietzsche. She began her collection of Nietzsche's manuscripts as an adoring little sister, filing her brother's first literary attempts in her treasure chest. That trove grew to be the Weimar Archive, a lovely building Elisabeth established to house her brother's papers and her brother as well; he spent his last insane years living upstairs. Elisabeth raised money, negotiated publishing contracts, and managed a staff of workers (mostly Nazis after Hitler came to power) who catalogued his work. She published all of his collected works from 1892 on, plus eighty-one articles and a three-volume biography. She became known throughout Europe as a woman of letters and the guardian of Nietzsche's legacy, on a par with Cosima Wagner, who was similarly watching over the creative estate of her late husband, Richard. Elisabeth was nominated three times for the Nobel Prize.

But Franz Overbeck warned that Elisabeth was a different kind of sister: a dangerous one. It is Overbeck's review that has lasted. Why has Elisabeth been so completely vilified by scholars? As a devout Lutheran, a rabid anti-Semite, and a fierce nationalist who revered Hitler, Elisabeth was uniquely unsuited to represent a man who was anti-anti-Semitic and anti-patriotic, who wrote God's obituary and the script for demolishing everything she held sacred. Nietzsche's attempts to keep his mother and sister from knowing how far he had traveled from the hometown Christian virtue failed. Over the years Elisabeth avoided the increasingly dire contradictions between her morality and her brother's by twisting truth at every step to match her wished-for image of reality.

The Nobel committee would have made a big mistake if they had honored her because she edited as she pleased, changing letters to make them read the way she thought they should have been, rarely even bothering to cover her tracks. Biographers now refer to her politely as an unreliable witness, or with less restraint as a compulsive and pathological liar, singularly nasty, bigoted, and bloody-minded. Her compiled editions of Nietzsche's work, in particular *The Will to Power*, included passages from his notebooks that he might never have wanted published. Scraps of writing from a waste basket left in his room in Sils Maria found their way into his published works, freely edited. One of Elisabeth's worst failings was to put the archive in the service of Adolf Hitler.

Elisabeth's first meeting with Hitler took place in February 1932 in Weimar's National Theater, where a play about Napoleon co-authored by Benito Mussolini (who later donated money to the Nietzsche archive) was being staged, thanks in part to Elisabeth's machinations. Hitler, who had come to town accompanied by storm troopers, heard that Nietzsche's sister would be at the theater. He approached her box with an armful of red roses. While she was initially cool to him because she (rightly) assumed he would be defeated for the presidency by Hindenburg, she began to sing his praises after he took over a year later: "We are drunk with enthusiasm because at the head of our government stands such a wonderful, indeed phenomenal personality like our magnificent Chancellor Adolf Hitler."[20] His fascinating eyes seem to stare right through you, she recalled. When she died, Hitler laid a laurel wreath on her coffin.

The Nietzsche legend as created by Elisabeth had no place for syphilis, so it is ironic that word of his disease might never have reached the public if she had not attempted to cover it up. Her first blunder was to allow access to Nietzsche's medical records at Basel and Jena to the respected Leipzig neurologist and psychiatrist P. J. Möbius. If Elisabeth had hoped for a sympathetic portrait of the last illness from Möbius, she was sadly deceived. In 1902 he published *On the Pathological in Nietzsche,* in which he not only revealed the diagnosis, although by innuendo rather than by name, but far worse, suggested that the first indications of mental instability appeared as early as 1881 with the "lightning" inspiration for *Thus Spake Zarathustra.*

Elisabeth probably did not know the diagnosis at the time; if she had known it, she would not have given Möbius access to the records. Dr. Wille would have had no reason on Nietzsche's admission in Basel to tell the distressed mother the origin of her son's illness, nor would the doctors at Jena. Once the story was out, though, Elisabeth tried all the damage control she could devise. An aggressive pathographer, Möbius warned the public against the sick philosopher. Only those who are intellectually deaf, he warned, can miss the undertones of progressive paralysis in *Thus Spoke Zarathustra*. "If you find pearls do not imagine that it is all one chain of pearls. Be distrustful, for this man has a diseased brain."[21] The creeping onset of late syphilitic disease was superimposed on Nietzsche's already morbid mental state, declared Möbius. Elisabeth flew into a rage, calling his accusation a "disgusting calumny," not so much because he revealed her brother's disease as because he suggested that Nietzsche had been infected by a prostitute. Philosopher and psychologist Karl Jaspers credited Möbius with being the first to recognize the incisive transformation in Nietzsche beginning in the early 1880s, but he concluded that Möbius's insight did not gain approval because it was so encumbered with absurdity.

Möbius interviewed many of Nietzsche's friends from student days looking, unsuccessfully, for stories of any sexual activity. He concluded rather lamely that although Nietzsche's attraction for sex had been abnormally weak, "and he lacked the sex-urge which a healthy male needs in order to devote himself to a woman,"[22] he must have been curious enough to try sex at least once. Biographer R. C. Hollingdale had an opposite idea: that Nietzsche was "highly sexed and inordinately attracted to women," yet there is no record, or even hint, of his ever having gone to bed with a woman of his own class—or with any woman, we might add. That Nietzsche was inordinately attracted to women goes against all the known evidence.

Elisabeth did not give up in her attempts to cleanse the record of the ignoble diagnosis and its probable disreputable cause. If she could not stop the gossip about syphilis, she could at least put the prostitute rumor to rest. For this task, in 1923 she engaged one of Nietzsche's doctors, Health Commissioner Vulpius, who had assisted Binswanger at Jena. Vulpius's finding of an inflammation of the left iris had confirmed for him the diagnosis of progressive paralysis: "The right pupil was considerably wider open than the left one, which was extremely deformed, but both showed no reaction to light. Slight adhesions of the somewhat discolored left iris with the front lens capsule were mostly dissolved after the insertion of a grain of atropin into the corner of the eye."[23]

"I too was deeply moved upon meeting the shadow of a man whose writings I had studied with lively enthusiasm as a student," Vulpius recalled. "So it is understandable that I approached my patient not only with medical but also with psychiatric interest which in turn led Frau Dr. [honorary] Förster-Nietzsche to entrust me with writing a critique of her brother's medical history and the unsavory controversy connected with it."[24] Vulpius's cooperative and fanciful theory at least satisfied Elisabeth with an alternative to sexual transmission:

> The causal toxin must have once entered Nietzsche's system, namely without his knowledge. The most obvious and likely occasion for this assumption was his service as a volunteer medical corpsman in the 1870 campaign, and especially perhaps the final transporting of influenza and diphtheria patients under the most unfavorable hygienic conditions. To overcome his lively disgust and probably in the belief that he was thereby enjoying some disinfecting protection, he smoked in the ambulance. How easily a transmission of the poison could have taken place if he ever set down his cigar in order to help a patient in the crowded vehicle![25]

As far-fetched as the cigar theory sounds, spirochetes from a mucous patch in the mouth could be transferred on a cigar. Joseph Rollet, a doctor from Lyon, demonstrated that secondary syphilis is contagious in ways other than sexual by observing a glassblower with an infectious mucous patch in his mouth who infected a coworker when he passed a glassblowing pipe. By 1864 Rollet had fifteen such case studies, thus establishing the contagiousness of secondary syphilis. But Vulpius had no reason to think Nietzsche was infected in this way (perhaps he was humoring Elisabeth), and there is one sufficient reason why he was not: Nietzsche served as a volunteer medical corpsman only in 1870, whereas Möbius claimed to have in his possession letters from two Leipzig doctors who had treated Nietzsche for syphilis in 1867. This information about the Leipzig letters was provided by psychiatrist Wilhelm Lange-Eichbaum in a monograph published in 1946. (He had written "Nietzsche as a Psychiatric Problem" in 1931.) In this monograph he stated that a Berlin psychiatrist had told him about the treatment by these known doctors. Walter Kaufmann included this information in his entry on Nietzsche in the *Encyclopedia of Philosophy*,[26] although he noted that there was no proof of the existence of these letters. And according to Hollingdale, Richard Blunck, in a study of young Nietzsche "reproduces evidence which makes it impossible to doubt that Nietzsche was treated for a syphilitic infection by two Leipzig doctors during 1867."[27] In the clinical records Nietzsche is reported to have said he was infected twice in 1866, so treatment the following year fits a reasonable timeline for secondary syphilis. Although the information about the Leipzig treatment is not substantiated, there is no reason to doubt Möbius's word that he had these letters in his possession.

Elisabeth noted that Nietzsche had "cholera" twice in 1867, either incident being a possibility for a secondary syphilitic fever. Another possibility is that he was infected earlier and first treated only then. There was no sharp turn toward chronic illness in 1867. In fact, Nietzsche's medical history contains suspicious conditions much earlier. Between 1861 and 1866, for example, he complained of headaches; pains in the neck, chest, and throat; hoarseness; rheumatism; and spells of coughing, which has led to speculation about early meningitis following a syphilitic infection.

Elisabeth's next ploy was to get the syphilis diagnosis discredited. In May 1905 she assigned Peter Gast, who was working for her in the archive, the job of writing to Franz Overbeck, on his deathbed, requesting him to acknowledge that the diagnosis of syphilis found in the medical records at Jena was based on a remark he had made at the time of Nietzsche's admission. Overbeck angrily answered at once that Professor Binswanger had told him in February 1890, after swearing him to secrecy, that there was no doubt in his mind about the syphilitic origin of Nietzsche's paralysis. "I have kept Binswanger's confidence, except in your case, Mr. Gast."[28] This correspondence was another of Elisabeth's blunders. By trying to erase the diagnosis, she unwittingly documented a confirmation. When she asked Ida Overbeck to obtain a deathbed confession, Ida refused and soon after sued Elisabeth for libel for accusing her husband of losing a manuscript of the missing part of the *Will to Power* in Turin. In 1922 Binswanger stated that although the origins of Nietzsche's disease could not be known, the diagnosis of progressive paralysis could not be doubted. According to present science, Nietzsche had a syphilitic infection of the central nervous system.[29]

Indefatigable Elisabeth also attempted to explain away Nietzsche's paralysis as an effect of drugs. A "Javanese soporific," thought to be liquid hashish, was given to him in the summer of 1881 by a Dutchman, who told him never to take more than a few drops in a glass of water. Elisabeth tried it and it had an exhilarating effect, but she came to dislike the feeling and implored her brother to be moderate in its use. In 1885 Nietzsche admitted he had taken a few drops too many and had flung himself to the ground, exhilaration passing over into a spasmodic laughter. According to Elisabeth, Professor Wille at Basel told her that Nietzsche was experimenting with soporifics not yet tried by science. All of this was revealed only after Möbius's book was used by Elisabeth to promote the theory that Nietzsche's paralysis was a "hashish paralysis."[30] She also suggested that the sleeping medication Nietzsche took left him excited in the morning. Despite Elisabeth's best efforts, the diagnosis would not disappear.

One of the most frequently quoted theories for where Nietzsche was infected with syphilis is also one of the least likely. In February 1865, while a student at the University of Bonn, he took a short vacation by himself to Cologne. A porter who was asked to take him to a restaurant brought him to a brothel instead. Nietzsche recounted this story of the adventure to his friend Paul Deussen: "I found myself suddenly surrounded by half a dozen apparitions in tinsel and gauze, looking at me expectantly. For a short space of time I was speechless. Then I made instinctively for the piano, as being the only soulful thing present. I struck a few chords, which freed me from my paralysis, and I escaped."[31]

"According to this story and everything else I know about Nietzsche," Deussen wrote, "I am inclined to believe that the words which Steinhart dictated to us in a Latin biography of Plato apply to him: *mulierem nunquam attingit*" (he never touched a woman).[32] Nietzsche's unambiguous antipathy to these prostitutes might lead to the conclusion that the Cologne brothel is the last place where he might have come in contact with syphilis. Yet this very brothel has entered the popular literature as the most probable place of infection, with numerous biographers stating it as fact.

The reason for this twist is to be found in Thomas Mann's novel, *Dr. Faustus*. The protagonist, Adrian Leverkühn, is modeled on Nietzsche. The brothel episode as recounted to Deussen is a key scene. "That up to then he had 'touched' no woman was and is to me an unassailable fact," says the narrator. But Mann changes one detail: in his story, Adrian is touched on the cheek by one of the prostitutes. In Nietzsche's account of the episode, repulsion is key, but in Mann's fiction, repulsion switches to obsessional attraction. Adrian travels in search of the woman with the fatal touch and *chooses* to be infected with the "exhilarating but wasting disease," even though she warns him away. "And, gracious heaven, was it not also love, or what was it, what madness, what deliberate, reckless tempting of God, what compulsion to comprise the punishment of sin, finally what deep, deeply mysterious longing for daemonic conception, for a deathly unchaining of chemical change in his nature was at work, that having been warned he despised the warning and insisted upon possession of this flesh?"[33]

In an essay on the inspiration for *Dr. Faustus*, Mann reveals the reason why his fictional Nietzsche/Leverkühn waited an entire year after the brothel encounter before looking for the prostitute. After saying that Nietzsche was "twice infected" with syphilis, he wrote: "The medical history preserved at Jena gives the year 1866 for the first of these misadventures. In other words, one year after he had fled from the house in Cologne he returned without diabolic guidance, this time to some similar place and contracted the disease (some say deliberately, as self-punishment) which was to destroy his life but also to intensify it enormously."[34]

But Thomas Mann was guessing, as was R. C. Hollingdale in turn: "How he contracted it remains strictly a matter for speculation, although the problem is surely not a very difficult one: a young man in Nietzsche's situation could hardly have come in contact with the disease anywhere but in a brothel." Angus Fletcher expresses the scholarly confusion: "Nietzsche's own account of this experience was ambiguous or changeable, and finally unreliable. Did he touch the woman at the brothel, or only the piano?"[35] But there is nothing ambiguous in Nietzsche's statement: "I struck a few chords, which freed me from my paralysis, and I escaped." Scholarship has come full circle to fault Nietzsche for that which he did not say.

More details about Nietzsche's private life when he was a student come from a most unexpected source: Carl Gustav Jung. Jung pursued Nietzsche's life story, especially that which pertained to his sexuality and his disease, with the tenacity of a private investigator, gathering information from confidential interviews with people who had known Nietzsche personally. In his memoir *Memories, Dreams, Reflections*, Jung tells how Nietzsche's experience was central to his own personal journey, in particular the critical descent into his own unconscious. He never published what he learned, except for a few scraps in the memoir, but he did speak of it to others, and so there are notes to be found in transcripts of conversations: in the minutes of the Wednesday meetings of Freud's Vienna Psychoanalytic Society, and in course notes (1,544 published pages)·taken at a seminar that Jung conducted in English on Nietzsche's *Zarathustra* between 1934 and 1939.[36]

In the memoir Jung related that his interest in Nietzsche had started when he was a medical student. He delayed reading Nietzsche because of a "secret fear" that he might be like him, that he might be forced to recognize that he too was a "strange bird" with a morbid second personality, a thought that threw him into a cold sweat. Nietzsche could afford to be a "sport of nature" because he was published and spoke many languages, whereas Jung, with only his Basel dialect felt vulnerable to criticism.

Although Nietzsche had taken a permanent leave of absence from Basel for his health nineteen years before Jung began his investigation, there were still people who had known him and were able to recall unflattering tidbits, such as the way he pretended to be a nobleman. Nietzsche's stylistic exaggerations got on the nerves of the Basel academics.[37] In the *Zarathustra* seminar Jung remarked that Nietzsche walked around Basel in a gray top hat, dressed to imitate Englishmen who came to Switzerland. "He did not wear a veil, but otherwise he was a complete English gentleman from the storybook, a perfectly ridiculous sight. That was adorning himself! For nobody in Basel ever dreamt of walking about like that."[38]

In the *Zarathustra* seminar, Jung recounted (from the correspondence between Nietzsche and Overbeck) a dream that Nietzsche had about a toad:

Now in this correspondence, he mentions the fact that Nietzsche always suffered from a peculiar phobia that when he saw a toad, he felt that he ought to swallow it. And once when he was sitting beside a young woman at a dinner, he told her of a dream he had had, in which he saw his hand with all the anatomical detail, quite translucent, absolutely pure and crystal-like, and then suddenly an ugly toad was sitting upon his hand and he had to swallow it. You know, the toad has always been suspected of being poisonous, so it represents a secret poison hidden in the darkness where such creatures live—they are nocturnal animals. And the extraordinary fact is that it is a parallel to what actually happened to Nietzsche, of all people—that exceedingly sensitive nervous man had a syphilitic infection. That is a historical fact—I know the doctor who took care of him. It was when he was twenty-three years old. I am sure this dream refers to that fatal impression; this absolutely pure system infected by the poison of the darkness.[39]

Along with the fantasy improvisation on Nietzsche's dream, this passage contains two very important bits of information relating to the syphilis question: that Jung knew the doctor who treated Nietzsche and that Nietzsche was infected when he was twenty-three, which would be in 1867, the same date Möbius gave for the two treatments in Leipzig. It takes only a little digging to establish that Jung knew Otto Binswanger. Otto's nephew Ludwig Binswanger was a colleague of Jung's and a member of Freud's Wednesday evening group. Ludwig Binswanger had used Jung as a subject in his word association experiments. In February 1908 (the year of the two meetings of the Vienna Psychoanalytic Society concerning Nietzsche), Jung and Ludwig Binswanger visited famous uncle Otto together. The date is confirmed by a postcard that Jung mailed to Freud from Jena, signed by himself and Ludwig Binswanger.[40]

While talking about how Nietzsche maintained distance from his friends, Jung revealed a surprising personal connection with Franz Overbeck: "Overbeck always handled Nietzsche with gloves; I knew him. He was a typical, refined historian, a very learned man, and in all his ways exceedingly polite and careful not to touch anything that was hot; he appreciated the great genius in Nietzsche, but the man Nietzsche he handled most carefully."[41] Jung added that, when insane, Nietzsche produced the most shocking erotic literature, which Elisabeth destroyed, but Overbeck saw it and, Jung hints, discussed it with him: "there is plenty of evidence of his pathological condition."[42] Curiously, Jung did not specify what was so shocking that he would have deemed it pathological.

Jung corresponded with Elisabeth, although these letters were probably quite formal. And he had an opportunity to speak, at least on one occasion, with Lou Andreas Salomé, Nietzsche's sometime friend and confidant, when they both attended the Third Psychoanalytic Congress in 1911.

What Jung had learned through his private sleuthing about Nietzsche was revealed indirectly at the 1 April 1908 meeting of the Vienna Psychoanalytic Society. Paul Federn stated: "According to a reliable source, Nietzsche had at certain periods of his life homosexual relations and acquired syphilis in a homosexual brothel in Genoa."[43] In the 28 October 1908 meeting, Federn again mentioned a report that Nietzsche was homosexually active and was infected that way. Freud then gave the source of that report: "Jung claims to have learned that Nietzsche acquired syphilis in a homosexual brothel." Freud added, "Completely cut off from life by illness, he turns to the only object of investigation that is still accessible to him and which, in any event, is close to him as a homosexual, i.e., the ego."[44]

Freud was still alluding to this allegation in 1934 when he tried to dissuade his younger friend Arnold Zweig from writing a romanticized novel about Nietzsche: "First, it is impossible to understand anyone without knowing his sexual constitution, and Nietzsche's is a complete enigma. There is even a story that he was a passive homosexual and that he contracted syphilis in a male brothel in Italy."[45] Throwing doubt on Jung's rumor: unless Nietzsche took an unknown trip to Genoa as a student, he could not have been infected there when he was twenty-three.

Nietzsche's sexual history remains a mystery. Most biographers have portrayed him as chaste, at best unlucky at love, and possibly clandestinely involved with female prostitutes, although here with little to go on. Joachim Köhler's biography reveals a homoerotic Nietzsche, at home in the expatriate gay communities of Messina.[46] The intense, intellectual friendship of Lou Salomé with Nietzsche and his friend Paul Rée in the summer of 1882 reads differently if she is seen as the friend of two gay men and as Nietzsche's biographer-to-be, rather than as rejecting his amorous advances. Nietzsche wrote that he might consider marriage when he was on his way to meet Lou, but a two-year marriage at most, and

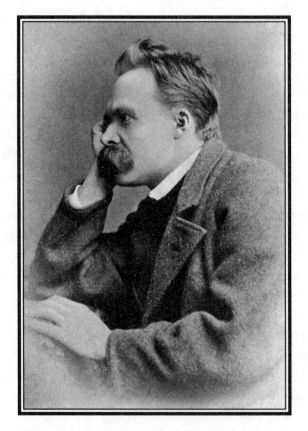

Figure 16.2   Friedrich Nietzsche (Bettmann/Corbis)

he did tell their mutual friend Malwida von Meysenbug that he would consider himself duty bound to offer Lou his hand in marriage if they were all to live together in Paris as they had planned. However, it is unlikely that his proposal meant more than that, and Lou's motivations for repeating a proposal story are unknown.[47] Nietzsche at one point suggested that Paul Rée should marry her, assuming that Lou might have been tempted. Details of ménage aside, Nietzsche had great plans for Lou, who was to be his disciple and heir who would carry on his work if he were destined for a short life.

That summer he confided to Lou the deep philosophical secret of the Eternal Return and his plan for Zarathustra, the illumination that Möbius called the first flash of pre-paretic consciousness. It was, perhaps, Nietzsche's later electric excitement and misery that led Möbius to see paresis approaching. Nietzsche wrote: "Each cloud contains some form of electric charge which suddenly takes hold of me, reducing me to utter misery."[48] He thought he ought to be in a Paris electricity exhibition. "Perhaps I am more receptive on this point, unfortunately for me, than any other man on earth."[49] He told Peter Gast in August 1881 that he felt "like a zig-zag doodle drawn on paper by a superior power wanting to try out a *new pen*."[50] "On my horizon thoughts have arisen, the like of which I have never seen before. . . . Sometimes I think the life I am living is really dangerous because I am one of those machines that could *explode*. . . . Each time I had wept too much the previous day while I was walking, and not tears of sentimentality but jubilation. I sang and talked nonsense, possessed by a new attitude. I am the first man to arrive at it."[51]

Lou was an avid listener; if anyone had heard them talking, she recalled, he would have thought two devils were conversing. But Nietzsche, angry at reports from Elisabeth of loose talk about him at the Wagner Parsifal festival in Bayreuth that summer, broke off the relationship. He came to regret that break later when he saw through Elisabeth's reports and realized that Richard Wagner was the one spreading tales, but the damage was done.

The Nietzsche period was a painful part of Lou's life, off limits when she joined the Freud group in 1911, although she may have discussed it in confidence with Freud. In 1895 Lou had published the first in-depth study of Nietzsche. Many reviews were splendid, but Elisabeth predictably accused Lou of revenging herself upon poor invalid Nietzsche when he could no longer defend himself.

Whether or not Lou knew of Nietzsche's syphilis (and how much Nietzsche related it to his own progressing illnesses) is unknown. But she certainly knew about it after Möbius's veiled revelation in 1902, just as it was common knowledge, avidly discussed, in the Freud entourage by 1908. When Lou attended the Third Psychoanalytic Conference in Weimar in 1911, she brought with her the charisma of having been close to Nietzsche in her youth. A picture taken of the attendees of that event on the lawn in front of the conference center shows Freud seated in the middle, with Jung crouching a bit not to look taller than Freud. Lou is wearing a fur wrap in the front row; in the back is her lover, the Swedish psychotherapist Poul Bjerre. In 1905 Bjerre had published *The Insanity of Genius* (*Der geniale Wahnsinn*), a book about Nietzsche that agreed with Möbius in suggesting that the first warnings of paresis were seen years before the final breakdown. Bjerre identified bacterial syphilis poison as the cause of the paralysis. (Had he heard in time for publication of Schaudinn's viewing of the spirochete that year?) Two conference attendees, Hans Sachs and Ernest Jones, visited Elisabeth Nietzsche on a break.

We can only imagine what conversations may have taken place about Nietzsche, his insanity, his genius, his sexuality, and his syphilis, as Freud, Jung, Lou, Bjerre, Hans Sachs, Ernest Jones, and others strolled together on the lovely lawns of the Weimar conference center.

In her published doctoral dissertation, Pia Volz has provided the most complete medical history for Nietzsche, including a long list of the various hypothesized diagnoses: epilepsy, apoplexy, hereditary mania, premature brain atrophy, paranoia, schizophrenia, and inadvertent self-poisoning. As usual with the mania and depression of syphilis, numerous scholars have suggested a bipolar disorder. Volz favors syphilis, a significant vote given the comprehensiveness of her research into Nietzsche's condition.[52]

Many explanations, from the plausible to the bizarre, have been proposed for where, when, why, and how Nietzsche was or was not infected, and what he knew about it. Here are some of the theories: he infected himself without sexual relations (Hildebrandt); he infected himself with prostitutes as a form of subconscious self-punishment (Brann); he was saddled with a false diagnosis (Sigfried Mandel); he thought he was cured (Angela Livingstone); he didn't know he had it (Walter Kaufmann); it was not syphilis at all but a repressed memory of childhood abuse (Alice Miller); it was only a miserable sexual accident (Otto Rank);

and all his ills were psychosomatic (Hildebrandt again). Novelist Stefan Zweig wrote darkly that Nietzsche mistook for illumination the poisonous germ of the waiting catastrophe. Rudolph Steiner, who visited Nietzsche at the end, had a vision of him as a reincarnated Franciscan monk who had spent his days kneeling in front of an altar until his knees were a mass of bruises; the pain tied him to his physical body so that in the next incarnation he had no desire to be in the body at all. Topping the list, Nietzsche himself once remarked that it was to Wagner's music that he owed his nervous decline.

When Pastor Karl Ludwig Nietzsche, a preacher's son and Prussian court preacher, baptized his first child, born on 15 October 1844 and named for King Friedrich Wilhelm IV of Prussia, whose birthday he shared, the father had no idea that he, his royal patron, and his new son would all end their lives mentally ill. In 1844 there was only jubilation at the birth of a first child to the pastor and his young wife Franziska. Two years later Elisabeth Therese Alexandra, named for three princesses, was born.

Family harmony was destroyed when revolution swept Europe in 1848. Pastor Nietzsche retired to the library in a deep depression following news that his king had given in to the demands of the revolutionaries. It soon became obvious something else was wrong when he suffered convulsions and loss of memory. In extreme pain, after eleven months of illness, with blindness and incoherence at the end, he died at age thirty-six. The cause of death was stated as "softening of the brain."

When he was four years old Nietzsche was taken to a professor of ophthalmology at Jena, who observed the unequal diameter of his pupils, a trait he inherited from his mother. Ronald Hayman noted that the circumstances of Pastor Nietzsche's death could argue for Nietzsche's having congenital syphilis, but despite his not speaking until very late, his headaches, myopia, and rheumatism, "the evidence is not conclusive."[53] Congenital syphilis is usually obvious because of lesions at birth, or the famous Hutchinson notched teeth, but it is possible for the child to be normal and for the disease to remain hidden until adulthood. Usually it first shows up in patients over the age of fifteen, although there are cases of congenital syphilis not appearing until age sixty. According to syphilologist Burton Peter Thom, in this form of syphilis "as in acquired syphilis, no organ or tissue of the body is exempt." But congenital syphilis seems very unlikely in Nietzsche's case.

Nietzsche left home to attend Schulpforta, a well-known Protestant boarding school, then the university in Bonn, and later Leipzig. Appointed at an unusually young age to a professorship of classical philology at the University of Basel, he was off to a promising career as a philologist when his health declined and he took a year's sick leave in 1876. Three years later, he requested a permanent leave of absence for the same reasons of health. For the next ten years he traveled from place to place in Italy and Switzerland in search of "clear skies" and relief from his agonies, living frugally on his pension and a small inheritance.

Although the question of when the warning signs of paresis first appeared has dominated the syphilis debate, a second issue of whether Nietzsche's physical torments before and during his decade of wandering were caused by syphilis has received little recognition. The assumption has been that if he had syphilis, it was latent, and his attacks, characterized by days of headaches, vomiting, and exhaustion, were typical migraines. Nietzsche's letters and notebooks are filled with reflections on pain as a reason to wish for death and conversely as an inspiration for life. (What initially endeared Lou to him was her youthful poem on this theme, "To Pain," which he set to music as "Prayer to Life.") Selected collections of his letters edit out the extent to which day-to-day physical pain dominated his correspondence. If his attacks were caused by syphilis, then his archive is the most profound and eloquent record of a syphilitic that exists.

In June 1875, Nietzsche complained to his friend Carl von Gersdorff in a letter: "The stomach would no longer be subdued even by the most absurdly rigorous diet. . . . Recurrent headaches of the most violent sort, lasting for several days. Vomiting that lasted for hours even when I had eaten nothing. In short the machine looked as if it wanted to break down and I will not deny that I have several times wished that this could be the end."[54]

Nietzsche spent the summer holiday that year in the Black Forest at the clinic of a specialist in diseases of the stomach. He was diagnosed with "gastric catarrh" with dilation of the stomach that kept significant blood from reaching the brain. A morning enema was prescribed and a diet of roast meat three times a day, raw eggs, and red wine. Leeches were applied to Nietzsche's head. His stomach was better by July, but the doctor there could obtain no such results with Nietzsche's other complaint: "a nervous disorder." That December Nietzsche wrote to his friend Rohde about the time he spent in bed in real torment, exhausted, with no appetite left for life. Nietzsche had an episode so severe that he feared brain damage was at the root of his troubles.

To Elisabeth he complained in 1876: "My dear sister; things are not right with me, I can see that! Continuous headache, though not of the worst kind, and lassitude. Yesterday I was able to listen to *Die Walküre,* but only in a dark room—to use my eyes is impossible."[55] He consulted a doctor in Naples who assured him he had no brain tumor, only treatable neuralgia.

In 1877 he wrote to his mother: "My head still seems to be short of blood; I have done too much thinking over the past ten years which, as is well known, has a worse effect than just 'doing too much work.'"[56] And to Elisabeth he wrote: "I was so unwell! Out of fourteen days, I spent six in bed with six major attacks, the last one quite desperate."[57] He added that he must leave Basel University if he were not to sacrifice his health entirely.

In May 1877 he went to Bad Ragaz for four weeks, seeing the doctor and taking remedial baths. Overbeck visited, and Nietzsche told him that it was out of the question for him to begin teaching again in the fall. In June he wrote to Elisabeth: "My head is in a far worse state than we thought. . . . any mental strain is immediately harmful. You cannot believe how weary and unwilling to work the head and eyes are."[58] In St. Moritz he tried drinking waters "as a remedy against deeply entrenched nervous illness."[59] His eyes now had to be within two inches of the paper he was writing on.

To Malwida von Meysenbug he wrote from four thousand feet above sea level: "I do lie sick in bed here as in Sorrento and drag myself around in pain, day after day; the thinner the air is, the more easily I endure it. I have not begun a treatment with St. Mortiz waters, which will keep me busy for several weeks."[60]

In September Nietzsche returned to Basel. One of his most troubling complaints, the condition of his eyes, points to syphilis. In October he consulted with Dr. Otto Eiser, who sent him to a colleague, an ophthalmologist, Dr. Gustav Kruger, who found bilateral inflammation of the inner layers of the eyes and diagnosed chorioretinitis which, after iritis, is the most frequent syphilitic affection of the eye.[61]

Another examination by Dr. Alfred Graefe in Halle yielded a further pessimistic opinion: Nietzsche must not read or write for several years; must avoid bright light; must wear blue sunglasses; must avoid spicy foods, coffee, and heavy wine; and must not exert himself mentally or physically. Eiser for his part prescribed quinine and wrote to Richard Wagner, who hypothesized that Nietzsche's eye problems were due to excessive masturbation. Eiser later suggested that *Human, All Too Human* marked the beginning of Nietzsche's mental decline. After seeing the two doctors, Nietzsche had extended his medical leave from the university for six more months. Eiser reported that Nietzsche told him he had engaged in sexual relations several times on doctor's orders and had been infected with gonorrhea (*Tripper*) twice but never had syphilis. Since the syphilitic chancre was difficult to distinguish from gonorrhea in 1867, when Nietzsche was supposedly treated, this comment may have meant that he was misdiagnosed then. Eiser was closely connected to the Bayreuth circle and tended to take patient confidentiality lightly, so Nietzsche may not have wanted to confess syphilis to him. Nonetheless, this comment indicates that Nietzsche thought he did not have syphilis despite the two alleged treatments in Leipzig. The scar on his penis, found when he was admitted to the asylum, argues the opposite.

Eiser's prognosis was pessimistic when Nietzsche consulted him in February. He told Overbeck that he had never discounted brain disease in Nietzsche's case; indeed, observations of a colleague, Rudolf Massini, who examined Nietzsche made it seem probable. Massini suggested that Nietzsche be relieved of part of his teaching duties because he was experiencing an intense over-stimulation of his nervous system. In September 1878, Nietzsche's publisher Ernst Schmeitzner recorded a dismal image: "Nietzsche had broken down and he looked frightful. He was in a state of collapse."[62]

In 1879 Nietzsche had a septic inflammation under his finger-nail, which got worse. He wrote home: "Monday bad, Tuesday the *attack*, Wednesday bad, Thursday *and* Friday new, very violent attack not wanting to stop, today shattered and exhausted."[63] Teaching caused him too much mental strain. On the worst days he mentioned attacks of cramp, which made him keep his right eye closed for several hours, and which spread all over his body.

He confirmed that his eyes were not good enough for teaching. A headache lasted six days. One night he thought he was dying. He took a cold water cure. He considered resting for five years. "You can have no idea of the convulsions in my head or the fading in my eyes."[64] "My life is more torture than convalescence. . . . If only I were blind! This stupid wish is now my philosophy. Because I should not *read* and I do—just as I should not *think*— and I do."[65] He returned to Basel and consulted an oculist, who confirmed the deterioration of his eyes.

On 2 May 1879, Nietzsche took a final health leave of absence from teaching, suggesting in parting that Basel's weather might be responsible for his headaches: "abominable, noxious Basel, where I have lost my health and will lose my life."[66] Elisabeth wrote that she hardly recognized her dear brother, so exhausted and prematurely aged was he.

Nietzsche finished *The Wanderer and His Shadow*, telling Gast that he knew mental effort would induce agonizing headaches. He wrote in small notebooks while walking, then transcribed them despite great pain. About twenty of the longer thought sequences ("unfortunately really essential ones") were lost in his pencil scrawl. "I have to steal and collect minutes and quarters of an hour of 'brain energy' as you call it, steal them *from* a suffering brain."[67] At Christmas, after three days of vomiting, he went into a coma. Afterwards, he thought he would die.

To Eiser he complained: "My existence is a *fearful* burden: I would have long thrown it over if I had not been making the most instructive tests and experiments on mental and moral questions in precisely this condition of suffering and almost complete renunciation. . . . On the whole I am happier than ever before. And yet, continual pain; for many hours of the day a feeling closely akin to sea-sickness, a semi-paralysis which makes it difficult to speak, alternating with furious attacks."[68]

In January 1880 he wrote to Malwida: "For my life's terrible and almost unremitting martyrdom makes me thirst for the end, and there have been some signs which allow me to hope that the stroke which will liberate me is not too distant. As regards torment and self-denial, my life during these past years can match that of an ascetic of any time; nevertheless, I have wrung from these years much in the way of purification and burnishing of the soul—and I no longer need religion or art as a means to that end."[69]

To Franz Overbeck (in Latin in the original) he wrote: "I am desperate. Pain is vanquishing my life and my will. What months, what a summer I have had! My physical agonies were as many and various as the changes I have seen in the sky. In every cloud there is some form of electric charge which grips me suddenly and reduces me to complete misery. Five times I have called for Doctor Death, and yesterday I hoped it was the end—in vain. Where is there on earth that perpetual serene sky, which is my sky? Farewell, friend." [70]

Again he wrote to Overbeck: "My dear friend, I think you haven't written to me in a long time. However, perhaps I deceive myself, the days are so long, I no longer know what I will do with each day: I've lost interest in everything. Deep down, an unmovable black melancholy. Also weariness. Most of the time in bed; it's the most sensible thing for me. I have become quite thin which is surprising. I have a good trattoria now and would like to build myself up again. But the worst is: I don't see any more why I should live even another half a year, everything is boring, painful, degoutant. I've suffered and sacrificed too much and have a sense of the imperfection, the mistakes, and the mishaps of my entire spiritual past life which is beyond all understanding." [71]

Nietzsche celebrated the New Year with one of the most violently painful attacks of his illness. In February he wrote from Genoa: "Fever, chill, sweating at night, acute headaches, constant chronic exhaustion, no appetite, dull palate."[72] He had reached a low point, saying he would rather kill himself than live through another such winter.

Nietzsche complained to Overbeck from Sils Maria: "Even my Genoese years are a long, long chain of self-conquests for the sake of that aim and not to the taste of any human being that I know. So, dear friend, the 'tyrant in me,' the inexorable tyrant, *wills* that I conquer this time too (as regards physical torments, their duration, intensity, and variety, I can count myself among the most experienced and tested of people; is it my lot that I should be equally so experienced and tested in the torments of the soul?)"[73]

In *Ecce Homo* he wrote: "In the midst of torments which accompany an uninterrupted, three-day cranial pain together with troublesome vomiting of phlegm, I possessed a dialectician's clarity *par excellence* and very deliberately thought things through for which I am not enough of an acrobat, not cunning and not cool enough under healthier conditions."[74]

At the end of 1888, Nietzsche was experiencing electrified energy, writing new work at white-hot temperature, fearing madness and death and reflecting continually on illness and pain as it both demoralized and instructed him. He thought of a future time when his work would be understood and appreciated. In all these things we see a parallel with van Gogh during that same year. Pure creative inspiration, mental illness, or paretic disinhibition: whatever the combination, the result in each case was astonishing.

17

Oscar Wilde
1854–1900

History is merely gossip.

—OSCAR WILDE

"**M**Y WALLPAPER AND I ARE FIGHTING A DUEL TO THE death. One or the other of us has got to go," Oscar Wilde quipped shortly before the wallpaper won. A deathbed photograph places him beneath the garish and motley red blotches of the victorious design, holding a rosary, the sign of his deathbed conversion to Catholicism. Present with him in his last weeks in the shabby room at the Hôtel d'Alsace in Paris in September 1900 were his dear friends Robbie Ross and Reggie Turner as well as doctors, medical assistants, a solicitous and generous hotel owner, and a stream of visitors. Wilde's friend Frank Harris was following the terminal drama at the Alsace through frequent correspondence. Food was delivered from a local restaurant. Oscar drank champagne.

Wilde was attended by an embassy physician, Maurice Edmund a'Court Tucker, pictured by Ross as "a silly, kind, excellent man," who made sixty-eight visits to the hotel room. But Tucker was not an otologist (he later became one), and when Wilde developed a nasty middle ear infection, a specialist (whose name re-

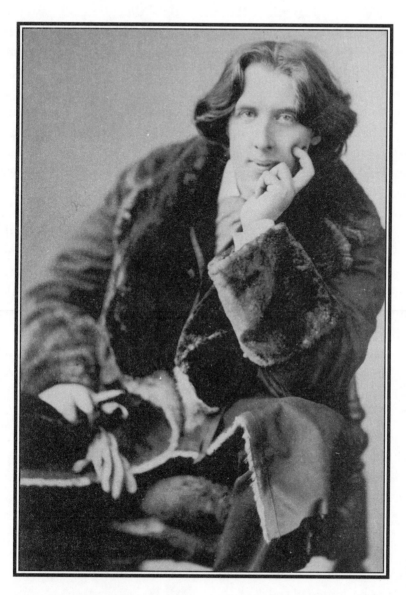

Figure 17.1   Oscar Wilde (Library of Congress)

mains unknown) was called in. Surgery was performed on 10 October. Wilde telegraphed Robbie Ross: "Operated on yesterday. Come over as soon as possible," and then: "Terribly weak. Please come."[1] Robbie arrived and joined Reggie Turner at a bedside vigil, including consultations with the various doctors as Wilde's condition became worse. They also worried with him about finances. Oscar, by his own statement, was dying beyond his means.

When meningitis threatened, they called in an eminent specialist, Dr. Paul Claisse, an academic physician from the Paris Faculty of Medicine. Some biographers have assumed Claisse performed the surgery, but he did not arrive on the scene until 25 November. Wilde was attended by a postoperative wound dresser named Hennion, who warned Robbie about underestimating the seriousness of Wilde's condition; the ear trouble, he said, was not of that much importance in itself but was a grave symptom. As the infection spread to the brain, Wilde's condition continued to decline. At the end he was in great pain, sometimes lucid, often delirious. He died at 1:50 P.M. on 30 November 1900.

Claisse and Tucker made an official statement confirming that the cause of Wilde's terminal illness was inflammation of the brain stemming from an ear infection:

> The undersigned doctors, having examined Mr. Oscar Wilde, called Melmott [Wilde's pseudonym], on Sunday, 25 November, established that there were significant cerebral disturbances stemming from an old suppuration of the right ear, under treatment for several years.
>
> On the 27th the symptoms became much graver. The diagnosis of encephalitic meningitis must be made without doubt. In the absence of any indication of localization, trepanning cannot be contemplated.
>
> The advised treatment is purely medical. Surgical intervention seems impossible.[2]

If Wilde's affection for Lord Alfred Douglas was "the love that dare not speak its name," syphilis may well have been his second secret: the disease that dare not speak its name. According to his close friend Robert Sherard, Oscar "knew himself to be syphilitic."[3] Years after his death, the correspondence and the publications of four friends—Sherard, Reggie Turner, Robbie Ross, and Frank Harris—revealed that they all knew his secret, and that the doctors present at the Alsace had diagnosed it as the cause of the ear infection that led to the brain infection that caused his death.

A month after Wilde's death Robbie Ross specifically linked Wilde's ear infection to the terminal brain inflammation: Wilde "caught a cold in the ear. The English doctor said it was of little importance, but the French doctor regarded it as a grave symptom. It was, however, the abscess which eventually produced inflammation of the brain."[4] Years later, in a letter to Sherard, Reggie Turner wrote very clearly that the doctors present at the Alsace diagnosed that grave symptom as a tertiary symptom of syphilis. "The ear trouble, which I believe began in prison," Turner wrote, "was only shortly before his death diagnosed as a tertiary symptom of an infection he had contracted when he was twenty. The doctor told him he would live many years if he took care of himself."[5] Consider how this reads with syphilis substituted for the euphemism: "The ear trouble, which I believe began in prison, was only shortly before his death diagnosed as *syphilis*."

The syphilis diagnosis first appeared in print twelve years after Wilde's death, in a biography by Arthur Ransome. Since it was dedicated to and probably overseen by Robbie Ross, it is not surprising to find the statement that Wilde's death "was hurried by his inability to give up the drinking to which he had been accustomed. It was directly due to meningitis, the legacy of an attack of tertiary syphilis."[6] Ransome's revelation was one of the rare times that syphilis was called by name. Note here that he does not say that the meningitis was an attack of tertiary syphilis, but the *legacy* of one—that is, the result of the ear infection. He removed the references to syphilis from the 1913 edition (and was praised by Sherard for doing so), giving as a reason that he wished to spare the feelings of those who might be pained by them. But the word had been published and subsequent biographers (H. Montgomery Hyde and Hesketh Pearson) repeated it.

In 1916 Frank Harris's biography (also looked over by Ross) told that syphilis inflamed the ear infection and was the cause of Wilde's recurrent skin rash as well. Like Turner, but with a flourish, Harris invoked euphemisms to avoid using the forbidden word:

> The local malady [the ear problem] was inflamed, as I have already said, by a more general and more terrible disease. The doctors attributed the red flush Oscar complained of on his chest and back, which he declared was due to eating mussels, to another and graver cause. They warned him at once to stop drinking and smoking and to live with the greatest abstemiousness, for they recognized in him the tertiary symptoms of that dreadful disease which the brainless prudery allows to decimate the flower of English manhood unchecked.[7]

Again, consider how differently the same paragraph reads if the euphemisms for syphilis are replaced by the word itself:

> The local malady was inflamed, as I have already said, by *syphilis*. The doctors attributed the red flush Oscar complained of on his chest and back, which he declared was due to eating mussels, to *syphilis*. They warned him at once to stop drinking and smoking and to live with the greatest abstemiousness, for they recognized in him the tertiary symptoms of *syphilis*.

All the tissues of the body were weakened by this dreadful disease, Harris added.

Three decades later, Wilde's most popular biographer, Richard Ellmann, concluded that syphilis was a key to understanding his subject:

> He [Wilde] never admitted having it, and many authorities deny it. Admittedly the evidence is not decisive—it could scarcely be

so, given the aura of disgrace, shame and secrecy surrounding the disease in Wilde's time and after—and might not stand up in a court of law. Nevertheless I am convinced that Wilde had syphilis, and that conviction is central to my conception of Wilde's character and my interpretation of many things in his later life.[8]

The conviction was "central" to his interpretation of Wilde's character, yet Ellmann tucked this key revelation away in a single, polite footnote, one of the more remarkable illustrations of how syphilis hides in the wings in biography.

The friend most responsible for the question being raised about infection in Wilde's earlier life is Robert Sherard, the fourth after Ross, Turner, and Harris to speak of syphilis. Most responsible—and most conflicted: Sherard revered Wilde, recalling their days together in Paris with damp-eyed nostalgia as he (over)wrote his way through three volumes: *The Story of an Unhappy Friendship, The Life of Oscar Wilde,* and *The Real Oscar Wilde.* His knowledge about the medical progression of syphilis has already been seen in a previous chapter in the discussion of his biography of Guy de Maupassant. There he went through linguistic contortions (recall "the Monster of infinitesimal size but Himalayan mischief"[9]) to say syphilis without using the word.

The great-grandson of William Wordsworth, Sherard left Oxford after one unsuccessful year (he was thrown out for debt) and went to Paris in 1883 to write a novel, which he did. There he met Wilde, who had returned from his triumphant American tour and was writing the *Duchess of Padua* in a suite of splendid rooms overlooking the Seine at the Hotel Voltaire. Wilde lived in dazzlingly high style, so elegantly dressed that he was parodied in the magazines. After initially being put off by Wilde's flamboyance, Sherard came to be devoted to "the most wonderful talker the world has ever seen"[10] and inspired by him: "It was for me a new and joyous life, an unending feast of the soul, and each day my admiration for my new friend grew more enthusiastic."[11] Financially flush at the time, Wilde could entertain his young friend lavishly. When not writing, they drank coffee with the Paris literary world.

Wilde's first homosexual lover was Robbie Ross, but that was not until 1886, after Wilde had married Constance Lloyd. There is a story that Sherard did not know the truth about Wilde until he observed him through a window making love with Robbie. Sherard believed firmly that homosexuality belonged in the domain of pathology. He defined his friend as the ideal gentlemen, "the purest man in word and deed,"[12] who was (alas) incidentally occasionally taken over (as if against his will) by this "allied madness," this "crouching demon." If the truth of his sexuality were known, Sherard feared, his literary work could be consigned along with the author to the "eternal night of eternal oblivion."[13]

If Sherard was discreet in print about Wilde's homosexuality, André Gide was not. It was Gide's story in his autobiography about Wilde in Algiers that finally infuriated Sherard enough to reveal the syphilis secret as the lesser of two evils. Using his title Chevalier de la Légion d'Honneur, he came galloping to Wilde's defense in 1934 in *Oscar Wilde Twice Defended from André Gide's Wicked Lies and Frank Harris's Cruel Libels*. "Heavens!" exclaimed outraged Sherard. "The task of shooing hyenas away from the graves of the illustrious dead."[14] This is the story Gide told.

In 1895 he and Wilde were in a café in Algiers. A "marvelous youth" came over to their table and began to play the flute, soon joined in the music by the boy who served the coffee. Gide recalled his own admiration of the boy: "His large black eyes had the languorous look peculiar to hashish smokers; he had an olive complexion; I admired his long fingers on the flute, the slimness of his boyish figure, the slenderness of his bare legs coming from under his full white drawers."[15] Outside, Wilde whispered in Gide's ear: "*Dear*, would you like the little musician?" Gide thought his heart would fail him. Yes, he said with a choking voice. Later that day Wilde took him to a house in a populous part of town where he showed Gide into a tiny apartment of two rooms. A guide appeared with the two youths, each with his face hidden by a burnoose. Wilde sent Gide to one room with the flute player

Mohammed, then retired to the other room with the boy who poured the coffee. Gide recalled: "No scruple clouded my pleasure and no remorse followed it. But what name then am I to give the rapture I felt as I clasped in my naked arms that perfect little body, so wild, so ardent, so somberly lascivious?"[16] In an episode two years later, this time without Wilde, Gide observes his friend Daniel having sex with the same boy, Mohammed. This time the feeling is quite different. He sees Daniel as a huge vampire feeding upon Mohammed's corpse, and he feels like screaming in horror. The gentle boy Mohammed is now hard, restless, and degraded. He has given up hashish for absinthe.[17]

Sherard told the following story. Wilde had been infected with syphilis at age twenty at Oxford "thanks to the idiotic system which arises from British hypocrisy." (Does he mean prostitution? Recall Harris's swipe against the "brainless prudery" of the English as the cause of syphilis.) In 1886 a fresh and virulent outbreak of the infection chased him from his marriage bed. That "was undoubtedly the teterrima causa of all his subsequent mental, moral and physical aberrations." Sherard also defends Wilde against a charge by Dutch doctor G. J. Renier who "would have us believe that kindly, humane, fatherly Oscar Wilde did deliberately, knowing himself to be the potential conveyer of this loathsome contagion, sexually debauch a child thirty years younger than himself." Wilde may have been homosexual and irresponsible, Sherard concluded, but he was definitely not a sodomite or a criminal. He adds that an eminent critic told him that no proper biography of Wilde could be written without the collaboration of an "expert syphilogue."[18]

In an unpublished letter to Arthur Symons, Sherard regretted what he had left out of his passionate defense:

> I ought to issue a P.S. to *Andre Gide's Wicked Lies*. I ought to have pointed out the enormity of the charge agst Oscar considering the fact that he knew himself to be syphilitic, and so, supposing that he had committed the outrage with which Gide (and Renier) charge him it would mean that in debauching an

Arab child he would willfully have exposed his victim to a terrible infection and disease. Kind, humane Oscar Wilde.[19]

Sherard appears not to have known that syphilis was not infectious in the later stage. Since he thought there had been an infectious relapse with Constance in 1886, he might have believed the danger continued in later years. Melissa Knox (who currently argues the pro-syphilis side of the Wilde debate) commented that Wilde might no longer have been so kind and humane when he went to Algiers in 1895: "Paresis destroys these qualities." But Wilde didn't have paresis; he probably didn't even have neurosyphilis. At most he had a mild case of slowly progressing syphilis that was only approaching the advanced stage when he died.

Thirty-five years after Wilde died, Sherard visited biographer Boris Brasol, sharing with him various details that subsequently showed up in Brasol's biography as the most complete summary of the story of Wilde's early years of infection:

> Oscar Wilde . . . while at Oxford had contracted syphilis for the cure of which mercury injections were administered. It was probably due to these treatments that Wilde's teeth subsequently grew black and became decayed. Before proposing to Miss Constance Lloyd, Wilde went to see in London a doctor who assured the poet that he had been completely cured and that there was no pathological obstacle to his marriage. However, shortly after the birth of Vyvyan, Wilde discovered that syphilis, which apparently had been altogether dormant, had broken out in his system. He clearly realized that if he were to continue marital intercourse with his wife, a syphilic child might have been born.[20]

In a letter to Arthur Symons in May 1937, Sherard recalled: "I cannot remember where I got the story of the infection of Oscar at Oxford at age 20, but it was after I had written my attack on

Harris [the final section of the Gide pamphlet]. It satisfied me so completely that though I had it well in mind when last year I revised that ms. and omitted any reference to it. I have since regretted this omission."[21] In another letter to Symons that month, Sherard wrote that Constance's mention of illness "at the time made me think the damned thing had come out again while they were cohabiting . . . later information and reflection satisfied me that she was referring to the damage to her health caused by his year-long marital neglect of her."[22]

To Symons in April 1935 Sherard finally used the forbidden word, referring to "the syphilis he [Wilde] contracted at Oxford when he was 20, which broke out again in 1886 and destroyed his married life."[23] Later Sherard wrote that he was not sure what the cause of Oscar's death was and so "were I writing his life anew, I could with an easy conscience toward my public omit all reference to a disease which is still looked upon by the hypocritical and the ignorant as a proof of depraved character."[24]

Symons had been diagnosed with tertiary syphilis himself, so Sherard had a correspondent who was knowledgeable about the disease. His was a most unusual case, and probably a misdiagnosis. In August 1909, James Joyce wrote to his brother: "Arthur Symons has G.P.I. [general paralysis of the insane.]"[25] London neurologist J. S. Risien Russell had confirmed the diagnosis and arranged for Symons to be admitted to an English asylum when he was transferred from an institution in Bologna. Symons claimed to be the pope, a millionaire, and the duke of Cornwall. He felt "all on fire with a life that tingles in every vein and dilates the nostrils"[26]—a fair description of syphilitic ecstasy—followed by a decline to "a gibbering, grimacing lunatic" when he was suffering from pneumonia. Russell gave him two years to live and waived his fee. But Symons fooled everyone. He recovered completely, outliving his entire literary circle and dying at age seventy-nine.

According to Sherard, it was at Oxford (Magdalen College) as an undergraduate that Wilde contracted syphilis, from the one and only campus prostitute, whose name was "Old Jess."[27] Richard

Ellmann speculated that the most probable time was March 1878 while Wilde was finishing the prize-winning poem "Ravenna." "It was at Oxford that an event occurred that was to alter his whole conception of himself," Ellmann wrote. "Wilde contracted syphilis, reportedly from a woman prostitute."[28]

In a most bizarre mixing of historical bedfellows, the *Lancet* published a letter to the editor suggesting that Old Jess might be the same woman who infected Lord Randolph Churchill![29] The social circles intersected once again years later when Lord Randolph's son Winston successfully sued Wilde's lover Bosie for libel; Bosie served six months' jail time at Wormwood Scrubs.

Soon after the alleged Old Jess episode, Wilde became seriously ill and spent several days in bed, surrounded by flowers. He wrote to a friend that he was wretched and ill and expected as soon as possible to be sent somewhere out of Oxford. His convalescence took place at the Royal Bath Hotel. He consulted Reverend Sebastien Bowden, a priest known for converting the well-to-do. Bowden wrote to him of his "temporal misfortune" adding: "Let me then repeat to you as solemnly as I can what I said yesterday, you have like everyone else an evil nature and this in your case has become more corrupt by bad influences mental and moral, and by positive sin."[30] Wilde's grandson, Merlin Holland, argues that this temporal misfortune had to do with Wilde's receiving an inheritance that was less than he expected, but this doesn't explain the rest of Bowden's statement about corruption and positive sin. Wilde considered joining the Church, but at the time of his planned conversion, he sent a large bouquet of lilies instead. In "Taedium Vitae" he wrote of "that hoarse cave of strife/Where my white soul first kissed the mouth of sin." Ellmann speculates that this may be the poem advertised by a bookseller as being to the prostitute who infected him.

In her biography of Wilde, Barbara Belford (a proponent of the no-syphilis argument) deemed it unlikely that he would have joined other randy young lords in visiting the prostitutes in and around High Street: "Bragging about visiting a brothel is the kind of outrageous fabrication that Wilde would use to interrupt a conversation during his period of self-mythologizing."[31] But why would visiting a brothel be an outrageous fabrication? Wilde was very attracted to women at that time (Constance was not the first woman he considered marrying), and later statements make it clear that prostitutes appealed to him, at least later on. While in Paris he told Sherard about these experiences, including one with a well-known woman of the streets, Marie Aguétant, who was later murdered. "What animals we are, Robert."[32] Arguing against Wilde having Baudelaire's disease, Belford concludes that Ellmann was trying to give his subject "some heterosexual patina to make him more sympathetic"[33] when he opted for the syphilis-from-a-prostitute theory—although it would seem that his initially joyous marriage to Constance and two lovely children establishes his heterosexual interests then well enough. Wilde was certainly less interested in female prostitutes later in life. Upon his release from prison the poet Ernest Dowson took him to a brothel to stage a public event to prove his "rehabilitation." Afterwards, Wilde confided to him that the first in ten years would also be the last; the experience reminded him of cold mutton.

Oscar wrote passionate letters to Constance in the early days of their courtship: "Dear and Beloved, Here am I, and you at the Antipodes. O execrable facts, that keep our lips from kissing, though our souls are one. . . . The air is full of the music of your voice, my soul and body seem no longer mine, but mingled in some exquisite ecstasy with you, I feel incomplete without you."[34] And she adored Wilde: "Prepare yourself for an astounding piece of news!" she told her brother. "I am engaged to Oscar Wilde and perfectly and insanely happy."[35] Their wedding on 29 May 1884 at St. James's Church was carried off in grand Wildean style. Constance's dress, designed by him, as were the dresses of the bridesmaids, was rich creamy satin with cowslip tint, a square low bodice, and a high Medici collar. They honeymooned in Paris, where Wilde took walks with Sherard and expounded on his new happiness, embarrassing his younger friend with rhapsodies about his bride's virginity.

Back in London the couple moved into the showcase "House Beautiful" on Tite Street. They had two healthy children, Cyril in 1885 and Vyvyan in 1886. Wilde edited *Woman's World* from 1887 to 1889. He published a book of children's stories, *The Happy Prince and Other Tales,* followed by *The Picture of Dorian Gray*, his only novel, and several collections of stories published in 1888. In the next years he achieved both fame and fortune as a playwright, delighting London with *The Duchess of Padua, Lady Windemere's Fan*, and *A Woman of No Importance*. In 1895 his theatrical career reached its peak with *The Importance of Being Earnest* at the St. James Theater and *An Ideal Husband* in Haymarket Theater. The Prince of Wales congratulated Oscar on one of his opening nights. Constance's gorgeous gowns were described in detail in the press.

But during this time all was not blissful in the House Beautiful. Constance's ideal husband had become repulsed by her during her pregnancies: "I tried to be kind to her; forced myself to touch and kiss her; but she was sick always, and—oh! I cannot recall it, it is all loathsome. . . . I used to wash my mouth and open the window to cleanse my lips in the pure air." Nature was disgusting; it befouled the altar of the soul. Instead, he preferred the red roseleaf lips of "My Own Boy," Bosie.

If 1895 was the height of Wilde's success, it was also his downfall. His flaunted infatuation for Lord Alfred, Bosie, infuriated Alfred's father, the marquess of Queensberry, author of the Queensberry rules of boxing, who sent a calling card to Wilde's club with this accusation scribbled on the back: "For Oscar Wilde, posing somdomite." Poor spelling aside, the wording is notable: Queensberry did not accuse Wilde of sodomy, but of posing. When Wilde recklessly filed a charge of libel, the defense had no problem finding numerous boy prostitutes who were happy to testify against him.

Queensberry was acquitted, and the English judiciary system was forced to bring charges against Wilde for a crime usually ignored at the time. The constabulary waited until 4:00 P.M. when the final ferry had departed for Calais before taking Wilde, dazedly drinking at the Cadogan Hotel, into custody. He was convicted of a law that made "commission of any act of gross indecency with another male person" punishable by up to two years. The law, Section 11 of the Criminal Law Amendment Act of 1885, became known as the Blackmailer's Charter.[36] On the first round the jury was hung, but on the second a verdict of guilty was proclaimed. He was sentenced to the maximum, two years at hard labor.

Wilde's legal troubles tore Constance's life apart. The House Beautiful was sold in bankruptcy and all the family possessions auctioned before Wilde was sentenced. Friends had scrambled to rescue manuscripts. While Wilde was ruining his hands picking oakum in jail, Constance changed the family name to Holland and moved away from London. When Oscar was released from prison, he traveled on the continent under the name of Sebastian Melmoth. Constance still had some private income, and she provided her husband with an allowance.

The story of Wilde's two years in prison is painful to read.[37] Locked in a thirteen-by-seven-foot cell, sleeping on a bed of planks, restricted from talking to other prisoners, and worse, at times given nothing to read and no writing implements, he constantly feared that he was going mad. He asked his visitors if they thought his brain was all right. In a petition to the home secretary asking to be released early to head off sure insanity, he called his cell a tomb for those not yet dead. To Harris he described the feeling of being so isolated with nothing to read: it was as if the mind was being ground away between the upper millstone of regret and the nether millstone of remorse. He complained of quivering in every nerve with pain, wrecked with tides of hysteria, unable to sleep or eat.

When Wilde was released from prison in 1897, he learned that Constance was suffering from a progressing spinal paralysis. Hardly able to write by hand, she found a typewriter but had difficulty using it. She engaged a German governess to take care of the children when she became unable to do so herself. Her doctors advised her to walk ten minutes a day, but even that was difficult. Her left arm was semi-paralyzed. Oscar was distressed at her serious condition. It would clearly be impossible for her to bring the boys and join him in France as he had hoped. He wrote: "I don't mind my life being wrecked—that is as it should be—but when I think of poor Constance I simply want to kill myself."[38] Oscar wrote to Robbie from Naples that he was joining Bosie because when he was alone, he felt suicidal. They lived in a villa overlooking the bay of Naples. When he communicated to Constance that he was again living with Bosie, she exclaimed that this was the letter of a madman and stopped his allowance. When he broke with Bosie, she restored it—and then arranged for it to be continued if she died before him. She wrote to Vyvyan, with difficulty by hand: "Try not to feel harshly about your father,"[39] a letter some have taken to indicate that she foresaw her imminent death. She went into a nursing home in Genoa for an operation, the second one, to relieve her intense pain. The operation was not successful; she died on 7 April 1898.

Although the family story was that Constance's spinal paralysis was the result of a fall down the stairs at Tite Street, some have questioned that event. The suspicion of syphilis remains. An infectious relapse in 1886 was improbable, assuming Wilde was infected at Oxford, but she could have been infected earlier, at the time of her marriage, within the range of expected relapses, although at the far end of that range, six years. (Jonathan Hutchinson gave seven as the outside limit for infectious relapse.) Perhaps she did find him guilty. Sherard recalled seeing a letter to Wilde from Constance that said: "And you know that you made me ill."

In her novel *The Case of the Pederast's Wife*, Clare Elfman fictionalized what is known about Constance at the time, beginning with an assumption that Wilde had syphilis, and questioning the fall down the stairs as the cause of her spinal problem. But she uses these circumstances as a starting point for a story in which Constance's disabilities are hysterical in nature, caused by repression of hostile feelings toward her husband.

Given the details of Constance's neurological disorder, tabes dorsalis would have to be considered in any differential diagnosis. Until more information is available about Constance, however, the question must be held in abeyance. Her life and health require further study.[40]

Was the red flush that first bothered Wilde in the summer of 1899, the one that Frank Harris "attributed . . . to another grave cause," a manifestation of tertiary syphilis? A key letter about this condition and about his general ill health at that time, originally thought to be his last correspondence before his death, has been redated to be several months earlier, 28 February 1900. "My dear Robbie," he wrote:

> I am very ill and the doctor is making all kinds of experiments. My throat is a lime kiln, my brain a furnace and my nerves a coil of angry adders. . . . I see that you, like myself, have become a *neurasthenic*. I have been so for four months, quite unable to get out of bed till the afternoon, quite unable to write letters of any kind. My doctor has been trying to cure me with arsenic and strychnine, but without much success as I became poisoned through eating mussels, so you see what an exacting and tragic life I have been leading. Poisoning by mussels is very painful and when one has one's bath, one looks like a leopard. Pray never eat mussels.[41]

At Easter Wilde seemed to get better during a trip to the Vatican. He credited the pope with the cure: "When I saw the old white Pontiff, successor of the Apostles and Father of Christendom pass, carried high above the throng, and in passing turn and bless me where I knelt, I felt my sickness of body and soul fall from me like a worn garment, and I was made whole."[42]

Although Wilde attributed the leopard spots to mussel poisoning, the skin condition did not clear up quickly as a rash from mussel poisoning would have done. Macdonald Critchley analyzed the varieties of mussel poisoning and concluded that none of them pointed to chronic dermatitis.[43] And the rash was recurrent, which it would not have been with mussel poisoning. Wilde wrote to Harris: "I'm all right, Frank, but the rash continually comes back, a ghostly visitant."[44]

Late syphilitic rashes took so many forms and were so difficult to distinguish from other rashes that even syphilologists recommended calling in a dermatologist for a consultation. So important was the proper identification and treatment of skin lesions in late syphilis that dermatology and syphilology became sister disciplines, often practiced by the same doctor. John Stokes wrote that cutaneous lesions were of great value to the diagnostician both to arouse suspicion in cases not otherwise indicating syphilis and to clinch a diagnosis in a dubious case.[45] Although they were not as serious as the deep ulcerative lesions that sometimes occurred in tertiary disease, skin rashes were among the most terrifying harbingers of late syphilis because they were visible to the world. When Wilde showed signs of meningitis at the end, Paul Claisse was called in to consult, presumably because he had published on that topic. But Claisse had also published papers on dermatology and tertiary syphilis, so an expert in late syphilis was on board who could have rendered the opinion on all aspects of Wilde's disease, including the red flush being due, not to eating mussels, but to the other "graver cause" mentioned by Harris.

Because Wilde complained of the skin rash being itchy, Richard Ellmann eliminated it from consideration as a clue to syphilis, and subsequent writers have cited Ellmann and moved on to look for other possible causes, including allergy to hair dye[46] and vitamin deficiency dermatitis from overuse of alcohol. Wilde was drinking excessively; Dupoirier, proprietor of the Alsace, reported more than a liter of brandy a day, and substantial amounts of absinthe as well.

But Ellmann was wrong about the itchiness ruling out syphilis. Although the general constitutional rash of early syphilis is not itchy, the localized rashes of tertiary syphilis are often very itchy and even painful. In Wilde's case, the itchiness, rather than eliminating syphilis, tended to reduce the numerous possible lesions to a few. Under "itching syphilids" John Stokes lists two forms of late benign lesions, the follicular and the psoriasiform.

There is not enough information to know which syphilitic rash Wilde may have had, but because there are several itchy, blotchy, recurrent, localized late rashes in the textbooks,[47] and because of Harris's note that the doctors suspected the rash was caused by syphilis, we must consider Wilde's leopard spots after his bath a strong suspicion arouser. Of artistic note, though not of diagnostic value: several illustrations of the specifically itchy late rashes in the syphilis texts look remarkably like the spots of a leopard.

If Wilde did have a syphilitic rash, it may have been rather good news. According to *Jacobi's Atlas of Dermochromes*, late cutaneous eruptions rarely lead to general paralysis or tabes,[48] which seems consistent with the progression of syphilis in Wilde's case, and a key point to consider in asking why so many scholars have been reluctant to consider that Wilde might have had syphilis. Nineteenth-century neurosyphilis was so dramatic that other, less ostentatious manifestations of the disease have been forgotten. Wilde never showed any of the warning signs of paresis: grandiosity, euphoria, or bizarre, uncharacteristic behavior, although his letters of 1897–1900 show considerable mood swings. One suspicious sign was the degeneration of his handwriting, an early sign of approaching paresis. He noted that his previously beautiful Greek script had become a scrawl. Certainly Wilde was witty and sharp at the end, although this does not rule out paresis since mental acuity right before onset of paresis was common. A case can be made that his mental state was not what it had been, or that his judgment was at times faulty, perhaps as early as when he took Queensberry to court, which has seemed to many to be reckless and self-destructive. But other circumstances might have had a deleterious effect on his later mental state, in particular the horror of his incarceration and his excessive drinking. If there had been any possibility for late syphilitic euphoria, it would probably have been effectively doused by a liter of brandy a day. Around the time of his imprisonment, Constance said that he had been mad for three years. But she may have been equating homosexuality with madness, as others did at the time.

In his last years, Wilde showed a general decline together with several conditions that arouse suspicion of syphilis. Whereas at Oxford he was physically active, engaging in swimming, lawn tennis, riding, and hunting, he later took cabs to go even short distances. Ross noted that his friend had an "odd elephantine gait." He also had gout and recurrent headaches, although again, his alcohol consumption could have caused a splendid headache, and he often could not get out of bed until late in the day.

Problems with his eyes while he was in prison are more specific. Wilde described himself, the prisoner, in the third person: "He is conscious of a great weakness and pain in the nerves of the eyes, and objects even at a short distance become blurred. The bright daylight, when taking exercise in the prison-yard, often causes pain and distress to the optic nerve, and during the last four months the consciousness of failing eyesight has been a source of terrible anxiety, and should imprisonment continue, blindness and deafness may in all human probability be added to the certainty of increasing insanity and the wreck of reason."[49] Would gas lighting in his cell have been sufficient to cause these problems, as has been suggested?

In *The Picture of Dorian Gray*, a young man lives a life of carefree sin and aesthetic pleasure, forever youthful, while in the attic his portrait, in a kind of Faustian bargain, shows progressive decay with each crime. Was this novel Wilde's confession of the anguish of secret syphilis, his expression of the knowledge that the disease was causing interior destruction, and his guilt at the possibility of infecting others? If Sherard was correct in saying that Wilde knew himself to be syphilitic—and at this point there is more than enough reason to believe he did—then Dorian Gray becomes one of the most poignant portrayals of the fears of the secret syphilitic. He wrote it while he was "grievously ill" with a nervous fever during the early years of infection when such a fever might indicate a relapse. Was Wilde indicating that he had been cavalier about his disease when he wrote from prison to Lord Alfred in *De Profundis*: "I took my pleasure careless of the lives of others and passed on"?

Richard Ellmann had no doubt that Dorian Gray was Wilde's parable for secret syphilis. He suggested that Wilde chose mercury over religion as the specific for his dreadful disease "as the spirochete began its journey up his spine towards the meninges."[50] (While the metaphor is apt, Ellmann is off base medically; spirochetes do not go on a pilgrimage up the spine looking for what one writer called their favorite organ of dessert, the brain; they reach the central nervous system in the earliest stage of the disease.)

Dorian locks the door behind him and surveys his portrait:

> He could see no change, save that in the eyes there was a look of cunning, and in the mouth the curved wrinkle of the hypocrite. The thing was still loathsome—more loathsome, if possible, than before—and the scarlet dew that spotted the hand seemed brighter, and more like blood newly spilt. Then he trembled. Had it been merely vanity that had made him do his one good deed? Or the desire for a new sensation, as Lord Henry had hinted, with his mocking laugh? Or that passion to act a part that sometimes makes us do things finer than we are ourselves? Or, perhaps, all these? And why was the red stain larger than it had been? It seemed to have crept like a horrible disease over the wrinkled fingers. There was blood on the painted feet, as though the thing had dripped—blood even on the hand that had not held the knife. Confess? Did it mean that he was to confess? To give himself up, and be put to death? He laughed. He felt that the idea was monstrous.[51]

The red stain that creeps on his skin like a horrible disease reminds us of the red stain that crept across Wilde's skin in his last year. Earlier, while in prison, Wilde wrote of "vices . . . embedded in his flesh" which spread over him "like a leprosy, feeding on him like strange disease."

> Was he always to be burdened by his past? Was he really to confess? Never. There was only one bit of evidence left against him.

The picture itself—that was evidence. He would destroy it. Why had he kept it so long? Once it had given him pleasure to watch it changing and growing old. Of late he had felt no such pleasure. It had kept him awake at night. When he had been away, he had been filled with terror lest other eyes should look upon it. It had brought melancholy across his passions. Its mere memory had marred many moments of joy. It had been like conscience to him. Yes, it had been conscience. He would destroy it.

Dorian slashed the painting with a knife. The servants heard a cry of agony. The police came. When they entered, they found hanging upon the wall a splendid portrait of their master as they had last seen him, in all the wonder of his exquisite youth and beauty. Lying on the floor was a dead man, in evening dress, with a knife in his heart. He was withered, wrinkled, and loathsome of visage. It was not until they had examined the rings that they recognized who it was.

In 1959 Terence Cawthorne set out to debunk the Wilde syphilis hypothesis, which to that point had not been seriously questioned, in an address to the History of Medicine Section of the Royal Society of Medicine. In so doing he introduced into the literature an error that has persisted to the present. He said: "with the exception of Frank Harris, none of his [Wilde's] biographers who have dealt with the cause of his death have doubted that neurosyphilis was responsible for his terminal illness."[52]

But none of Wilde's biographers had ever suggested neurosyphilis, nor had anyone suggested that syphilis of any kind was the cause of the brain inflammation. As reviewed above, the literature is consistent on the point that the brain inflammation was the *legacy* of the ear infection. Recall that Turner wrote: "The ear trouble, which I believe began in prison, was only shortly before his death diagnosed as a tertiary symptom of an infection he had contracted when he was twenty." So although doctors Tucker and Claisse, friends Turner, Ross, and Harris, and a long line of biographers including Ellmann (who put the argument back on course with his acceptance of death from meningitis) have all agreed that the meningitis followed from the ear infection, a number of medical writers have digressed in Cawthorne's wake to discount neurosyphilis as a cause of the brain inflammation (rightly) but then to conclude (wrongly) that if Wilde didn't die of neurosyphilis, he did not have syphilis at all. J. B. Lyons wrote: "Richard Ellmann offers neurosyphilis as the cause of death, a diagnosis that hardly accords with the clinical picture which Ellman himself and others describe."[53] But of course, Ellmann never mentioned neurosyphilis.

How could Wilde's ear trouble have been a symptom of tertiary syphilis? The focus of medical attention returned to the ear on the 100th anniversary of Wilde's death when the *Lancet* published an article by two South African doctors, Sean L. Sellars, an otologist, and Ashley Robins, a psycho-pharmacologist. Since there was no medical record of Wilde's ear surgery and the name of the surgeon remains a mystery,[54] they studied what was known of the postoperative condition and from a careful study of the surgical procedures of the time, deduced that the operation performed in the dim light at the Alsace was probably radical surgery to evacuate the diseased mastoid (the region behind the temporal bone of the ear) and middle ear tissue and debris.[55]

Following this article, every major London newspaper reported its contents and the authors were interviewed by numerous press agencies and radio and television stations. Why would such an arcane bit of literary trivia published in a medical journal attract attention? Because it appeared to scotch the syphilis rumor once and for all. And that was news. A headline in the *Guardian* proclaimed: "Chronic ear disease, not sex, killed Wilde." Merlin Holland told a BBC interviewer that "around 25% of Victorian men had syphilis and he may have had it too—we'll never know—but one thing that's almost certain is that he didn't die of it."[56] This statement from Holland is key, since it shows that he is not opposed to the syphilis argument but is rightly opposed to drawing conclusions from the hypothesis that go beyond the facts.

Sellars and Robins hypothesized that the ear condition might have been a cholesteatoma, a growth of skin tissue within the middle ear that destroys bones within the middle ear and mastoid. It leads to chronic purulent infection that can extend to the brain with potentially lethal consequences. Perforation of the eardrum, foul discharge, deafness, and pain are features of the disease.[57] Cholesteatoma was quite common in those days. If they are correct about the nature of the surgery, and if those present at the Alsace linked the ear condition to syphilis, could the excised material have been a syphilitic tumor, a gumma?

Syphilis texts tell us the answer is yes: the common, destructive, rubbery, syphilitic tumors can be found anywhere in the body, including the brain *and mastoid*, and they cause complications when they become infected. A purulent middle ear infection was cause for grave concern when tertiary syphilis was suspected—because it could point to a syphilitic tumor in the mastoid. And if such a tumor was found, a radical mastoidectomy was called for to head off a lethal brain infection. In short, Wilde's ear infection could very well have been caused by a syphilitic tumor, and a doctor in 1900 (especially Claisse, who wrote about tertiary syphilis) would have considered a syphilitic gumma in a differential diagnosis of Wilde's condition.

Syphilologist Burton Peter Thom neatly summarized the condition, quoting a colleague who "was of the opinion that many cases of prolonged middle ear suppurations were due to syphilis. With his opinion I am in accord. In tertiary syphilis the bony structures of the middle and inner ear are involved and the deafness resulting from the destruction of the delicate bony framework including the ossicles is usually beyond recall. *Should a gumma of the mastoid become infected and a pyogenic [pus-forming] meningitis threaten, relief by surgical interference is necessary*"[58] (emphasis added).

Is there any way of knowing if the mystery doctor who performed the surgery on Wilde found cholesteatoma or a syphilitic gumma? Given the inadequate lighting in the room at the Alsace and the lack of a surgical microscope, it might not have been possible for the surgeon to make a diagnosis prior to surgery. Would a surgeon have been able to differentiate even during or after surgery, lacking a laboratory to test a tissue sample? According to

William Allen Pusey: "With gummas concealed deep in the body, the great difficulty in the past has been the uncertainty in establishing their syphilitic character by purely clinical means."[59]

If Turner's statement is true, that the doctors gave syphilis as a reason for the ear surgery, then the scales tip toward a suspected gumma. But even if the tumor was caused by syphilis, and the infection from the tumor spread to the brain, the final cause of death was a superimposed bacterial infection that caused a terminal brain inflammation.

When the Tucker-Claisse statement about Wilde's medical condition surfaced and was sold at auction at Sotheby's in 1982, scholars asked why, if the doctors thought syphilis was a factor in Wilde's terminal condition, was that not mentioned in their final statement? In the nineteenth century, the taboo against mentioning syphilis by name extended to the medical profession. It was the norm to document the actual cause of death without mentioning a long-standing concomitant syphilitic infection, in respect for the reputation of the deceased. Syphilis expert Joseph Earl Moore wrote that the mortality rate from syphilis was often hidden under a cloud of inaccuracies when physicians were disinclined to give it as a cause of death, fearing publicity for the patient, further hurt to a sorrowing family, or risk of losing insurance. Further, since syphilis masqueraded as so many other diseases, it often remained undiscovered as a cause of death. Sir William Osler concluded (based on British statistical tables of 1915) that syphilis was so underreported that it ranked first instead of the apparent tenth among killing infections. In a high-profile case such as that of the notorious Oscar Wilde, such discretion would be expected.

Clare Elfman dramatized a cover-up in *The Case of the Pederast's Wife*. This fictional conversation takes place between the two doctors at the Alsace:

"Meningitis, then?"

"Oh, yes," he said thoughtfully, "we will certainly put meningitis on the death certificate when the time comes. You can tell his family. Rest assured." He leaned closer. "But my friend. Between us . . . "[60]

Wilde's earlier ear infection in Reading Gaol does not rule out a gumma, nor does the fact that he was seen by at least seven physicians while in prison, none of whom diagnosed syphilis. These doctors bungled the previous ear infection; one even referred in his notes to the wrong ear. Wilde stigmatized them as brutal, coarse, and worse—indifferent to the comfort or health of the prisoners in their charge. They would have had no reason to suspect syphilis, nor is it probable that Wilde would have revealed the old diagnosis in an already hostile environment. One other hypothesis should be mentioned in passing: that the deafness Wilde mentioned while in prison might have been from syphilitic damage to the eighth cranial nerve.

Who knew what when about Wilde and syphilis? More to the point, who can be believed? The chronology of revelation is particularly tortuous and made even more complex by the way the contentious cast of characters in Wilde's story continually accused one another of lying or sued for libel. Wilde himself started it off, of course, by so disastrously suing the marquess of Queensberry. Bosie unsuccessfully sued biographer Arthur Ransome for libel. Robert Sherard berated André Gide and Frank Harris (but then everyone accused Frank Harris of embellishing the facts) and called Robbie Ross's *Oscar's Last Days* pathetic.

In "Biography and the Art of Lying," Merlin Holland called Sherard a fatuous fabricator and fanatic, concluding that he was a totally unreliable source about the syphilis (another hyena to be shooed from the grave of the illustrious dead?). Yet elsewhere in the article he comments that Sherard's spaniel-like devotion to the memory of Wilde was an embarrassment. Why, then, would Sherard make up such a story about his hero? And why would the other three friends, at widely varying times, agree? The sense that comes from reading the various revelations in order is more of a secret held to the last moment, then given up reluctantly. There is no glue here to hold a conspiracy theory together. And Holland bases his repudiation of Sherard's veracity on backwards logic: If Wilde died of meningitis, he did not die of syphilis. If he did not die of syphilis, then "Sherard's recreation of his syphilitic history no longer has any proper foundation."[61] But one can die of anything and still have had syphilis, so the cause of death does not rule out a prior infection.

Did Oscar Wilde have syphilis? The possibility raises many questions that have been hotly fought out in the Wilde literature. Did a prostitute, possibly named "Old Jess," infect him when he was a student at Oxford? Did Robert Sherard lie in spreading this story? Did treatment with mercury rot Wilde's teeth? Did a doctor assure him that he was no longer infectious and therefore safe to marry Constance? Did he ever tell Constance that he had syphilis? Did he have an infectious relapse that resulted in her eventual spinal paralysis and death? Was he so sick in the last months of his life because his disease was progressing? Was the pattern of leopard spots on his body in his last year the rash of tertiary syphilis? Did the doctors think his terminal brain infection was caused by an infected syphilitic gumma or tumor or by cholesteatoma?

The *Picture of Dorian Gray* may have been a secret parable for the disease that destroyed his body while he faced the world without a mark. The indications favor a syphilitic condition throughout Wilde's career, in which case Dorian Gray expresses a running, lacerating awareness of it that must be the basis for further understanding of his life's work.

PART III
The Twentieth Century

Karen Blixen (Isak Dinesen)
1885–1962

> I myself was the lightest thing of all, for fate to get rid of.
>
> —KAREN BLIXEN

WHEN SHE WAS TWENTY-EIGHT, KAREN DINESEN traveled to East Africa, married her cousin Bror von Blixen-Fineke, thus gaining the title baroness, and started a coffee plantation of 1,500 acres near Nairobi. She lived much of her life in British East Africa, growing coffee beans, hunting lions, and writing stories using the pen name Isak Dinesen. Her collections include *Seven Gothic Tales* and *Winter's Tales*. *Out of Africa*, an autobiographical work, was made into a popular film starring Meryl Streep and Robert Redford. Although she was nominated twice for the Nobel Prize, it went instead to her husband's friend Ernest Hemingway (Bror was the model for the white hunter in Hemingway's "The Short Happy Life of Francis Macomber") in 1954, and three years later to Albert Camus.

Blixen married Bror at the beginning of 1914 and came down with syphilis at the end of the year, probably due to his adventures in the Masai community where the disease was epidemic, although he might also have been infected by one of the women in their circle of friends. She described the jealousy she felt upon discovering his various infidelities to be like a claw grabbing her heart, or as if she had been shaken and tumbled by a wild animal. In such a situation there are two things to do: shoot the man or live with it. She chose to live with the jealousy and the syphilis. She later wrote to her brother, Thomas Dinesen, on 5 September 1926: "If it didn't sound so beastly I might say that, the world being as it is, it was worthwhile having syphilis in order to become a 'Baroness.'"[1]

At first she thought the fever, insomnia, and weight loss pointed to malaria. In February of the following year, still suffering from insomnia, she took too high a dose of a sleeping medication. Bror found her in a stupor. After vomiting for two days, she consulted an English physician in Nairobi who confirmed a case of the Pox "as bad as a trooper's" and prescribed mercury tablets for a year. She experienced inflammation of the mouth and gums while continuing to lose weight.

In March she returned from a two-month safari in the mountains with a high fever. On her doctor's orders, she returned to Europe for treatment. Several Paris specialists in venereal disease convinced her that the long and painful treatment would best be accomplished at home. One of them told her he doubted very much if she would ever be cured, an idea that stayed with her all her life. In June she returned to Copenhagen, where she consulted Dr. Carl Rasch, professor of skin and venereal disease, who took over her care then and for the next decade. He confirmed syphilis with a positive blood Wassermann test, and also saw signs of mercury poisoning. He treated her with seven injections of Salvarsan. A second Salvarsan series was planned, but she quit the "infernal cure" (which by then was known not to be a cure after all, although it lessened the effects of syphilis) after only four injections. Arsenic drops taken by mouth caused hair loss (she wore a turban) and darkening and thickening of the skin. Two regimens of mercury salve (despite the previous mercury poisoning) in 1919 marked the end of her treatment for syphilis.

Syphilis for Karen Blixen was "life's bitter secret." When she returned to Europe for treatment, she chose to be in the general ward of the hospital to keep her diagnosis from her family, although she told her mother first and the others eventually found out. Several of her African friends knew, but found it contradicted by her robustness between episodes; some accused her of making it up. Her syphilis became public knowledge sixteen years after her death when one of her doctors, Mogens Fog, published an article in the third yearbook of the Karen Blixen Society, *Blixenia-nia*. Fog diagnosed tabes dorsalis as the cause of her gastric crises, her chief complaint over the years. Other doctors had considered her extreme stomach pain to be the result of mental overwork. Fog found a letter of 13 January 1922 describing a severe attack of gastric pain to be the first episode. Weakened knee and ankle reflexes and diminished sensitivity on her abdomen helped confirm the diagnosis. In 1956 Blixen had surgery for a perforating ulcer, another sign of tabes.

Although Karen Blixen's initial diagnosis of syphilis has not been questioned, the progression of her disease has elicited some debate, as many of her complaints that point to syphilis were not considered to be related to her disease during her lifetime or in the subsequent medical literature. Over the years she was sick with many conditions that puzzled her doctors and either defied diagnosis or were diagnosed as other illnesses but could have been related to syphilis: Spanish flu, sunstroke, blood poisoning, malaria, amebic dysentery, gallstones, mysterious tropical fevers, an enflamed jawbone, inflammation of the spine, and ulcers. Because of the healthy periods when she was able to swim, bicycle, and garden, she herself wondered how many of her illnesses should be attributed to syphilis and whether there was a psychological reason for her pain.

On numerous occasions Blixen felt that she would die at any minute, only to recover completely. In April 1922 she recalled in a letter to her mother, Ingeborg Dinesen, "so clearly lying in bed in the hotel in Zurich looking out over the square and the town clock, thinking that I was quite certainly going to lay my bones to rest there in Zurich, and that it was only a question of how many hours I had left to look at that clock in.—And look! Now I'm as fit an anyone in the world, and all that agony is utterly vanished and forgotten and seems to have existed only in a dream."[2] The following year she wrote to her brother Thomas: "I came straight from a spell in the hospital when I really believed that I was about to die, and resumed work on the farm without a week's convalescence."[3] She often minimized her condition, telling her mother in April 1923: "There is probably nothing to worry about, one can't always be in perfect health, and actually I think it is one of the easiest diseases to deal with if one keeps a watch on it."[4]

On 29 June 1924 Blixen complained of a new pain: "It is beastly cold here at the moment and—whether on account of this or not I don't know—I am afflicted with a kind of lumbago that sometimes almost drives me mad. I think there is something the matter with my nerves; I do not mean that I am 'nervy,' but now and then I get such terrible pains, like a toothache in various places, my heels, hands, ears—but one must always have something wrong with one."[5] Her descriptions of the toothache pain suggest the type of pain in the extremities that announces tabes dorsalis. Although she was anticipated and feared insanity as her syphilis progressed (she once said she feared being a megalomaniac like Nietzsche), she did not link these attacks with her disease, guessing instead that she had lumbago or inflammation of the spine. Nor did her doctors at the time notice that her pain fit the pattern of tabes dorsalis. She wondered if there might be a psychological component. Biographer Judith Thurman, with hindsight, concluded with certainty that syphilis and not her psyche caused her suffering.

Blixen described her disease as a Faustian bargain; her soul was the devil's in exchange for the ability to tell stories. She was a child of Lucifer and the songs of angels were not for her, nor was a normal physical life, a great sacrifice for a young woman. In the early days of her syphilis, she had still hoped to have a child with Bror. One doctor assured her they were both getting better by the day and would be able to become parents. When she was thirty-seven, she became pregnant by her lover, Denys Finch Hatton, possibly for the second time. She wired him using the name Daniel, their code word for a child. He quite clearly was not interested, wiring back: "Strongly urge you cancel Daniel's visit." She may have had a miscarriage.

Bror Blixen had a mild case of syphilis, and after the initial infection remained healthy until his death in a car crash, with the exception of one relapse in 1924. He had filed for divorce and, while the divorce was pending, went elephant hunting in Uganda. Karen wrote to her brother in April 1924: "There is little doubt as to what is wrong with him, he himself realizes that it is his old illness; he writes that to start with his whole body became covered with sores, and now he has a kind of inflammation in all his joints, which are quite stiff and swollen, as well as constant high fever and a kind of paralysis."[6] There were no hospitals, he had no money, and their friends would not want him to be around their children in this condition, so she could think of no other place for him to go except back to her farm, assuming he could be moved. "I cannot let him lie there and die like a dog."[7]

There are stories that Bror traveled with a double cot in his tent because so many of the wives of other hunters wanted to sleep with him. Bror infected and divorced his wife, depleted her wealth, and used their house for orgies with the Masai when she was in Europe; the last has been questioned by Bror supporters, who have said that he would have found it beneath his station to consort with the Masai. One detail seems to characterize him above the rest: he used his wife's best crystal for target practice.[8]

By the 1930s, Blixen's balance was impaired and she had difficulty walking. Her stomach problems continued, with sudden bouts of vomiting and abdominal pain so severe that at times she sat on the floor howling like an animal. Syphilis texts tell of the extreme gastric pain of tabes. John Stokes wrote: "It is of agonizing intensity, grinding or spasmodic, and soon reduces the average patient to sobbing helplessness."[9] Twice surgeons severed nerves in her spinal cord to relieve some of the pain. Numerous operations left her "sliced through on all my flanks and edges." Were all these surgeries necessary? Concerning the gastric pain of tabes, Rudolph Kampmeier wrote that a careless physical examination in cases of abdominal pain may lead to mistaken diagnoses and needless operations. "We have seen one patient who had undergone eight abdominal operations because of tabetic root pain."[10] John Stokes reported a patient with five abdominal scars from useless surgeries in a case of a tabetic with gastric crises, calling this "unbelievable persistence of error. . . . If emphasis be placed upon the *signs* of tabes elicited in history and examination, rather than upon the blood serologic reactions and spinal fluid examination, both of which may be negative, this mistake will almost never happen."[11]

Blixen also tried heat treatment using an experimental steam box, recalling the nightmarish contraptions that were used hundreds of years before to sweat patients during mercury treatments. After four or five hours, she became too claustrophobic to continue. This extreme heat was developed as an alternative to another popular treatment for late syphilis, fever induced by giving the patient malaria. In 1927 Julius Wagner Jauregg won the Nobel Prize for his discovery that patients in the late stage of syphilis improved when they came down with malaria. Another treatment, the "Electronic Cabinet of Kettering," was developed at General Motors as an alternative to malaria treatment by the scientist who invented the electronic ignition for automobiles. In this contraption, carbon light bulbs were used to raise the body temperature to within a fraction of the lethal point. The French novelist Colette tried an experimental treatment, weekly hot baths to raise her temperature to 104 degrees Fahrenheit, recommended by a leading syphilologist. She took ether for her pain and never admitted that she had contracted syphilis from her husband. The Native American sweat lodges reached a temperature sufficient to accomplish the same goal, leading to speculation that they may have been beneficial for syphilis sufferers.

On her high-profile American tour in 1959, Blixen was too weak to dress herself and had to be carried by her secretary. When

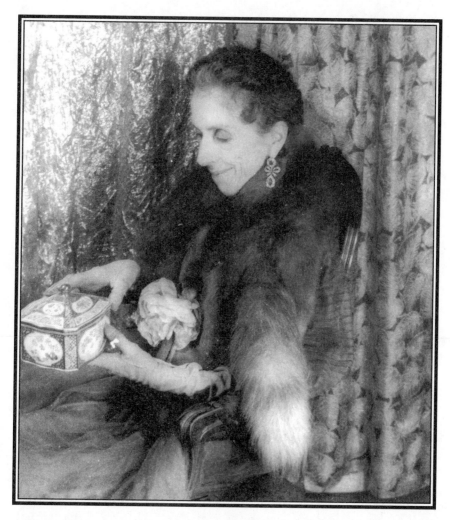

Figure 18.1   Karen Blixen (Library of Congress)

a gardener carried her home one day, her delicate skin turned black and blue. Her doctor told her she had all the symptoms of a concentration camp prisoner. She died on 6 September 1962 at the age of seventy-seven. The cause of death was emaciation. At the end she lived on fruit and vegetable juice, royal jelly, oysters, and dry biscuits. "And by the time I had nothing left, I myself was the lightest thing of all, for fate to get rid of."[12]

In 1995 Danish physician Kaare Weismann questioned the tabes dorsalis diagnosis, hypothesizing instead that Blixen may have been suffering from chronic heavy metal poisoning.[13] Weismann points to Blixen's anemic, wasted state at the end of her life as being a result of this poisoning, but since weakness and weight loss are signs of tabes, this is not a definitive argument. Tabes or not, the mercury, arsenic, and Salvarsan must have had a deleterious effect on her health, as did her amphetamine use.

Weismann's argument against tabes is based mainly on her conclusion that Fog diagnosed the condition on a single symptom, the gastric crisis. But there are a number of textbook indicators of tabes besides the gastric pain: the mysterious "toothache" pains in Blixen's hands, heels, and ears; the difficulty managing stairs; weakness and loss of weight; weakened ankle and knee responses; and finally, the perforating ulcer that required surgery. Weismann discounts the gastric crisis altogether as a symptom of tabes but does not provide an adequate argument to discount the vast syphilis literature to the contrary. Gastric crises were first identified in tabes by the well-known physician Jean Martin Charcot in 1874.

After her initial positive Wassermann, Blixen had seven lumbar punctures, all resulting in negative Wassermann reactions. Weismann concludes: "It is inexplicable how the spinal fluid was normal in 1920 and 1925."[14] Syphilologist R. H. Kampmeier provides an answer: "Unlike general paresis, the clinical picture of rather marked tabes dorsalis may be associated with a negative spinal fluid, with or without positive blood tests for syphilis."[15] John Stokes agrees: In cases of tabes "the negative spinal fluid in progressive cases, especially with trophic changes and crises, is too commonly misinterpreted in general diagnosis, especially where a surgical issue seems to be involved."[16]

That Karen Blixen was infected with syphilis in 1914 is rarely contested. How much of her pain over the years may be attributed to syphilis and how much was caused by the many toxic drugs she took, or even other illnesses, is, of course, debatable. She did not show any of the personality changes that warn of approaching paresis, although like anyone diagnosed with syphilis, she feared the possibility.

Blixen spent a year working on *Last Tales* with "a foot and a half in the grave." It was rejected by the English Book Society and the Book of the Month Club, possibly, it has been suggested, because of "The Third Cardinal's Tale," a story about a woman who gets syphilis. It had first been published alone as a splendid coffee table book with elaborate illustrations. In this story Lady Flora Gordon, an enormously wealthy Scottish noblewoman descended from kings, is described by the narrator, Cardinal Salviati, as commanding in presence, not ugly, just large: Her teeth can be compared with those of his dapple gray horse; her hands and feet are the size of the angels in his chapel. At the end of Lady Flora's story, the cardinal adds an epilogue, describing the last time he saw her. It was when he was visiting the Bath of Monte Scalzo, a spa for the cure of the migraines and rheumatisms of syphilis, although he does not use the word. Instead he just says that the patients at Bath are people who had spent an hour with Venus and ten years with Mercury, quoting the famous line, the motto of the spa: *Hora cum Venere, decem annu cum Mercurio.* Lady Flora had been treated with quicksilver. She was now very thin and a wig had replaced her brilliant red hair. She tells the cardinal the story of how she was infected.

FROM "THE THIRD CARDINAL'S TALE"

Lights were burning in front of St. Peter's figure. In the dusk it looked very big. I gazed at it for a long time, knowing that this was our last meeting. When I had stood so for a while one of the candles flickered a little; it looked as if the face of the Apostle changed, as if his lips moved faintly, and parted. A young man in a brown cloak came into the church, went by me and kissed the foot of the statue. As he passed me I felt a smell of sweat and stable, a smell of the people. I first paid real attention to him after he had passed me, because he stood still so long with his mouth against St. Peter's foot; in the end he walked on. He was slight of build, with a perfect gracefulness in all his movements. His face I never saw. I know not, Cardinal, what in this moment drove me to follow his example. I took a step forward and, like him, kissed St. Peter's foot. I had thought that the bronze would be ice-cold, but it was warm from the young man's mouth, slightly moist—and that surprised me. Like him, I held my lips against it for a long time.

Four weeks later, as I was staying in Missolonghi, by the Bay of Patras, I discovered a sore on my lip. My English doctor, who accompanied me, at once diagnosed the disease and named it to me. I was not ignorant, I knew the name.

I stood, Your Eminence, before the glass and looked at my mouth. Then I bethought myself of Father Jacopo. To what, I thought, does this bear a likeness? To a rose? Or to a seal?[17]

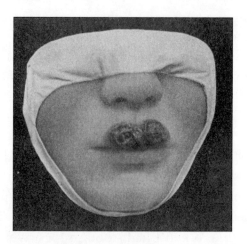

Figure 18.2   Syphilitic lesion on upper lip

James Joyce
1882–1941

He sent out Christy Columb and he came
back with a jailbird's unbespokables in his
beak.

—JAMES JOYCE, *FINNEGAN'S WAKE*

IN JAMES JOYCE'S *ULYSSES*, LEOPOLD BLOOM WARNS THAT
the Nighttown area of Dublin was "a regular death-trap for
young fellows of his age."[1] The author of *Ulysses* had his own experience with this death-trap. In 1904 James Joyce visited Nighttown and came home with a venereal disease. "Let me hear about
your dingus," Joyce's friend Oliver St. John Gogarty wrote to his
friend Jim on 13 February 1904, lecturing him at the same time
about the necessity of chastity. A month later he wrote: "Congrat-
ulations that our holy mother has judged you worthy of the stigmata. . . . If I would venture an opinion—you have got a slight
gleet from a recurrence of original sin. But you'll be all right.
When next mounting be careful not to wish eternal blasting as the
process is intermittent."[2]

That same day he wrote to Dr. Mick Walsh on behalf of his
friend, introducing him thus: "Mr. Joyce is the name of the tissues
surrounding the infected part if you will dam him you will delight

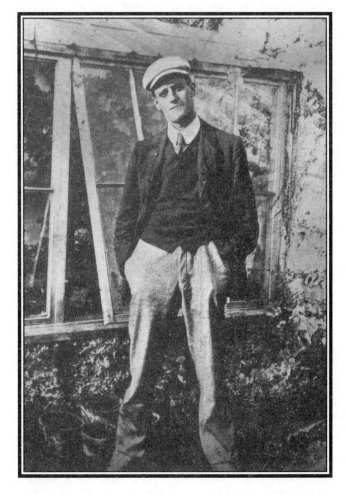

Figure 19.1   James Joyce, 1904 (Hulton Archive/Getty Images)

me. He may have waited too long and gotten gleet."[3] In May, Gogarty sympathized with the "so long neglected ladies," continuing: "without faith we cannot be healed. Good luck old man: Give this 'to Elwood Poxed,'" including with the letter this poem:

In the house where whores are dwelling
Unless it is wrapped in a glove
A little Hunterian swelling
Poxes the part that they love.

Gogarty's postscript adds: "Thas a poem as yet in the head of the father, Chaos—to Elwood/the end would be/scalded when he pissed/And now he prays to Mercury/Who was an atheist."[4] At about the same time, Gogarty noted that the canker (chancre?) had attacked Art.

Gogarty and Joyce were roommates briefly in 1904, the year after Joyce had dropped out of medical school. Gogarty lasted the course and became an otolaryngologist, as well as being a poet, novelist, and satirist. In a clever ballad, his syphilitic sailor Sindbad was so full of mercury that he was knocked unconscious when he stood near a heater. In 1906 Gogarty wrote an essay on venereal disease in which he called infection venereal bad luck.

Gleet is a chronic inflammation of the urethra due to gonor-rhea. Some biographers have assumed that Joyce's infection from Nighttown was nothing more than a minor case of the clap, but Gogerty's references to "Elwood Poxed" and mercury suggest syphilis, as does his noting that the condition was recurrent. Gog-arty might be giving us the answer in the little Hunterian swelling: Joyce may have had both. Poor Dr. John Hunter was well known in the literature then for a bungled self-inoculation exper-iment. Hypothesizing that two diseases could not exist simultane-ously in the same organ, in 1767 Hunter used a lancet to inoculate himself with pus from the lesion of a prostitute. Unfortunately, she was doubly infected, as was he shortly afterward. Some historians tell another story, that Hunter inoculated an experimental subject with the double misfortune. Joyce may have been similarly un-lucky. (In *Ulysses* Joyce wrote of "pox and gleet vendors" and "the snares of the pox fiend.")

On 3 June Joyce reassured Gogarty about Elwood's fate and plans: "Elwood's nearly cured. I have a rendezvous with Annie Langton." Whatever happened to poor Annie Langton is not known, but the future of another woman he met that month, his life partner and the mother of his children, Nora Barnacle, is known. Nora's biographer, Brenda Maddox, describes how, on their first date, Joyce had taken Nora to a deserted harbor area where "to Joyce's grateful astonishment, she unbuttoned his trousers, slipped in her hand, pushed his shirt aside, and, acting with some skill (according to his later account), made him a man."[5] This special event took place on 16 June 1904, the day on which all the action takes place in *Ulysses*. Joyce and Nora left Dublin to begin life together in Zurich in October 1904. On their third day of traveling, Joyce wrote his brother Stanislaus with the news: As of that morning Nora was no longer a virgin, though doubt about whether she really had been before continued to torment him.

J. B. Lyons, opposing the Joyce-syphilis theory, argued that the initial infection was venereal but not syphilitic because even "the least gallant lover" would not have engaged in sex at that time, and we know he did with Nora. Hopefully Joyce thought that Elwood was cured—of whatever he thought the ailment to be. Jim and Nora did not spend a happy time together in Zurich. He had diverse pains and complaints at that time that point to secondary syphilis: rheumatism, tonsillitis, colitis, and "nerves." Nora Barnacle also spoke of "nerves" and "nervous breakdown." They both mentioned depression, anxiety, insomnia, and fits of weeping.[6] On 28 December 1904, Joyce wrote to Stanislaus about cramps in his stomach and problems with vision, uveitis, and glaucoma. Since syphilis is most contagious in the early months, Nora would have been at risk. She and Joyce had two healthy children, but when she was pregnant with Lucia, she took an "ugly arsenical medicine," a strong clue to syphilis. A pregnant woman would hardly take arsenic for any other reason. Joyce took arsenic later in his life as well for a large boil on the arm.

Richard Ellmann, Joyce's best known biographer, downplayed the Nighttown episode and delicately evaded the word gonorrhea in his 1959 book: "On March 13, he [Joyce] was out all night and not long after he had to write Gogarty, who was away at Oxford, to give him the name of a physician who would cure a minor ailment contracted during a visit to Nighttown."[7] But the minor ailment was not so minor.

One of Ellmann's students, Kathleen Ferris, was puzzled when she noticed that he had neglected to include some significant materials about Joyce's health in his extensive biography, in particular information about syphilis. Finding enough clues to warrant continuing, Ferris followed her leads and eventually put together a compelling argument that Joyce had a severe case of tabes dorsalis. She was fortunate to be able to check her hypothesis with a fine syphilologist, Rudolph Kampmeier, author of the 1943 text *Essentials of Syphilology*.[8] With his consultation, Ferris published *James Joyce and the Burden of Disease* in 1995, boldly calling her former professor's work "incomplete and misleading," claiming that he had suppressed evidence in order not to alienate Joyce's friends and family, who had lent him generous support and literary access. Having no such constraints, Ferris made full use of that evidence. In the five decades that had passed since Joyce's death, she argued, "there has remained a great untold segment of Joyce's life that none of his biographers has explored."[9]

Ferris was the first to put together all the pieces of the puzzle and establish the pattern of acquired syphilis running through Joyce's adult life, from infection, secondary illness, and signs and symptoms of developing tabes dorsalis, to death and autopsy. Then she took the next step, tracking the pox as a major theme in Joyce's work. She postulated that it was a significant subtext and a personal confession of shame and guilt. She catalogued the many references to syphilis in Joyce's work, and concluded that Leopold Bloom and Stephen Dedalus both showed some of the same symptoms of syphilis that their author had.

Scholars had to take notice. In a review, Hugh Kenner conceded that Ferris had done a fine job of establishing the syphilis diagnosis (she had good medical advisers and her catalogue of symptoms was in order), but he looked askance at her attempt to make syphilis "*the governing theme* of the masterworks." Noting an instance where he feels she is overreaching, he complains: "Oh sure. And that is how she goes on and on, turning our century's architectonic prose wonder into a huge blur of code centered on the author's disease—which he likely had, but did not have *always* on his mind."[10]

But did Ferris overstate it? Imagine a man living with the shame and secret of syphilis, fearing that he may have infected his wife and daughter, fearing too the inevitable dismal progression and outcome to insanity (although his disease took the route instead to tabes dorsalis), semi-blind, in constant pain, bent, unable to walk without a cane. Then ask if perhaps Kathleen Ferris was right to emphasize how much it was on Joyce's mind. Given that perspective, the number of references to the Pox noted by Ferris in the work does not seem excessive.

Did Ellmann miss syphilis or, like Kenner, just consider it of only moderate concern in Joyce's life? Ferris's text points clearly to a conscious decision, but perhaps Ellmann found mentioning syphilis to be not that critical, and not mentioning it a fair return for the documents made available to him. In his Oscar Wilde biography he boldly called syphilis central to Wilde's life and work, but his pronouncement fell to the bottom of the page in a mere footnote.

J. B. Lyons, a friend of James and Nora Joyce, posed and denied the question of syphilis in a lecture subsequently published in a book of essays with the title *Thrust Syphilis Down to Hell and Other Rejoyceana*. The question was, he pronounced, well, ill-mannered: "There is nothing to suggest that Joyce had syphilis."[11] As between congenital or acquired syphilis, Joyce, he was glad to say, had neither. Lyons confidently excludes iritis in Joyce's case because "after two to eight weeks the iritis subsides and does not recur,"[12] which is incorrect. According to Stokes: "The commonest lesion of relapse or progression involving the eye is iritis."[13] Lyons notes that doctors found no syphilis in Joyce's daughter, but no syphilis in Lucia would not rule out syphilis in Joyce, nor guilt that she might have inherited it from him, and as will be seen later, there is speculation about Lucia. Lyons argued that the postmortem did not show signs of syphilis; against this J. D. Quin argued that lymphocytic infiltrate around the vasa vasorem could indicate syphilis.[14] All in all, Lyons has sparse reason to discount syphilis as against Ferris's strong case for it.

Ferris was the first to track syphilis in Joyce's life, but she was not the first to suggest that he had it. Florence Walzl spoke on more than one occasion to the International James Joyce Foundation, promoting her thesis that Joyce suffered from syphilis, but she drew little attention. In 1974 she coauthored an article with Burton A. Waisbren suggesting that Joyce rewrote "The Sisters," the first story in *The Dubliners*, specifically to give the dying priest, Father Flynn, paresis. The authors suggest that Joyce scholars have missed the priest's diagnosis because many of them were unaware that "paralysis," a word used in the story, was synonymous with paresis, or general paralysis of the insane. Furthermore, they argue that Joyce used paralysis as a theme throughout the whole series of stories to represent the psychological paralysis of his country, citing this letter: "My intention was to write a chapter of the moral history of my country and I chose Dublin for the scene because that city seemed to me to be the center of paralysis."[15]

In "The Sisters" a boy listens to adults discuss the death of a priest who had tutored him. The boy knows that something was wrong mentally with the old man. The story appeared in *The Irish Homestead*, an agricultural journal, on 13 August 1904. A diary entry made by Stanislaus Joyce on that day, 13 August, describes his brother Jim's idea: "He talks much of the syphilitic contagion in Europe, is at present writing a series of studies on it in Dublin, tracing practically everything to it. The drift of his talk seems to be that the contagion is congenital and incurable and responsible for all manias."[16]

Waisbren and Walzl track the details of the rewrite to show how Joyce added the symptomatology of paresis, based, they hypothesize, on medical knowledge. Their case is well made. Joyce had been a medical student in 1902 and 1903. In 1904 he lived with Gogarty, his closest friend, and drank with Trinity medical students in the pubs. The authors suggest that if Joyce had been planning to add the theme of paresis to the story, he would have consulted the key text of the time, William Osler's *The Principles and Practice of Medicine* (4th ed., 1902), which they confirmed was in the Royal College of Physicians of Ireland at the time. Their conjecture is borne out by their comparison of the changes in the story to details about paresis in Osler. For example, they compare "the facies [the appearance of the face indicative of a specific disease or condition] has a peculiar stolidity" (Osler) with "the heavy grey face of the paralytic" (Joyce). One by one they match changes in the priest's malady with Osler's description of paresis. Finally, they connect the priest's death with his moral change: "One last set of revisions needs special comment. Whereas in the original version the words *paralysis* and *paralytic* were never used, they are now repeated three times in contexts where they are specifically associated with evil and guilt."[17]

But one connection the authors do not make: in the spring of 1904, Joyce had his venereal misadventure in Nighttown, and Gogarty deemed him "worthy of the stigmata." Joyce, then, was writing the results of his research about the horrors of paresis into "The Sisters" and applying paralysis to Dublin and Ireland and Europe during the first months of his own infection.

Joyce's father was suspected of having had syphilis. In an appendix to his Joyce biography, Stan Gêbler Davies cited an article published in the *Irish Medical Times* of 9 May 1975 by Dr. F. R. Walsh of Kilkenny, who wrote that Joyce's father had confessed to having had a syphilitic chancre that he cauterized with carbolic acid when he was a medical student in 1867. Walsh counted that of Dr. Joyce's ten children, two were stillborn, two died a few days after birth, and two did not live beyond adolescence. Davies suggests that John Joyce, that amiable ruffian, may have "carried in his blood an agency which, untreated, blinded—perhaps even helped to kill—James Joyce."[18] In 1975 it was well-known that syphilis was not hereditary, as Davies suggests, but syphilis could have been passed congenitally by Joyce's mother. However, there is nothing to indicate congenital syphilis in Joyce's case, and so acquired syphilis from 1904 remains most likely.

Congenital syphilis was again suggested in connection with Joyce's ongoing miseries with his eyes. In a letter to Harriet Shaw Weaver, Joyce wrote that Dr. Hartmann, a young French ophthalmologist, said that his eye trouble could only have proceeded from congenital syphilis. Dr. Arthur Collinson, one of Joyce's ophthal-

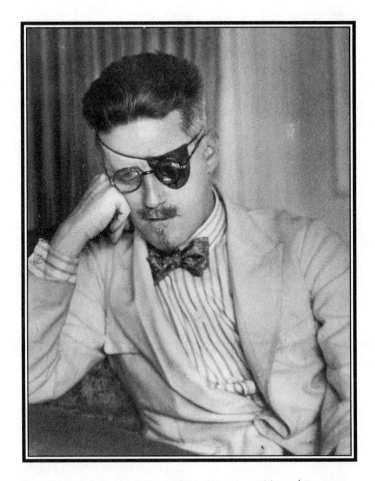

Figure 19.2   James Joyce, 1926 (Bernice Abbott/Commerce Graphics Ltd., Inc.)

mologists in Paris and younger partner of the doctor who performed surgery on Joyce's eyes, said syphilis was the suspected cause. The first surgery performed on his eyes was an iridectomy that removed bits of the iris to enlarge the pupil.

In 1916 Ezra Pound wrote to Joyce, who had sent a photograph of himself, that he found his eyes "a bit terrifying." Joyce later told Harriet Weaver that Pound had been able to see the pathological condition of his eyes from the photograph. Did Pound know of or suspect Joyce's syphilis? He followed Joyce's illnesses carefully, and once even referred a doctor to treat him.

Joyce also had glaucoma and cataracts, compounded by inflammation. Dr. Alfred Vogt, a Swiss specialist, operated and restored some sight. Somber news came from Vogt later that Joyce's postponing visits for two years had allowed his right eye to calcify beyond saving, and now his left eye required two more surgeries. Walsh (in the *Irish Medical Times*) wondered why Dr. Vogt never tested Joyce for syphilis, which would have been routine then for someone with Joyce's eye problems; he concluded that it simply didn't occur to him that such an eminent man of letters could have syphilis. There is another possibility: that if Joyce had been tested for syphilis, the results of that test would have been highly confidential.

In 1906 Joyce wrote: "I presume there are very few mortals in Europe who are not in danger of waking some morning and finding themselves syphilitic."[19] The unlucky mortals so infected would have feared the progression of syphilis to paretic insanity, and Joyce's preoccupation with paralysis indicates that he did. His symptoms over the years, however, show that his disease progressed instead to tabes dorsalis, with agonizing gastrointestinal pain, damage to the eyes, nervous collapses, fainting fits, visual and auditory hallucinations, and shuffling gait.

Joyce's pain began early on. Stanislaus Joyce kept a diary of his brother's ailments between 1906 and 1908, cataloguing indigestion, stomach pain, back pain, neuralgia, and rheumatic pains that shifted from spot to spot. In 1907, from mid-July until September, Joyce was treated for a serious illness in Trieste. As a doctor, Gogarty would have been watching his friend carefully for signs of progressing syphilis. When Joyce wrote to him at this time, Gogarty responded that he was glad to see that he could write, as he had heard that his friend had "a grievous distemper" and was paralyzed.[20] Joyce had pains in his limbs and back. His abdominal pain was once so severe that Nora lamented: "Oh my God, take away Jim's pain."[21] Extreme pain often kept him from working for weeks at a time. At other times, weariness left him energy to work for only a few hours after he got up at eleven in the morning. He went from doctor to doctor, with no good diagnosis offered; one of them told him that the pains of the last seven years were psychosomatic, caused by nerves.

Lucia was born with no sign of syphilis, but when she later developed severe mental illness, Joyce considered it his fault. "Every day brought a new explanation for her disease," wrote Paul Léon: "The only thing which does not vary is the fact that he is the culprit."[22] Since syphilis was still thought to be hereditary, Joyce would have had reason to worry about his part in his daughter's mental illness.

Joyce was understandably irked when C. G. Jung wrote in an introduction to a book on *Ulysses* that it typified the schizophrenic mind at work, but he was mollified by a letter from Jung calling the last nonstop forty pages "a string of veritable psychological peaches." When Lucia set fire to her room and had to be taken away in a straitjacket, it was clear that she needed permanent clinical supervision, and Joyce eventually decided that Jung, someone he wouldn't consult himself, might help his daughter. As her twentieth doctor, Jung got her to speak with him openly at first, although later she became critical and saw him as "a big fat materialistic Swiss man try[ing] to get hold of my soul."[23] Jung found the creative similarities between the father and daughter fascinating. He met several times with Joyce to discuss her case.

Lucia's madness had aspects of both schizophrenia and paresis. Several clues point to paresis having been suspected, either by her doctors or by Lucia herself. Did Joyce and Jung discuss that possibility in their meetings? Lucia underwent a fever cure in 1934. Kathleen Ferris consulted a neurologist who concluded that the treatment Lucia received was "indeed the successor of Wagner-Jauregg's famous malaria fever cure for paresis."[24] And when Joyce came to visit her, Lucia told him not to pretend not to know what was wrong; she had syphilis, although, enigmatically, of her own fault, not his. Ferris quotes this statement (from the Ellmann collection) as having been made in the presence of a doctor.

Joyce returned to Zurich, where he and Nora had begun their life together almost forty years before. In January 1941 he was taken to the hospital on a stretcher when he developed severe stomach cramps. A perforated duodenal ulcer required immediate surgery. At first he refused, but finally he submitted. When he required a transfusion, he commented that the donors, two Swiss soldiers from Neuchâtel, were a good omen: he liked Neuchâtel wine. On 13 January, Nora was summoned to the hospital in the middle of the night, but she arrived too late: Joyce had died at 2:15 A.M. He was buried on a snowy day. When Lucia was notified of her father's death, she said:"What is he doing under the ground, that idiot? When will he decide to come out?"[25]

Of *Ulysses* Joyce wrote:"I've put in so many enigmas and puzzles that it will keep the professors busy for centuries arguing over what I meant, and that's the only way of insuring one's immortality."[26] Syphilis adds one more level of enigma, one more puzzle, as a theme in the work, and as a painful and terrifying reality in the author's life.

20

Adolf Hitler
1889–1945

> Combating syphilis should have been made to appear as *the* task of the nation. Not just *one more* task. . . . Everything—future or ruin—depended upon the solution to this question.
>
> —ADOLF HITLER

G IVEN THE IMMENSE NUMBER OF WORDS WRITTEN ABOUT Adolf Hitler—120,000 references in one bibliography—it would seem that by now each pebble of his life would have been picked over and examined in great detail. Yet no one has bothered to investigate and organize the many clues that point to the existence of a boulder dead center in the field: *syphilis*. References to syphilis found throughout the vast Hitler literature are usually limited to a brief, dismissive sentence or two. But if Hitler's life is looked at through the selective lens of a possible diagnosis of syphilis, one clue leads to another and then another until, when they are all assembled and looked at in order, a pattern of infection and progressive disease emerges. Syphilis must then be considered in our understanding of Hitler's career, his motivations, the events of World War II, and even the Holocaust.

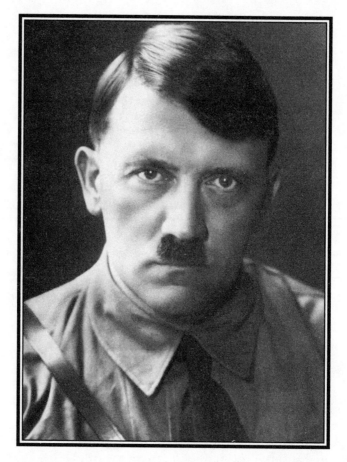

Figure 20.1   Adolf Hitler (Hulton-Deutsch Collection/ Corbis)

In 1936 Hitler hired a syphilologist, Theo Morell, to be his private physician. Hitler's presenting symptoms (shin lesions and extreme gastric crises) would have put any syphilologist on high alert. Morell apparently was so alerted. From a secret diary he began in 1941, we can construct a pattern of syphilis beginning with one of the most terrifying manifestations of late syphilis, disease of the heart. Hitler's medical portrait of the last years gives reason to re-open his case, with syphilis as a serious contender in any differential diagnosis.

Critical questions arise from the hypothesis that Hitler and Morell were covering up an approaching medical catastrophe in the bunker: Who else knew? How was the cover-up accomplished? What trail of documents supports syphilis in Hitler's case? What references to syphilis can be found in his writing? What clues to syphilis were present before 1936?

RUMORS OF INFECTION

A syphilologist reviewing Morell's case notes would begin by asking if there were any rumors of high-risk sexual activity, any significant changes in health or circumstances, or any references to treatment. Intimate friends of youth often reveal the syphilis secret years after a sufferer's death. In Hitler's case, Putzi Hanfstaengl, a friend from the days of the beer halls in the 1920s, published in his memoirs that Hitler was infected in Vienna in 1908. How reliable was Putzi? Did Hitler share this secret with his friend in the days before his ascent to power? Or was the offhand remark a fabrication? Putzi may have been getting his revenge against Hitler for having turned on him, but Simon Wiesenthal, the well-known Nazi hunter, found instances when Putzi revealed his personal knowledge of Hitler's syphilis in the early days, before revenge would have been a motive.

Rumors abounded in Hitler's own time that he was infected by a Jewish prostitute in Vienna. All fall into the category of hearsay, sometimes several times removed. Of what use is it to track such rumors? They certainly don't in any way "prove" that Hitler had syphilis; in fact, their very elusiveness almost detracts from the argument. And yet they add to the Hitler story from another angle: if rumors were plentiful that Hitler had been infected with syphilis as a youth, then his generals and SS operatives would have heard them and would have been warily watching his rapid physical and mental decline in the last years for the signs of tertiary syphilis. So they were.

The well-known and respected London syphilologist T. Anwyl-Davies revealed a story told to him by two men who claimed to have been infected by the same Jewish prostitute as Hitler. His witnesses would rightly be discredited in a court of law—their story was told over a bottle of wine late at night—but it remains of interest that this reputable British authority had gathered enough information to believe that Hitler was in the tertiary stage of disease at the end of the war. Wiesenthal, avidly on the trail of the Hitler-syphilis connection, acknowledged the hearsay aspect of what he unearthed and concluded: "As a criminal investigator, however, I would say that two sources at a considerable distance from each other have nevertheless come up with clues which conform astonishingly well. Clues which, if it were a criminal case, would induce me to follow them up."[1]

Wiesenthal's clues deserve following up. Why, he asks, has the question of syphilis drawn so little attention from researchers? He speculates that the old Nazis would bridle at the besmirching of their idol, while others would resist seeing complex events reduced to one person's pathological degeneration. He puzzles at the same time over his own curious reluctance to see Hitler as a syphilitic. Hitler's physical and mental condition in the bunker at the end of the war invites us to circle back to the beginning. The search for syphilis in Hitler's story begins, then, with Putzi Hanfs-taengl and the rumors of infection.

Putzi befriended Hitler after he heard him mesmerize a beer hall audience in 1922. He invited Hitler to his rich home, lent him money to buy two American presses to print the Nazi newspaper, and entertained him on the piano. Having played for pre-game rallies when he was a student at Harvard, Putzi translated the Harvard football chant "Fight! Fight! Fight!" to "Sieg Heil! Sieg Heil! Sieg Heil!" Hitler, imitating a Harvard cheerleader, marched around the Hanfstaengl living room giving the cheer that would be repeated on an elaborate scale at the Nuremberg rallies.

Putzi, who became Hitler's foreign press secretary, remained a loyal but unruly follower long after the rise to power. His story is the stuff of Hollywood Nazi movies. He escaped what he thought was a plot engineered by Hitler to have him shot while parachuting from a plane. On his escape route, he spent a number of hours being interviewed by C. G. Jung. He ended up in Washington writing psychological profiles of Hitler and the Nazi inner circle for his old friend from the Harvard Club, Franklin D. Roosevelt.

In 1957 he published *Hitler: The Missing Years*, an account of his observations of Hitler's degeneration from the popular orator whose eloquence gave him hope for a return to the comfortable and traditional values of his youth to a power-hungry demonic monster and murderer surrounded by ignorant fanatics and criminals: except, of course, Putzi himself. He observed that Hitler did not seem to have had "orthodox" sexual relations with any woman as long as he had known him. He speculated that Hitler was the repressed, masturbating type, an impotent man with tremendous nervous energy, of an uncertain and strange sexual constitution, both sadistic and masochistic. "I felt Hitler was a case of a man who was neither fish, flesh, nor fowl, neither fully homosexual nor fully heterosexual," he explained. "You can drink very weak tea, or very thin absinthe and you can suffer from very diluted sex-inversion." He added, almost casually: "Hitler's repressed homosexuality probably dated from the time when he caught syphilis in Vienna about 1908."[2]

While doing research for his book *Hitler Among the Germans* in the early 1970s, Rudolph Binion visited Putzi at his villa in Munich to identify some obscure names in the records of Hitler's early entourage. He recalled the meeting: "Putzi, if anyone, knew Hitler's sexual constitution because of his snoopiness and his closeness to Hitler when Hitler was less in the limelight than after the Putsch. He told me Hitler had contracted syphilis from a whore in Vienna because (hold tight!) he didn't know enough not to ejaculate.

"Whereas Putzi began by explaining Hitler's sexuality as post-syphilitic, he soon switched to talking about his own fear of ejaculating into prostitutes as a youngster: 'We had to hold it in, to pull back at the last moment,' he said with big eyes, muted, husky voice, and histrionic clutching of my arms, to evoke the psycho-moral ordeal his generation was pitiably up against, 'but Hitler was too green to know he should pull back in the nick of time.' It was all bizarre: an explanation of Hitler's trouble turned into a plaint over Putzi's (alias his whole generation's, including Hitler's) ordeal, and that with no trace of pride or contentment in having survived the ordeal triumphantly where Hitler had failed."[3]

How could Putzi or Hitler have believed that only ejaculation could result in infection? Only three years had elapsed since Fritz Schaudinn first viewed the pale spirochete of syphilis under his microscope and established a specific agent of contagion. Many biologically incorrect ideas about how syphilis spread were still part of the popular knowledge. The idea that ejaculating could result in infection arose from a centuries-old belief that syphilis could only enter a flaccid penis. François Ranchin, a member of the Faculty of Medicine at Montpellier in the seventeenth century, wrote a treatise on the Great Pox in which he warned that to avoid contamination by a "fallen woman" it is necessary "that the member be erect, not soft or limp, because otherwise it drinks the infection in like a sponge, and preservatives are almost useless."[4] Putzi's comment makes sense relative to the beliefs of the time.

In Landsberg prison after the Beer Hall Putsch, Hitler wrote thirteen pages in *Mein Kampf* about syphilis being the direst threat to the future of the race. A passage about prostitution seems especially confessional in light of Putzi's recollection: "And the upshot of it all is that the man who gets an unpleasant surprise later can, even by thoroughly wracking his brains, not recall his kind benefactress, which should not be surprising in a city like Berlin or even Munich. In addition, it must be considered that we often have to deal with visitors from the provinces who are completely befuddled by all the magic of the city."[5] Was Hitler, himself a visitor from the provinces, completely befuddled by the magic of the city? Did he get such an unpleasant surprise?

Wiesenthal asked himself: Could Hitler's pathological state of mind in the last years of the war be the result of tertiary syphilis? In *Explaining Hitler*, an attempt to get at Hitler's nature through a review of the conclusions of his biographers, Ron Rosenbaum finds Wiesenthal's quixotic search in the 1980s for a spectral spirochete of syphilis to explain Hitler's psyche to be just another instance of the elusive grail of Hitler studies: the search for an explanation for his anti-Semitism. Rosenbaum cries foul when Wiesenthal speculates, based on third-hand gossip, that the source of the infection was a prostitute in the Viennese underworld, specifically a Jewish prostitute: how unfair to put the whole weight of the Holocaust on the frail shoulders of "that poor woman of the streets if she'd ever existed."[6]

Wiesenthal published the results of his Hitler-syphilis sleuthing in 1989, two decades after he had first heard the Munich city councilor, Herr Fackler, offhandedly call Hitler syphilitic. The source was, once again, Putzi, who had told Fackler that during the First World War Hitler had almost faced a court-martial while stationed in Flanders. The charge, "self-disablement," referred to contracting syphilis to escape active service. According to Hanfstaengl, Hitler avoided the trial by proving that his syphilis had been contracted earlier.

Wiesenthal's second source was further removed. Edmund Ronald, a physician working in a hospital in Seattle in 1952 or 1953, had met an Austrian colleague whose father claimed to have treated young Hitler for syphilis contracted from a Jewish prostitute. The story went that sometime after 1938 German agents had confiscated the doctor's index cards and medical records having to do with Hitler. Another informant of Ronald's was more substantial: he had interviewed Professor Bodo Spiethoff, the first chairman of dermatology and syphilology at the University of Jena, who claimed that Hitler had consulted him for syphilis. And in a letter published in the *International Herald Tribune* in 1977, Ronald wrote that according to the eminent London venereologist Anwyl-Davies, Hitler had to have anti-syphilitic treatment on and off for twenty years because he caught syphilis from a Jewish prostitute in Vienna.

Anwyl-Davies, well-known for his research on the effects of mercury and bismuth on blood tests and for a monograph on the variable location of the female cervical chancre, was not difficult to find. But he was a dead end until a random reference about Hitler having a rosy rash while in the men's hostel in Vienna footnoted Alan Wykes. Wykes was the author of a series of books on World War II, including two about Anwyl-Davies and his story of Hitler's syphilitic rash, *The Doctor and His Enemy* (1966) and *Hitler* (1970).

Anwyl-Davies related the following story to Wykes during interviews in 1963. Two men, referred to as "Stefan" and "Daniel" to protect their identities since they were still living at the time, returned to their lodging at the Men's Home at 27 Meldemannstrasse in the northeast part of Vienna on an April evening in 1910. There they got into a fight over a prostitute with their fellow lodger, Adolf Hitler. They had told this story to Anwyl-Davies in 1933 when they were staying at the Hotel Royal in Stuttgart, in somewhat better circumstances than in the days of Vienna, although the Men's Home was then a state-of-the-art hostelry with private rooms and common kitchens where lodgers cooked together. The two men struck up a conversation with the English doctor, in the course of which they mentioned having known Hitler, whose picture was on posters at the hotel. Later, sharing a bottle of wine, they asked his profession; when he revealed that he was a venereologist, they confessed that they had both been infected with syphilis when they were youths, and added that their compatriot Hitler had been as well.

Anwyl-Davies shared another bit of interesting information with Wykes: that a specialist friend of his had reported a conversation with a German eye specialist named Viktor Krückmann, who had treated Hitler when he was hospitalized at Pasewalk for blindness from British gas. It was then that syphilis was discovered and given some "rough-and-ready" treatment, which was of little use at that time, eight years after infection. According to Wykes again, Krückmann wrote in 1965 about his diagnosis: "It is a nervous complaint often indicative of the tertiary stage of syphilis. I advise that this man should be examined for evidence of that disease and treated accordingly. He will recover his sight."[7] According to Krückmann, Hitler received treatment for venereal disease then, and Nazi leader Wilhelm Frick subsequently destroyed the records.

Although Paul Ehrlich's (supposed) magic bullet, Salvarsan, had been introduced in 1909, it was unlikely that it would have been used on anyone in Hitler's circumstances, Anwyl-Davies noted, meaning that Hitler would most likely have been treated with mercury. In *Mein Kampf*, Hitler referred to "the invention of a remedy of questionable character and its commercial exploitation"[8] that was of little use against the plague of syphilis. Was he referring to Salvarsan?

Wykes mentioned that in the early stages of his power, Hitler was treated by a physician named Conti for stomach disorders, headaches, and insomnia. In 1933, Dr. Leonardo Conti was special commissioner for medical affairs in the Prussian government. Later, in his position as Reich health leader and state secretary for health in the Reich Ministry of the Interior, he was present at meetings with Hitler to discuss legal and ethical issues of the euthanasia program.

It was Anwyl-Davies's hypothesis that *Mein Kampf* expressed Hitler's need for a vicious revenge: "It would not be enough for such a revenge to be aimed at the single member of Jewish society who had infected him: the entire race had to be persecuted in castigation."[9] Anwyl-Davies found symptoms typical of advanced syphilis at the end of Hitler's days in his mania and lunatic ravings, as well as the palsy of his left hand and leg, continual itching, insomnia, and head and stomach pain, as reported by his valet Heinz Linge. (The diaries of Theo Morell, which would have given Anwyl-Davies clues to symptoms of advanced syphilis, were as yet unpublished.) If Hitler had not committed suicide, he would have died soon enough, since his final ravings indicated that the cortex as well as the base of the brain was being attacked, and that would have led inevitably to general paralysis of the insane. A führer in a madhouse would not have served his vision of himself as messiah of the German people. Young Hitler had been "an idle and pusillanimous crackpot," Anwyl-Davies concluded, and would have stayed a nonentity except for the influence of syphilis—here expressing the belief that syphilis changes the personality from the early stages on.

Did Anwyl-Davies ever pass on his knowledge, Wykes wanted to know? He did not, assuming that British Intelligence, MI5, must have known, although he confirmed later that he was wrong. A queer partnership it would have been, Wykes mused, a venereologist in cahoots with military strategists.

In his second book, Wykes told the story in more detail.

Stefan and Daniel recalled a quarrel that resulted from Hitler trying to "appropriate" a Jewish prostitute they called "Hannah" (not her real name) when the other two men had already paid for her services for that evening. They bashed him over the head and in the ribs and tossed him, screaming, along with his paints and brushes, into the street. Hannah, who worked in doorways near the train station and sometimes had as many as four clients an hour, joined them at the men's home after they bribed the janitor with cigarettes to ignore the "no women" rule. They noted that a faint rash, previously observed on her body and thought to be heat rash or flea bites, was no longer visible.

When Hitler returned a week or two later, their anger had passed and they let him back in. They noticed when he took off his clothes to be deloused in the oven that he too had the pink flush. They had it as well, along with other unpleasant manifestations of disease and a general feeling of being ill, and so they consulted a doctor who alarmed them with a diagnosis of syphilis and treated them with mercury ointment. They were "maliciously heartened" to think that Hitler might have been infected on the very night of their argument.

If a diagnosis of syphilis rested on the testimony of two men claiming to remember, over a bottle of wine late at night, an unpleasant event of their youth associating them with the new dictator, the investigation would end there. As sterling as Anwyl-Davies's reputation as a venereologist was, the two men may have been having a bit of fun with him. It is, at best, dodgy hearsay evidence.

This statement made by Anwyl-Davies might have been aimed at Hitler in the later stages of disease: "The effect of cerebral syphilis on a nature already afflicted with megalomania is always to increase the confidence that every kind of opposition can be overcome, to see the path ahead lighted by Messianic triumphs when in fact ruinous disasters lurk in the shadows."[10]

Hitler was so intensely and successfully secretive about his sexual life that there is still no clear evidence of any sexual encounter, and biographers have variously speculated that he was chaste, impotent, heterosexual, homosexual, bisexual, sadistic, masochistic, and a pederast. Scholars have put him in and out of bed with many of his entourage, including his niece Geli Raubal, his companion Eva Braun (observant servants noted no sexual activity there), any number of men (Lothar Machtan's theory in *Hidden Hitler*), and even Richard Wagner's grandchildren, this last attributed to a Wagner great-grandchild in a *New Yorker* article.[11] Most agree that Hitler had an abnormally low libido, but again, this is only speculation.

In the Vienna years Hitler was fascinated with prostitutes and, according to his then friend Gustl Kubizek, talked for hours with him about sex, taking him twice to the "sink of iniquity," a street where prostitutes sat in lit windows enticing customers. After one of these expeditions, Kubizek recalled, Hitler lectured him on the evils and dangers of prostitution. Most scholars assume Hitler was only theoretically interested in sex in his Vienna years. Ian Kershaw, for example, concluded "with near certainty that by the time he left Vienna at the age of twenty-four Hitler had had no sexual

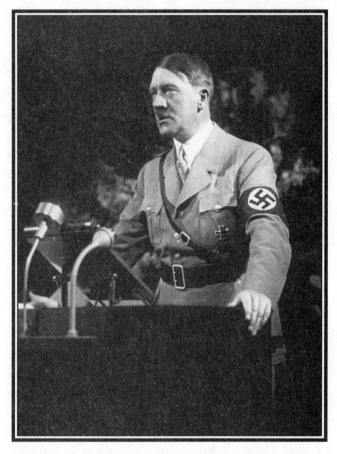

Figure 20.2   Adolf Hitler speaking at Nuremberg rally
(Corbis)

experience,"[12] but how can we be so sure that he didn't slip at
least once?

Why did Hitler wait until the final hour to vow "till death do
us part" with Eva Braun and then celebrate their honeymoon
with a double suicide? Hitler had given his vows to the state previously; he married only Germany, but why? Could it be because
he believed that he was infected with a disease, hereditary to the
tenth generation, that caused degeneration and insanity?

Wiesenthal's second syphilologist, Professor Bodo Spiethoff,
was, like Anwyl-Davies, well-known in the field of syphilology.

He experimented with a new drug, stovarsol, for the florid stages of syphilis, and he studied the use of liver extract to prevent liver injury. A quick search on the Internet located him on the home-page of the University of Jena, where he had joined the clinic in 1919 as the first specialist in dermatology and syphilology (the last year that Nietzsche's doctor at Jena, Otto Binswanger, was there). After he left Jena, Professor Spiethoff had been a Nazi activist. Hitler biographer Robert Waite wrote that rumors were rife in German medical circles that Spiethoff's treatment of Hitler was for mental disorders arising from syphilis.[13] He reports that medical authorities at Jena could find no record of Hitler's treatment, but that is explained if, as Wykes alleged, Spiethoff's consultation records were confiscated and impounded by Wilhelm Frick. If Frick confiscated Spiethoff's records, he knew in detail of Hitler's treatment for advancing syphilis, a point that will soon become relevant.

MEIN KAMPF: THE PLACE OF SYPHILIS IN HITLER'S POLITICAL AGENDA

Joachim Fest writes that "a curiously nasty, obscene odor" emanates from the pages of *Mein Kampf*, strongest in the "incredible and revealing chapter on syphilis."[14] Hitler wrote a long, passionately crusading section against syphilis in *Mein Kampf*, blaming previous leadership for losing the battle against a disease that, if not checked would in a few generations' time destroy the human race. Hitler's ideas in these pages were a combination of incorrect medical assumptions, prevailing folk knowledge, and anti-Semitism, mixed with one part cold reality: Syphilis numbers had increased drastically after World War I, and the epidemic showed no sign of slowing down.

Hitler's political agenda was clear, but the possibility that he knew himself to be infected, and therefore knew it was too late for him, adds to the shrillness of his provocation. Did he write those pages with the secret knowledge that his body harbored the syphilitic poison, and in the belief that his blood and bloodline were contaminated forever? Was he thinking of himself when he wrote: "Finally, however: who can know whether he is sick or healthy? Are there not numerous cases in which a patient apparently cured relapses and causes frightful mischief without himself suspecting it at first?"[15] Historians have tended to dismiss *Mein Kampf* as a poorly written, immature, and irrational piece of work. David Irving, for one, has never read it. (He said he was only interested in the Hitler of the war years.) If reviewed in the context of what was to follow, *Mein Kampf* contains a deadly logic and chilling blueprint for the Holocaust.

In Landsberg Prison in 1924 Adolf Hitler was transformed from a leader of the failed Beer Hall Putsch to a national hero. Fans sent him so many sausages and strudels that prison officials had to provide an entire room for his food. He began holding court and dictating his memoirs to cell mate Rudolf Hess to be typed on paper donated by his loyal follower, Richard Wagner's daughter-in-law Winifred. The working title, *Four and a Half Years of Struggle Against Lies, Stupidity and Cowardice,* was ultimately changed to *Mein Kampf* (My Struggle). Ten million copies were eventually distributed, the state providing a copy to each newly married couple. Second only in sales to the Bible, *Mein Kampf* made Hitler a rich man.

In *Mein Kampf* Hitler expressed three incorrect notions about syphilis that were part of the prevailing folk wisdom. The first was that syphilis could be inherited for many generations. The "syphilitic taint" passed to the germ, the sperm or the egg, in a single syphilitic sexual encounter and resulted in familial degeneration, insanity, and retardation—the sins of the father avenged to the tenth generation. The second erroneous idea was that syphilis spoiled the blood. Even medical texts of the time warned that healing the chancre and taking medicine for a few weeks or months would not cure the blood of the syphilitic poison. The third and most dangerous erroneous idea was that syphilis was a Jewish disease, and the Jews were responsible for its spread.

Blaming the spread of disease on the Jews had a long history. In 1348 when the Black Death killed millions of Europeans and rotting bodies were piled in the streets, Jews were accused of poisoning wells as part of an international conspiracy to kill Christians. Jewish communities were attacked, and thousands of Jews were burned alive as a result. When the Naples syphilis epidemic broke out, the Jews were blamed for being carriers of the disease from Spain. In Hitler's overheated rhetoric they moved, with deadly consequence, from being carriers of disease to being synonymous with it. He begins the syphilis section in *Mein Kampf* by blaming Jewish newspapers for spreading poisonous ideas, using a metaphor: "This poison was able to penetrate the bloodstream of our people unhindered to do its work, and the state did not possess the power to master the disease."[16] In the next sections, he links syphilis with the Jews, mixing metaphors about infection with the realities of the epidemic.

In "Blood Sin: Syphilis and the Construction of Jewish Identity" (*Faultline*, 1992), Jay Geller investigated this perception of the Jews as the source of the blood-poisoning syphilis, the widespread belief that Hitler expressed and amplified in *Mein Kampf*. This association was boosted by the fact that Jewish doctors, prohibited from practicing the more respected specialties, dominated the ranks of dermatology and syphilology. And discoveries about syphilis in science were often associated with Jewish researchers: Ehrlich, Neisser, and Wassermann.

Young women, Hitler wrote, were at risk in marriage to youthful Aryan husbands poisoned by prostitutes. That much at least was fact insofar as a young man of the time was routinely expected to go to a prostitute, no matter how dangerous, for his sexual initiation. But behind the prostitution business Hitler saw the Jew: "the cold-hearted, shameless, and calculating director of this revolting vice traffic in the scum of the big city. . . . The relation of the Jews to prostitution and, even more, to the white-slave trade, could be studied in Vienna as perhaps in no other city of Western Europe, with the possible exception of the southern

French ports. If you walked at night through the streets and alleys of Leopoldstadt, at every step you witnessed proceedings which remained concealed from the majority of the German people."[17] Leopoldstadt was a congested Jewish community where syphilis was rampant.

"The struggle against syphilis and the prostitution which prepares the way for it is one of the most gigantic tasks of humanity," Hitler wrote.[18] If the battle against syphilis was not fought to the end, there would be few images of God in five hundred years—"unless you want to profane the Almighty."[19] He charged prewar leadership with "total capitulation" resulting in a "syphilization of our people" and declared that the entire nation must be made to understand that "the question of combating syphilis should have been made to appear as *the* task of the nation. Not just *one more* task . . . Everything—future or ruin—depended upon the solution to this question."[20]

The spread of syphilis between the wars had increased dramatically, causing concern throughout Europe. The same erroneous ideas about hereditary syphilitic degeneration stated with such fervor by Hitler in *Mein Kampf* were current not just in Germany but also in other European countries. In *The British Medical Journal* of 19 August 1905, for example, Lieutenant-Colonel Lambkin, medical officer in charge of the London Military Hospital for Venereal Diseases, wrote: "To grapple with the treatment of syphilis among the civil population of England ought to be the chief object of those interested in that most burning question, the physical degeneration of our race." Even as exceptional a syphilologist as Alfred Fournier believed that syphilis was hereditary and linked it, in 1904, to species decline: "It emerges from recent research that syphilis can because of its hereditary consequences, debase and corrupt the species by producing inferior, decadent, dystrophic and deficient beings. Yes, deficient beings, according to the degree of their intellectual debasement, retarded, simple-minded, unbalanced, insane, imbecilic, or idiotic."[21]

The belief that syphilis was hereditary was one of the reasons behind Hitler's plan in *Mein Kampf* to eliminate "the mental defectives" to keep them from propagating "equally defective off-spring." This plan would represent the most humane act of mankind, sparing millions from undeserved suffering, he argued, but only if "systematically executed. . . . The determination to proceed in this direction would oppose a dam to the further spread of venereal diseases. The passing pain of a century can and will redeem millenniums from sufferings."[22] He proposed that what must be done to solve the problem required "truly incisive and sometimes almost unbearable obligations and burdens" as well as "ruthless measures and surgical operations."[23] He suggested years of preparation to focus the determination of the entire nation until it was willing to take exceedingly hard measures requiring the greatest sacrifices, meeting nearly impossible demands. He called for the whole attention of the people to be focused on this one question, the elimination of syphilis, as if life and death depended on its solution, even if it took the last ounce of energy.

Hitler titled the syphilis sections of *Mein Kampf*: Syphilis, Blood Sin and Desecration of the Race, the Task of Combating Syphilis, Sound Mind–Sound Body, Sterilization of the Incurables, and Prostitution of the People's Soul. After *Mein Kampf*, syphilis disappeared without explanation from Hitler's public language, but it might be expected that what he called *the* task of the nation, its eradication, would not disappear from his mind or plan. He told his lawyer, Hans Frank, that he regretted these pages; they were too self-revealing. The word syphilis disappeared; instead Hitler used the language of blood poison and infection when speaking of the Jews. Throughout the speeches are references to the Jewish poisoners of the blood and national body. Over and over he repeated this metaphor, interchangeably using images of the Jewish bacillus, the Jewish virus, the Jewish cancer: "Jewish blood poisoning and race poisoning"; "the deadly Jewish poison"; "the world poisoner of all peoples, international Jewry"; "How many diseases have their origin in the Jewish virus"; "a bloodiest tribunal to punish our people's poisoners"; "Consider that this blood poisoning can be removed from our national body only after centuries, if at all"; "This contamination of our blood, blindly ignored by hundreds of thousands of our people, is carried out systematically by the Jew today"; "The greatest danger is and remains for us the alien racial poison in our body. All other dangers are transitory."

In February 1942, Hitler publicly made one of his most alarming pseudoscientific statements. He said that the discovery of the Jewish virus was one of the greatest revolutions undertaken in the world, comparable to that of Pasteur and Koch in the past century. How many diseases are traced back to the Jewish virus? Hitler railed; health will be regained only when we eliminate the Jew.

This identification of the Jew with the sexually transmitted poison of syphilis was popularized in Julius Streicher's race-hate rag, *Der Stürmer*. A brutal schoolteacher who physically attacked Jews, Streicher, like Hitler in the early days, was rarely seen in public without his whip. When Streicher first heard Hitler speak in a beer hall, he thought he saw a halo around his head. He quickly turned over to Hitler the membership of his anti-Semitic group. At its height in 1935 *Der Stürmer* claimed a print run of 700,000 issues, with special editions at the time of the Nuremberg rallies running to two million. Hitler said it was the only newspaper he read front to back, and Streicher was one of the few men he addressed with the familiar "du" (although relations were not always peaceful between the two). Streicher's language was filled with sadistic images, as were the pages of his newspaper, where for twenty-two years (it folded in February 1945) it featured lurid images showing Jewish men defiling pure Aryan maidens, committing ritual murders, and conspiring.

Streicher wrote that the semen of a man of another race contained "alien albumin" that was absorbed by a woman's body in a single sexual act, thus destroying forever her ability to bear healthy German children. Hitler wrote similarly in *Mein Kampf*: "This contamination of our blood, blindly ignored by hundreds of thousands of our people, is carried out systematically by the Jew today. Systematically these black parasites of the nation defile our inexperienced young blond girls and thereby destroy something which can no longer be replaced in this world."[24] Streicher became a key propagandist of National Socialism, delivering rabble-rousing speeches and publishing incendiary copy. Hitler put him in charge of the boycott of Jewish businesses in 1933. He was tried at Nuremberg and hanged with nine other Nazi war criminals on 16 October 1946. As he approached the gallows, he shouted "Heil Hitler."

HITLER'S LATE MEDICAL AND PSYCHOLOGICAL CONDITION

In the spring of 1936 Hitler sent his private plane to fetch Dr. Theo Morell to cure his photographer, Heinrich Hoffmann, of a case of gonorrhea. Morell had a thriving practice on a fashionable street in Berlin where he treated the rich and famous, especially actors and actresses, for venereal disease. He was once invited to be the private physician for the Shah of Persia. Morell cured Hoffmann and the two men became friends, celebrating their friendship in Venice. On Christmas Day, Morell and Hoffmann were with their wives in the private bowling alley of Hitler's mountain estate, the Berghof, when Hitler asked to speak privately with Morell. When he offered Morell a villa in return for treatment the doctor accepted, choosing to neglect his lucrative practice to treat his führer.

Why did Hitler, who could have retained any doctor, choose Morell? Why did a public idol, who changed his white silk shirt twice a day, choose a notoriously unkempt and smelly man to watch over his health? The urgency of Hitler's request, the magnitude of his fee, and the presenting symptoms suggest that he chose Morell, a syphilologist, for the simple reason that he feared the progression of syphilis. A villa was excessive payment for curing a skin condition and a stomachache. But was any fee too great for a man in Hitler's position to contain and keep secret the horrors of late syphilis? Morell appealed to Hitler as well because he was willing to try alternative medical practices. He had an upscale, prestigious practice. And, unlike the majority of doctors treating venereal disease at the time, he was not Jewish.

When Simon Wiesenthal began tracking rumors of Hitler's infection, he asked Albert Speer, Hitler's architect and chief of war production, if he had heard them. Speer said no but did note that the entire entourage was puzzled when Hitler hired Morell, a specialist in dermatology and syphilology, as his private physician. According to Speer, Morell discreetly removed the plaque identifying his specialty when he signed on with Hitler.

Hitler's escort surgeon, Karl Brandt, and others in the entourage had been encouraging Hitler to have a full medical workup in a hospital, which he refused to do on the grounds that it would not serve his public image to be seen as a sick man. Meanwhile he did what he could to treat himself by taking a variety of self-prescribed medications and by changing his diet to eliminate rich desserts in favor of simple vegetables and cereals.

In 1936 when Hitler first interviewed Morell, his stomach cramps, with bloating and belching, and, of concern to his staff, excessive flatulence, were incapacitating. Lesions on his shin were severe enough to prevent him from wearing a boot. Skin lesions were particularly troubling to the secret syphilitic because late eruptions (as opposed to the rash of the early infection) announce progression of the disease—and because they are visible to the world. Syphilis of the stomach was rare, but days of grinding, spasmodic pain and vomiting followed by nervous exhaustion resulted when the abdominal ganglia or the vagus nerve were damaged.[25] With syphilitic gastric and visceral crises, the average patient was reduced to convulsive, sobbing helplessness. John Stokes compared the attacks to the state of nervous collapse of a "hypersensitive woman in childbirth."[26] Syphilologist James Kirby Howles wrote that with syphilitic visceral crises, strong men became hysterical and wept uncontrollably.[27] In 1944 (according to John Toland), Hitler experienced pain so severe that he held back the urge to scream.[28]

Morell's initial treatment appeared to be successful. Albert Speer quoted Hitler as saying: "What luck that I met Morell. If I hadn't I would have been dead long ago. He has saved my life. Wonderful, the way he has helped me," and: "It would be an in-

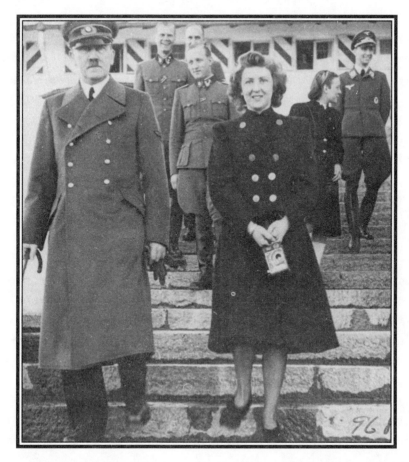

Figure 20.3   Adolf Hitler (walking with a cane) and Eva Braun
(Bettmann/Corbis)

conceivable tragedy if anything should happen to Morell. I could
no longer live without him."[29] Morell promised relief in a year;
within six months the eczema was gone, and so was the gastrointestinal pain, although the apparent recovery was only temporary.
Hitler paid Morell four times the salary of a general and gave him
lavish open-ended research grants. Although doctors then and
since have debunked his aggressive and unconventional treatments, Morell was often successful. Hitler referred friends to him,
including Mussolini and Göring.

Morell was forty-nine years old when he became Hitler's doctor. He had graduated from the Munich Medical School and had been an army physician in World War I. As a ship's doctor he learned folk remedies in the tropics. His polypharmaceutical approach has earned him harsh criticism from other doctors and accusations that his wild overmedicating may have caused some of Hitler's many symptoms. His medications—administered with literally thousands of injections—included Mutaflor, bacteria from the feces of Bulgarian peasants; Eupaverin, an anticonvulsant made from poppies; Nux vomica containing belladonna; and Homoseran, derived from human placenta. Hitler was a willing patient, actively involved with Morell in his treatment.

Hitler was intensely secretive and kept no diary or intimate correspondence that revealed concerns about his health. On 7 August 1941 Morell began the diary of his führer's daily medical treatment on small sheets penciled in blue. This log of details of Hitler's health, both mental and physical, in those years gives such a clear picture of advancing syphilis that we have to wonder if Morell was leaving a record to vindicate his unconventional treatment in years to come.

Did Hitler and his *Leibarzt*—personal physician—pull off one of the greatest cover-ups in medical history?

When Morell began his diary, Hitler was complaining of giddiness and a troublesome feeling over his left temple. He complained for several days of buzzing in the ears, a symptom he had experienced for years. Morell applied leeches to his temple to alleviate the buzzing. "Hitler sat in front of the mirror and watched fascinated as the leeches quenched their thirst on his blood."[30] That month as well he had a fever with shivering, chills, and vomiting. Morell called the episode encephalitis, an inflammation of the brain tissue. A second similar episode occurred in December. In March 1942 a note from Goebbels recorded that Hitler told him he was suffering from "the most violent dizzy spells."[31] Morell noted another significant medical event in July 1942 when Hitler was in Vinnitsa, his headquarters in the Ukraine:

"Brain edema with impairment of vision in right eye and high blood pressure (over 170 mm)."[32] He called it a Russian headache, noting that it was not unlike meningitis. Hitler complained of impaired vision in his right eye. He was experiencing tremors and weakness in his left leg.

Over the next three years, Hitler was progressively incapacitated, with old symptoms recurring and new ones added. He complained of pressure on both sides of the head, insomnia, more dizziness, and throbbing headaches that lasted for days. He experienced jerkiness of the leg and a hand tremor. His speech lost volume. He had agonizing flatulence and contractions of the intestines. Pustules and furuncles appeared on the back of his neck. Morell administered electric warming pads and moist compresses to the stomach and liver, set up oxygen for him in his room, and sent him to a field hospital in Rastenburg for a skull X ray that showed inflammation. His face became flat and lacking in expression. His skin took on a reddish tinge. He was apathetic, lost in details; his memory was increasingly impaired. He had an episode of jaundice. His housekeeper, Anni Winter, described him as weak, with scarecrow arms that shook uncontrollably. He showed signs of premature aging. Saliva dribbled from the corner of his mouth.

Fritz Redlich, retired dean of the Yale School of Medicine and author of *Hitler: Diagnosis of a Destructive Prophet,* a work of fifteen years and the most complete medical analysis of Hitler to date, classified as "diagnostic loose ends" a few of Hitler's enigmas. How many of these diagnosis-defying conditions fit the pattern of syphilis?

> The etiology of the [Parkinson's-like] syndrome is uncertain.
> . . . The gastrointestinal diagnostic picture is quite inconclusive.
> . . . The hepatic pathology, with atypical findings and three diagnoses . . . is even more puzzling. The ophthalmological examinations . . . make a satisfactory evaluation difficult. The etiology of tinnitus is rarely established, and Hitler's tinnitus was no exception. . . . The photosensitivity of skin and eyes also has not been satisfactorily explained.[33]

The possibility that Hitler was suffering from late syphilis suggests that his various illnesses can be looked at again from the perspective of this diagnosis. Matching the dozens of signs and symptoms of Hitler's physical state in those last years with a classic text of syphilology suggests a compelling likelihood that almost every part of his body was advertising a progressing late syphilis.

Although Hitler had complaints with most of his major organs during that time, each of which can be analyzed for consistency with a diagnosis of syphilis, the one part of his body that points us most directly to syphilis was his heart. The three most feared manifestations of tertiary syphilis were insanity, paralysis, and heart disease, in particular, death by rupture of an aneurysm. Stokes defined cardiac syphilis as "ubiquitous, insidious, disastrous": a manifestation of disease that should take precedence in treatment over all others and last for several years. "Until teacher and textbook turn . . . to habitual suspiciousness in observation, and to an acute analysis and ferreting out of veiled beginnings, syphilis of the heart and aorta will remain the great burying ground of the disease and the clinician's perpetual Waterloo at the hands of the postmortem pathologist."[34] (See Appendix B.)

There was nothing in Hitler's medical condition that by itself would point to syphilis of the heart. A number of excellent cardiologists have reviewed his history and seen nothing abnormal for a man of his age.[35] And yet if we look at Morell's observations from the viewpoint of a syphilologist who saw this condition frequently in daily practice, we see a characteristic pattern of disease and treatment that cannot be ignored.

The diaries provide more than enough reason to suspect that what Morell found with his stethoscope was the first indicator that Stokes and others found when syphilitic heart disease was suspected: *the clear, altered tympanic quality of the aortic component of the second sound.* Stokes found this particular music of the heart to be the most important of the early warning signs of syphilitic aortitis. He described this sign in terms not merely of accentuation but also of a pure, clear musical quality. "The words used to describe the musical quality of the sound vary from the hollow tap of an Arab drum to the German 'clang.' 'Amphoric' is often used, and 'tambour' is to our minds the best term."[36] Other syphilologists agreed. When Joseph Earle Moore sent a list of features of a physical examination meant to identify syphilis in the prospective subjects of the Tuskegee Syphilis Study in 1932, one of the fifteen signs to look for was "the presence or absence of an accentuated tympanic, bell-like aortic second sound."[37]

Stokes warned that extremely careful listening and exquisite technique were necessary to detect early syphilis of the aorta. Morell apparently had that acute sense and technique, because he identified this characteristic sign of early aortic damage in Hitler's heart over and over, and so noted it in the journal: 9 January 1940—"Second aortic sound today only weakly accentuated"; 7 August 1941—"Pulse normal at 72–76 per minute, regular and full; second heartbeat accentuated"; later that same evening— "Heartbeat somewhat accelerated, second heartbeat accentuated"; 23–24 September 1944—"Heart findings inconclusive except that as usual the second heart beat accentuated, with pure sounds, regular heart action"; 19 October 1944—"His heart tones are pure and weak, with a strong accentuation of the second heartbeat."[38]

At the end of the war, when Morell was interrogated by the Americans, he made a clear statement about having found the altered second sound in Hitler's heart. "Under auscultation accentuation of the second aortic sound was heard in second intercostal space in the right parasternal line."[39]

After the altered second sound, the next indicator of syphilitic aortic damage, what Stokes called the "grave electrocardial sign," was the appearance of T wave negativity, abnormal in 85 percent of patients with syphilitic aortitis. Again, Morell paid close attention to alterations in Hitler's T waves. He took electrocardiogram readings at least once a month, and often every week. Hitler himself sometimes asked for one. They secretly packed a portable machine when traveling together to various headquarters. The Hestons puzzled over the "unusual frequency" of these secret electrocardiograms and concluded they were "meddlesome and even bizarre."[40] They also found it strange that Morell would be so secretive about Hitler's heart condition. Even Hitler's valet did not know about these tests.

Morell did find T-wave negativity in Hitler's EKGs. He confirmed it by sending them—again anonymously referring to the patient as the "gentleman in the foreign ministry"—to a specialist, Dr. Karl Weber, first in August 1941, then in May 1943, and finally in December 1944. In the 1943 report Weber noted unquestionable deterioration "inasmuch as the ST depression has become clearer and the T1, which was at that time still clearly positive, is now negative. The T11 which was still clearly positive then now virtually coincides with the base line."[41] In 1944 he found "flattening of T in all three Leads," adding, "these changes for the worse should not surprise us."[42]

The medication of choice in the 1940s for late cardiovascular syphilis was iodide salt, either potassium or sodium. In 1937 Stokes wrote: "Of late a German revival of non-specific therapy for syphilis has brought various iodid[e] derivatives to the front of the literature. . . . Many drugs have been used over the centuries but none except potassium iodide has been able to hold its place as of permanent value in treatment of the disease."[43] "In the treatment of cardiovascular syphilis, the iodides deserve a high though in many respects intangible place. They should be used invariably and from the outset in every case of actual syphilitic vascular disease."[44]

Anwyl-Davies guessed that "The Magic Bullet," Salvarsan 606, would not have been used on someone in Hitler's circumstances with syphilis in 1910, but why would it not have been an obvious choice for Morell to use years later? Stokes gives the answer: "The arsphenamines are intrinsically toxic for the syphilitic cardiovascular patient; this is most true of [Salvarsan] 606."[45] With cardiovascular disease associated with syphilis "iodide is sovereign and should be used alone for some time before mercury or arsphenamine is considered."[46]

Most of the medications Morell tried on Hitler were used infrequently, but a few appear with regularity in the diary. One of the most often injected substances was Septoid, a solution of 3 percent iodine in the form of various iodine salts: potassium iodide. Morell's use of Septoid was aggressive and always linked to Hitler's heart condition and the altered second sound: "Second heartbeat accentuated. . . . Fetched Septoid and injected 10 cc. intravenously. Later that day: "second heartbeat accentuated . . . Intravenous shot of 10 cc of twenty percent glucose solution and 10 cc of Septoid. . . . "Took his blood pressure. It's 170–180mm! Gave him two intravenous shots of 10 cc Septoid. . . . Blood pressure 156 mm/110 mm, pulse regular, no complaints. Injections as usual. Intravenous of glucose and Septoid. . . . Injections as always (10 cc twenty per cent Glycovarin and 100 cc Septoid intravenously). . . . I made an electrocardiogram! I and II lead: isoelectric T—strong muscle current. Subsequently a series of injections of twenty percent glucose occasionally with added iodine (Septoid 10 cc)."[47] He wrote to Weber that he had been giving "the gentleman in the foreign ministry" repeated glucose and iodine injections, frequently administering courses of these injections two or three times a day.

In the fall of 1941, Morell began injections of Strophanthin, rapid-action digitalis. The Hestons were perplexed: "In the use of digitalis we find an intricate puzzle, for there was no evident reason for giving Hitler digitalis at all. . . . Morell said that he gave digitalis because of the electrocardiograph reports of Dr. Karl Weber, but those reports provide no medically competent reason according to standard practice then or now."[48] Such a medically competent reason is provided by Stokes and others,[49] who recommended treating ambulant syphilis patients having low cardiac reserve with powdered digitalis over long periods of time.

Stokes lists symptoms of early syphilitic aortitis as chest pain, shortness of breath, palpitation (rapid beating or fluttering of the heart), indigestion, dizziness, cough, insomnia, edema, weakness, angina pectoris, paralysis of the vocal chord, night terrors,[50] and hoarseness. Hitler is reported to have experienced them all except perhaps palpitation. Although each sign and symptom by itself could be explained by other conditions, the pattern strongly indicates early syphilitic heart disease. The aggressive treatment with Septoid suggests that Morell agreed.

Hitler stopped taking walks. He complained to Dr. Hans-Karl von Hasselbach of having a weak heart. In July 1941, when he had a fight with his foreign minister, Joachim von Ribbentrop, he suddenly turned pale and fell into a chair clutching his heart. Edwin Giesing, the specialist called in to treat Hitler's ears after the unsuccessful assassination attempt of 20 July 1944, attributed the tiring of Hitler's voice to a slight weakness of the vocal cord muscles (paresis of internus muscle).

Once cardiac syphilis has advanced to the point where damage can be identified with a stethoscope, the patient usually has only a few years left to live, however aggressive the treatment. Hitler's repeated insistence that he did not have much time left may have been correct. Historians who suggest that Hitler accelerated the war effort beyond reason at the end, or that he rushed the Holocaust ahead of his military schedule, may find a reason in the expectation that his heart might at any moment balloon with a fatal aneurysm.

The irrelevance of the negative blood Wassermann test, which Morell recorded anonymously for "Patient A," will be discussed later; for now, it is worth noting only that it is especially inconclusive in cases of cardiac syphilis. Stokes observed "the well-recognized occurrence of complete serological negativity in vascular syphilis,"[51] and again that "a low index of suspicion and uncritical acceptance of a single diagnostic standard like the blood Wassermann test permits syphilis to escape detection by the physician in his observation of cardiovascular disease."[52]

In the middle of February 1944 Hitler complained that he was seeing everything as if through an opaque veil. Earlier he had felt a light stabbing pain in his right eye. Morell referred him to an opthalmologist, Professor Löhlein, who (on 2 March 1944) reported finding diffuse turbidity in the vitreous humor (the jellylike substance between the retina and the lens) of the right eye. Löhlein's next report, on 7 April 1945, shortly before Hitler's suicide, again showed the vitreous to have a slight, delicate turbidity, sluggishly mobile, with a residue of hemorrhage and a lack of macular reflex. He suggested 2 percent yellow mercury ointment.

Giesing observed that Hitler had experienced turbidity in the vitreous humor for about eight years and that this cloudiness in the liquid of the eye was typical of a syphilitic condition. He pondered whether Hitler might have had congenital syphilis, noting that he did not have the characteristic notched teeth (known as Hutchinson's teeth after Jonathan Hutchinson) of the syphilitic child. Oddly, he did not consider acquired syphilis. What late syphilitic condition of the eye was Giesing considering when he reviewed Hitler's medical reports?

Morell noticed that Hitler had a fine hand tremor in 1941. Over the next years he developed tremors in his left arm and left leg. His posture became stooped. He required help in sitting and in raising his legs. The Hestons described his shuffling gait: "a normal though short swing and step of the right leg and foot and then the dragging of the left foot up to the right by rotating the pelvis forward, with the left toe staying in contact with the floor."[53] Hitler had difficulty speaking and he began to write in small script. Although these are all signs of late syphilis, they also suggest Parkinson's disease, raising the possibility that both affected Hitler. Arguments for Parkinson's do not exclude syphilis and vice versa.

Although Parkinson's disease is now generally accepted in Hitler's case, it has generated enough controversy that a more complete differential diagnosis including syphilis is called for. The Hestons opted for amphetamine toxicity that "led to a total syndrome that had Parkinsonian elements" to describe some of the late signs and symptoms, noting that none of the six physicians who treated Hitler at the end of the war suggested Parkinson's; indeed five of them (Giesing, Morell, Hasselbach, Brandt, and Ludwig Stumpfegger, Hitler's last staff doctor) specifically rejected it.[54] When the Hestons demonstrated a Parkinsonian tremor to people who had known Hitler in the last years, they were told that it was not like Hitler's tremor. Maser makes a strong statement against:

"An evaluation of Morell's neurological findings, however, disposes once for all of the allegation that Hitler suffered from Parkinson's."[55] The Hestons said they would have welcomed an alternative diagnosis that could be supported by the evidence. Does syphilis fit all criteria?

At the beginning of April 1945, Walter Schellenberg, Himmler's intelligence chief, paid a visit to his friend Max di Crinis, head of psychiatry at the Charité hospital in Berlin and an SS physician specializing in neurology. When King Boris of Bulgaria became terminally ill shortly after a meeting with Hitler, it was Crinis who was flown in to treat him. Crinis diagnosed Hitler with Parkinson's based on observing his tremors in newsreel footage and he passed this opinion on to Schellenberg. They discussed sending medication to Hitler to be administered by Stumpfegger.[56] Schellenberg reported all this to Himmler, who forbade discussion. On 8 April 1945 Morell began electro-galvanic therapy. On 15 April, he called Hitler's tremor a variety of *paralysis agitans*. He began injections of Homburg–680 and Harmin, both extracts of deadly nightshade; since these remedies were used for treatment for Parkinson's, it is possible that Morell suspected that condition at the end.

Tip-offs to approaching paresis—paranoia, grandiosity, depression, mania, violent rages, and sudden criminal behavior—are of limited usefulness in Hitler's case, given both his character and the circumstances of war. One of the reasons Simon Wiesenthal gave for suspecting tertiary syphilis with Hitler was his paranoia. Fritz Redlich agreed with the paranoia: "paranoid delusions were Hitler's most significant psychopathological complex. The attribute paranoid refers to persons who are extremely suspicious and believe that other persons or institutions are persecuting them."[57] But of course other persons and institutions were persecuting Hitler. He was not hiding in the airless bunker because he was delusional, but because the Allies, one bungling assassin after another,[58] and even some of those close to him were out to kill him. Even Albert Speer had a plan to murder Hitler. Giesing considered administering a drug overdose. In his diary Giesing confessed that at that moment, he did not want such a man to exist having the power of life and death. Hitler's valet interrupted Giesing before he could act on his impulse. When the assassination attempt of 20 July failed because Hitler chanced to put a heavy oak table between himself and the assassins' bomb just before it exploded, he jubilated at the sign that he was invincible; providence was indeed protecting him. Death in that case, he said, would have been liberation from cares, sleepless nights—and a severe nervous ailment.[59]

And how is it possible to diagnose pathological grandiosity in a man who came within a few steps of conquering the world? Or depression in someone losing a world war—or taking high doses of potassium iodide, which often had to be discontinued because of the depression it caused? Speer noted that Hitler often had tears in his eyes. He was elated for the last four or five months of 1942, leading Morell to consider that he was suffering from a manic depressive disorder, which is diagnostically indistinguishable from, and often mistaken for, syphilitic mania and depression. But he was also taking amphetamines at that time.

Hitler in the last years was still extremely coherent, as the published notes of his late military conferences show. But were some of his actions suddenly uncharacteristically lacking in judgment? Speer did not obey his order to "kill all the prisoners" (he said it was the product of a sick mind), nor did anyone act on the scorched earth command that would have left Germany in ruins. The possibility exists that syphilis could have intensified Hitler's fanaticism, supercharged his brutality, distorted further his already twisted moral sense, and fueled his terrible temper. He had always terrorized his staff with his tantrums, but the rages accelerated at the end in both frequency and intensity. He shouted for hours, foamed at the mouth, and rolled on the floor. Some sources say he even chewed on the carpet.

Other more subtle indications of approaching paresis can be seen in Hitler's actions in the last years. To name a few: impulsiveness (the Hestons mention snap decisions with horrible human consequences); absorption in detail (Speer noted that Hitler no longer delegated well but took over more and more control of minute detail, with grave consequences); disorganized thinking (when addressing armaments industry representatives in 1944, he neglected transitions and became confused about syntax); transient false beliefs (he committed mythical new armies one minute and realized the lack of resources the next); and mental rigidity and repetition (the staff noted that he often said the same thing over and over).

Of Hitler's mental state Albert Speer wrote: "Thus began (still from the summer of 1942 on) a peculiar state of petrification and rigidity; apathetic uncertainty, agonized indecisiveness, an apparent inability to deal with all important problems and obstinacy when faced with them; and a permanent state of caustic irritability. Formerly he had made decisions with almost playful ease. Now he had to squeeze them out of an overburdened brain."[60]

Was Hitler referring to himself, and perhaps anticipating what was to come, when he told Hans Frank that a man could be mad for years without anyone knowing? Field Marshall Rommel had no doubt about Hitler's mental state after the final assassination plot: "this pathological liar has become completely insane!"[61]

In the last year of the war, Hitler hid in a bunker under sixteen feet of concrete and six feet of earth. A noisy pump circulated air scented by his own excessive flatulence and Morell's foul body odors. Few people except his staff, his generals, and those of the inner circle saw him in that last year. Albert Speer described his decline:

> Now, he was shriveling up like an old man. His limbs trembled; he walked stooped, with dragging footsteps. Even his voice became quavering and lost its old masterfulness. Its force had given way to a faltering toneless manner of speaking. When he became excited, as he frequently did in a senile way, his voice would start breaking. . . . His complexion was sallow, his face swollen; his uniform, which in the past he had kept scrupulously neat, was often neglected in this last period of life and stained by the food he had eaten with a shaking hand. . . . I too

was constantly tempted to pity him, so reduced was he from the Hitler of the past. Perhaps that was the reason everyone would listen to him in silence when, in the long since hopeless situation, he continued to commit nonexistent divisions or to order units supplied by planes that could no longer fly for lack of fuel. Perhaps that was why no one said a word when he more and more frequently took flight from reality and entered his world of fantasy.[62]

How did those responsible for the war effort feel about this dangerously declining Hitler as leader? The answer lies in the many assassination attempts launched and bungled beginning in the spring of 1943, each one adding to Hitler's grandiose self-definition as one protected by providence, on a mission from God. How many of the would-be assassins believed that Hitler was in the late stage of syphilis and might go completely mad at any moment? Given that in the 1940s syphilitic insanity was well understood, the question of who knew what when about an imminent syphilitic catastrophe in the bunker becomes part of the story of the relationship between Hitler and his High Command in the last months of the war. If the enemy, the German army, or the German people had ever heard such a rumor, the results could have been disastrous to the war effort, but such knowledge had to have been shared, albeit with utmost discretion, among those with power. How many clandestine meetings were there that have gone unrecorded? So far, we have considered only that Wilhelm Frick, confiscating Hitler's medical records, may have known that Hitler had syphilis. What about others?

HEINRICH HIMMLER AND THE SECRET DOSSIER

At the end of 1942 Theo Morell and Karl Brandt faced a dilemma. They knew Hitler was approaching syphilitic dementia, but what could they do with that ultra-sensitive information? What conflicts did they experience, and what fears for their own personal survival did they feel when together they signed a report to be delivered into the hands of Hitler's deadly henchman, whose intense devotion to Adolf Hitler was expressed in the motto "My honor is my loyalty"? SS Chief Heinrich Himmler had heard rumors that his führer had advanced syphilis and hence might die or, worse, become demented at any moment. A troubled Himmler confided this top secret to his trusted masseur, Felix Kersten, who in 1956 published a diary of their conversations.

Kersten was born in Estonia but became a Finnish subject after he fought in the Finnish war of liberation against Russia. He studied manual therapy with a Chinese doctor in Berlin. He had already developed a royal and aristocratic clientele when he began treating Himmler for intestinal spasms that sometimes left him unconscious. According to Hugh Trevor-Roper's introduction to Kersten's memoirs, Himmler's masseur held the keys to Himmler's physical salvation and became "the all-powerful confessor who could manipulate at will the conscience as well as the stomach of that terrible, impersonal, inhuman, but naïve, mystical, credulous tyrant of the New Order."[63]

The first of two crucial conversations recorded in Kersten's diary took place on 12 December 1942. "This was the most exciting day I've had since I first began treating Himmler," Kersten related. "He was very nervous and restless; I realized that he had something on his mind and questioned him about it. His reply was to ask me: 'Can you treat a man suffering from severe headaches, dizziness and insomnia?'"[64] Kersten replied that he could, but of course he must examine the patient first and know the cause of the symptoms. Himmler said he would reveal the name only if Kersten would swear never to tell anyone. Indiscreet Kersten vowed discretion.

Himmler took from the safe a black portfolio containing a blue manuscript. "Read this. Here are the secret documents with the report on the Führer's illness."[65] The twenty-six-page report had drawn freely on Hitler's medical record from Pasewalk, where he had been hospitalized in October 1918 for treatment for temporary blindness resulting from being hit with British gas. The report noted that certain of the symptoms associated with syphilis were manifest at Pasewalk and that further symptoms had appeared in 1937 (Morell's first full year of treating Hitler), proving that syphilis was continuing its ravages. In the beginning of 1942 such symptoms showed "beyond any shadow of a doubt" that Hitler was suffering from progressive paralysis. "Every sign of syphilis was present except fixity of pupils and confusion of speech."[66]

Kersten told Himmler that he could not treat mental illness and asked what was being done for Hitler. Himmler replied that Dr. Morell was giving him injections to check the progress of the disease and to maintain the patient's ability to work. There was, of course, no recognized remedy for progressive paralysis at that time.

Himmler appealed to Kersten: "This is no ordinary patient but the Führer of the Greater German Reich, which is occupied in a struggle of life and death that can only be won with the Führer, for he is the only person whose powers are equal to the task; he mustn't fail us." He continued: "We must try every medical means to keep him going. I refuse to believe that this is the end, that the Führer's mind will give way, the mind that has such mighty achievements to its credit. . . . When I reflect how the Führer was sent to us by Providence, I just can't believe that there's no way of saving him from the consequences of syphilis. And now comes Morell and declares that he can help the Führer. There's nothing in the facts of the case to contradict him, for when he's had the injections the Führer is astonishingly clear and logical, and his thoughts are as original as ever they were in the old days."[67] Hitler should have a thorough examination in a mental hospital, Himmler allowed, but of course he would never agree to that, and besides, how could it be kept secret? If the foreign intelligence service ever got wind of it, enemy radio would alert the German people, and the most disastrous defeat imaginable would result. The war must be won first. Himmler once again emphasized the need for secrecy and returned the document to the safe. "Now tell me," he implored. "What would you do, Herr Kersten?"[68]

The following week (on 19 December 1942), Kersten recorded his second conversation with Himmler about Hitler's syphilis. Himmler asked if Kersten had any ideas for helping Hitler. Kersten suggested the Wagner-Jauregg malaria cure, a fever cure for late syphilis that won the Nobel Prize for its originator, and added that Hitler should refrain from exertion. Kersten explained that the illness might weaken Hitler's judgment and impair his critical faculty, producing delusions and megalomania. Physically there could be "headaches, insomnia, loss of muscular force, trembling of the hands, confusion of speech, convulsions and paralysis of the limbs."[69] What a grave threat to the German people this illness was, Kersten said. How could Himmler possibly distinguish whether orders that could affect the fate of millions were being issued in a lucid interval or under the influence of the disease? According to Kersten's account of the report, Hitler had received the standard treatment of the time (most probably mercury) at Pasewalk in 1918, and his symptoms had disappeared.

Kersten suggested that Himmler take steps to remove Hitler from office. Himmler said he could not. Disastrous squabbling would result because there was no planned line of succession. Besides, how could he prove that Hitler's symptoms were not just the result of exhaustion? The conversation ended with Himmler's glum reflection that he would watch carefully and act when the time was right.

On 4 February 1943 General Berger, in charge of the SS Head Office, asked Kersten about rumors abroad that Hitler was suffering from syphilis and progressive paralysis. Himmler had dropped hints; did Kersten know anything? Kersten admitted to vague recollections of something of the sort. Berger suggested that Hitler's exposure to poison gas might have activated some hereditary syphilis. Better not talk about it, Kersten said; it was a dangerous subject. Berger concurred: "We'll keep our mouths shut and behave as if we had never raised the matter."[70]

Again ignoring his promise of secrecy, Kersten asked Rudolf Brandt, Himmler's private secretary, what he knew about the secret dossier. Brandt "went pale with horror. 'Good god!' he said, 'you don't know what danger you're in. You, a foreigner, to have knowledge of the greatest state secret in our possession!'"[71]

Rudolf Brandt was willing to speculate that only Martin Bormann and probably Hermann Göring knew. Kersten asked him who had written the report. Brandt said he shouldn't tell, but he revealed this much: It was someone with a "very deep sense of responsibility, a person about whose integrity there could be no question" who considered it his duty to inform Himmler. This man had recently had a long interview with him at field headquarters. Kersten also inquired how long Himmler had known the facts of the case. He had always known of rumors circulating, Rudolf Brandt said, and had violently rejected them until the appearance of this report. Now he no longer dared to doubt the facts.

David Irving dismissed both Kersten's conversation with Himmler and the black dossier: "According to this bogus source, a paralysis of syphilitic origin that had first shown in Hitler in 1937 recurred in 1942. The blood tests in this book [his *Secret Diaries of Hitler's Doctor*] disprove this completely. As Hitler's adjutant Julius Schaub states: "There was never any such 'Black Dossier' as Kersten alleges, nor any such progressive paralysis."[72] But the blood tests, as we shall see later, were anything but definitive. Furthermore, how could Hitler's adjutant, Julius Schaub, possibly have known what secret, treasonous reports were in Himmler's private safe? In the introduction to *Hitler's War*, Irving calls Kersten a fictionalizer and cites the twenty-six-page medical dossier, checked against the Morell diaries, as an example. If the Morell diaries are read as a log of the treatment of a secret syphilitic, however, the Kersten document is validated by the comparison. But more to the point, Kersten included in his journal entries details about Hitler's treatment at the Pasewalk hospital and the current state of Hitler's health that he could not have known unless there was a secret report.

If it is assumed that Hitler did not have syphilis, then the Himmler-Kersten conversations are idle fictions rightly dismissed.

When Morell's diaries are looked at as a record of developing syphilis, however, the dialogue between Kersten and Himmler falls into place with a conflicted Himmler groping for contingency plans while warily watching Hitler for a medical disaster at any time. If Himmler had this nervous expectation, who else in the Nazi elite did? Of those who made statements that Hitler was mad already, how many attributed his aberrations to the rumors of syphilis that had been circulating for years?

Kersten's published diaries, for whatever reason, left out the startling identities of the signers of the report. They were later discovered by a Catholic theologian, Achim Besgen, whose book *The Silent Command* (1960) elaborated on Kersten's published material. Besgen had reviewed the original diaries with Kersten's widow's permission. He summarized Kersten's conversations with Himmler about the black dossier much as Kersten had published them in his memoi, but added:

"The report bears the signatures of Dr. Brandt and Dr. Morell" (emphasis added). ("Der Bericht trägt die Unterschriften von Dr. Brandt and Dr. Morell.")[73]

That inconspicuous sentence, buried at the end of a paragraph in Besgen's book, establishes that Hitler's escort surgeon, Karl Brandt, and Morell risked their lives to reveal to the head of the all-powerful SS at the start of the Battle of Stalingrad that Hitler had syphilis that might at any moment result in death or madness. Only Brandt and Morell had the details of the progress of Hitler's disease, so why did Kersten not name them later in his published memoir? Did he, out of respect for dead colleagues, not want to reveal their breach of the medical secret? While Morell was doing everything possible to keep Hitler functioning, and the joint signature implies that Brandt was assisting him, they both evidently felt it necessary to alert Himmler, in charge of internal security, to be ready to meet the emergency when it arose.

Morell and Brandt were anything but close. Morell had supplanted Brandt as the one most responsible for his health. Brandt became Hitler's escort doctor in 1934, flying with him when he met Mussolini. He maintained an uneasy alliance with Morell until October 1944, when Hitler fired him over his complaint that one of Morell's prescribed pills contained strychnine. The break-up was initiated when Giesing noticed six black pills on Hitler's breakfast tray and, snooping through Morell's literature on Koester's Antigas Pills, found strychnine as an ingredient. Hitler was recovering from jaundice at that time. Brandt confronted Morell, asking to be included in the medical plan. Morell recorded the following:

> Talk with Brandt. He said, "Do you think anyone would believe you if you would say that you only follow orders? Do you think Himmler would treat you better than anyone else? Right now so many people are getting hanged, the whole matter would have been judged very coldly. If something were to happen to the Führer, can you imagine what would have followed? One wouldn't have held von Hasselbach responsible, but you and most probably I would have been. Therefore, it is best if from now on I always know what is going on."[74]

The question of whether Himmler would stand up for Brandt and Morell in the event of a crisis takes on a different meaning once we know that those two had informed Himmler of Hitler's progressing syphilis. On 16 April 1945 Hitler had Brandt arrested and sentenced to death because he had moved his family out of Berlin into the American zone for safety. After Hitler's suicide only days later, Albert Speer had Brandt released, but no sooner was he free of the Germans than the Americans picked him up.

In October 1944, with Hitler's other doctors all dismissed by then, Morell was left with the sole responsibility for the health of his führer—and with the knowledge that Himmler was looking over his shoulder. Himmler sent his own physician, Ludwig Stumpfegger, to join the medical staff in the bunker from October 1944 to the following May. It is fair to assume that Stumpfegger, sent by Himmler, was fully informed on the syphilis question, and that Hitler knew that Stumpfegger knew. But did Hitler know that Himmler knew?

At the Military Intelligence Service Center, where Hitler's captured doctors were given the task of writing Hitler's medical history after the war, Brandt was assigned Morell as a cellmate. In the consolidated interrogation report of 15 October 1945 (declassified in 1964), "Hitler as Seen by His Doctors," Brandt, Giesing, and Hasselbach described Hitler in terms of rosy health, with good memory, excellent concentration, and no paralysis. The stomach problems were obviously hysterical in origin. Hitler loved to be merry and gay, wrote Hasselbach. All but Brandt testified that Hitler had no psychiatric abnormality; Brandt alone spoke of Hitler's "psychopathic personality."[75] The doctors' descriptions contrast quite markedly with the portrait of Hitler in Morell's diaries or Speer's description at the end of the war. The Americans' questions seem particularly unimaginative, restricted as they were to physical descriptions of various parts of Hitler's body—what small scars he had and how he parted his hair—as distinct from larger questions of pathology, perhaps simply because the serious state of Hitler's health at the end was not yet suspected. It may have amused the doctors to manage this misinformation while awaiting their fate in captivity. Morell told journalist Tania Long of the *New York Times* that he had never given Hitler amphetamines. He was released after a short time and lived in Bavaria until he died in 1948. Brandt was executed on 2 June 1948 at Landsberg prison for his role in Hitler's euthanasia program.

THE PASEWALK PAPERS

Two questions about Himmler's black dossier linger. If Morell and Brandt signed the document showing that Hitler was currently experiencing the ravages of tertiary syphilis, what Pasewalk document supported it showing that he had "symptoms of secondary syphilis" when he was hospitalized after being blinded by English gas? And who was the man of unquestionable integrity who had the secret meeting with Himmler at field headquarters? The first question sends us back to Pasewalk hospital in 1918.

While sitting on a concrete bunker, Hitler was hit with British gas and temporarily blinded along with several other men. They escaped when one less disabled led the others, goose-marching as blind men, to a field hospital in Brussels. Hitler alone was sent deep into Germany, where he was checked into the Pasewalk hospital. He was experiencing lid cramps and such swelling that his eyes could not be pried open.

Hitler recalled the incident in *Mein Kampf*:

> In the night of 13 October [the correct date was 15 October 1918], the English gas attack on the southern front before Ypres burst loose; they used yellow-cross gas, whose effects were still unknown to us as far as personal experience was concerned. In this same night I myself was to become acquainted with it. On a hill south of Wervick, we came on the evening of October 13 into several hours of drumfire with gas shells which continued all night more or less violently. As early as midnight, a number of us passed out, a few of our comrades forever. Toward morning I, too, was seized with pain which grew worse with every quarter hour, and at seven in the morning I stumbled and tottered back with burning eyes; taking with me my last report of the War. A few hours later, my eyes had turned into glowing coals; it had grown dark around me.[76]

Hitler regained his sight, only to lose it again when news of armistice reached the hospital. "Again everything went black before my eyes; I tottered and groped my way back to the dormitory, threw myself upon my bunk, and dug my burning head into my blanket and pillow."[77] He told the story repeatedly for some years afterwards that a supernatural vision inspired him to become Germany's savior, after which he regained his sight for the second time. Hitler was discharged from Pasewalk at the end of November 1918, fit for field service. Later, at the Putsch trial he testified that he could only make out the largest newspaper headlines and feared he had lost the ability to read a book.

When Rudolph Binion read *The Eyewitness*, a compelling fictional account of Hitler's experience at Pasewalk, he wondered whether the author, Ernst Weiss, a Jewish doctor, might have drawn on real documents for his well-informed story and modeled the character of the psychiatrist who treated "AH" in "P" on a real doctor. Binion's search did eventually lead to that real doctor, Edmund Forster, and from there to Forster's dramatic odyssey.

In 1933 Forster had taken his records on Hitler to Basel and then to Paris, where he gave copies for safekeeping to collaborators on a German emigrant weekly, *Das Neue Tage-Buch*, including Ernst Weiss. On his return to Germany Forster was dismissed from the medical faculty at Greifswald, then interrogated by officials of the university for thirteen days—matching the time of the eyewitness's interrogation by the Gestapo. Thereafter, the fate of the eyewitness diverges from that of Forster, who, as was learned with skepticism in Paris, committed suicide. Binion interviewed Forster's elder son, who recalled that his father, like the narrator of the novel, had been fanatical about keeping Hitler's "medical secret" to himself. Even with Forster dead, German journalists in Paris found the information too dangerous to publish in any case.

Weiss divulged the medical secret in fictional form, but his novel survived his suicide only as a rejected entry in an American competition. Lost for years, it was finally published in Germany in 1963 as *Der Augenzeuge* (*The Eyewitness*). In 1977 Houghton Mifflin produced an English version, with a foreword by Binion identifying Forster behind the narrator. Meanwhile, Weiss, like Forster before him, had shot himself in Paris on 14 June 1940, as German soldiers occupied the city. Unknown to him, Thomas Mann and Eleanor Roosevelt had obtained an immigration visa and plane ticket to the United States for him.

In the novel the eyewitness is assigned to the hospital at "P," where he treats soldiers emotionally crippled on the field: nervous, sensitive, hysterical, neurasthenic. One of his patients, AH, is emaciated, blind, and highly excitable from lack of sleep, a fanatical agitator requiring disciplining. Gassed by a grenade, his eyes "burned like glowing coals." [78] Weiss here and later drew wording from Hitler's own account of the event recalled in *Mein Kampf.* At night he gathers soldiers around his bed and incites them to hatred, blaming the Jews for Germany's failure.

The eyewitness hypnotizes him and instructs him to will himself to see, and then to be able to sleep. It works. "I had played fate—God—and had given the blind man his eyesight."[79] AH rises to power, mesmerizing audiences of thousands with a message that dejected and demoralized Germany too can recover by a miracle cure. The eyewitness keeps his case notes and buries them deep in a moor.

Weiss's narrator questions whether AH's racial hatred could be blamed on an erotic experience that he then links with syphilis by supposing that it would forbid future sexual activity by contaminating the blood:

> The blind hatred of the Jews returned again and again—it was the mysterious core of his soul. I knew well that I had cured him forever from his hysterical blindness, for a time from his hysterical sleeplessness, but not ever for a second from his hatred of the Jews. Had he fallen prey perhaps to a Jewish woman, a *Judt*, in his time of misery in Vienna? Was his chastity voluntary or compulsory? Could he no longer give himself to a woman of his race, of his German blood? Did this torture him, did this make him sleepless, did this make him loveless, insatiable, and did this give him his monstrous, fanatic power? Did he have this splinter under his fingernail so that he struck out with such a brutal fist?[80]

A man in a party uniform asks to speak to the eyewitness. He demands the papers on AH. The eyewitness refuses, then takes the papers from the moor and puts them in a fireproof safe. But the papers bother him in his house. He mails them to himself to general delivery at a distant post office, where they will be held for three months. Finally he decides he must hide them in Switzerland. He drives to Basel, where at the Federal Central Bank he rents a safe deposit box. Lured back supposedly to save his wife, he is arrested, interrogated mercilessly for thirteen days, and beaten almost to death. Still he will not give in: "Don't let them make you divulge your secret," he tells himself. "Hold fast!"[81]

Allowed to escape, the eyewitness is reunited with his wife. When he goes to the safe deposit box, it is empty; his holding out against torture was in vain. She had paid for his release with the papers, at the urging of their friend Helmut. And yet, even though the Gestapo now has the medical records of Patient AH, still they do not have the medical secret. The eyewitness describes the circumstances:

> One day he [Helmut] did begin to speak about matters to which there had been passing references—that he had paid for my rescue with a kind of disgrace. To be sure, he had given the notes, which I had put into the safe deposit box—down to the last sheet—to the Secret State Police, but not even they were received with favor. The most important part was supposed to be missing, that is, the part concerning relationships with women. It is true that in the long conversation in P. I had discovered much that has been kept from public knowledge. But even in 1918 I had not written a word of that. I still know it all. It is a case of too great importance. But you will look in vain for anything here. This secret, too, I wrote down in hieroglyphics which no one but me can decipher.[82]

What was the eyewitness's, and presumably Forster's, medical secret that concerned AH's relationships with women? In the introduction to *Explaining Hitler*, Ron Rosenbaum expresses the yearning behind his own search for an explanation of Hitler's psyche, the Holocaust, the nature of evil—his wish to find a Swiss safe deposit box with the document containing Forster's revelation: "the secret of Hitler's sex life hieroglyphically entombed in a safe-deposit box by the Pasewalk mesmerist."[83] Rosenbaum concludes with a plaintive wish for that lost key that could make sense of Hitler: "Yes something is missing . . . something here on earth, something we can contain in our imagination, something safely containable within the reassuring confines of a box in a Swiss bank. Something not beyond our ken, just beyond our reach, something less unbearably frightening than inexplicable evil"[84]— the apocryphal grail, he calls it, of Hitler explanation.

Syphilis was the secret in the Pasewalk report given to Heinrich Himmler in 1942. Was it also the non-apocryphal secret hidden in the mesmerist's safe deposit box in Basel?

One part of the report in Himmler's black dossier had to do with Hitler's current medical condition as reported by Morell and Brandt. The other part had to do with Hitler's having signs of syphilis at Pasewalk. How might a copy of the Pasewalk medical report have found its way into Himmler's hands? If at first it seemed impossible to track the medical records of an unknown soldier treated at Pasewalk hospital during World War I, especially after Hitler had given Frick the order to confiscate and destroy them, it soon became obvious that there were numerous possibilities for this information to have been retrieved and delivered to Himmler in 1942. In fact, there were a number of possible sets of health records kept (and multiple copies of some of them): Forster's case records, the summary hospital record, and the report that was issued to the military when Hitler was released as cured. Forster made two copies of his records for safekeeping by the German exile circle in Paris, one of which went to Ernst Weiss. And of course, he may also have left a third copy in a safe deposit box in Basel, as recorded in the novel.

The Gestapo seized various records over the years, raising the question of who within the Gestapo did the seizing—problematic for Hitler given how many people within his own organization were his enemies and how disturbing a report that the führer had syphilis would have been to the upper levels of the SS. Who could be trusted? According to Walter Schellenberg, Reinhard Heydrich, chief of the Security Police, gathered all of Hitler's health records, which had been transferred to Himmler after Heydrich's assassination in 1942. If this is true, then Himmler had information about Hitler's health before receiving the black dossier, adding weight to the possibility that he commissioned Brandt and Morell to write an opinion.

A copy of the Pasewalk report was included in the records of the Putsch trial. According to Binion, a political enemy of Hitler's from the Putsch days, Wilhelm Hoegner, had a copy of a document on Hitler in Pasewalk from the Putsch trial until the Gestapo seized it in 1933.[85] Göring ran the Gestapo then, but Himmler was in charge of the police in Bavaria when the Hoegner copy was seized. According to Binion, copies of Forster's formal case record were kept under cover by Wilhelm Canaris (chief of the Wehrmacht's secret service) and Himmler himself. Evidently General von Bredow had one, too, when he was shot in the Röhm Purge of 1934. In short, there were so many copies of medical records on Hitler from Pasewalk in existence that it would be surprising if at least one copy had not eventually made its way to Himmler.

Returning to Himmler's report, we still have the mystery of the identity of the third man. If Himmler already had a copy of Hitler's medical records, he might have approached Brandt and Morell directly for an update on Hitler's health. But Kersten had read the report bearing the signatures of Karl Brandt and Morell, and yet he still asked Himmler's secretary, Rudolf Brandt, for the identity of "the man whose integrity could not be questioned." Who at that time would have had copies of the Pasewalk documents, could have approached Brandt and Morell for an update report on Hitler's current health, and would have been the man of responsibility and integrity able to bring the information to Himmler?

Three men in Hitler's entourage at the time are known to have had Hitler's past health records in their possession: Reinhard Heydrich, Wilhelm Canaris, and Wilhelm Frick. Heydrich is out because he had already been assassinated and his papers transferred to Himmler. According to Walter Schellenberg, Admiral Wilhelm Canaris, former chief of the Wehrmacht's secret service, had a copy of Hitler's confiscated Pasewalk record. Canaris met frequently with Himmler in 1942 and, as a key figure in the resistance against Hitler and the planning of the 20 July 1944 assassination attempt, would have had good reason for wanting Himmler to be aware of Hitler's dangerous condition. Without suspecting Canaris himself of conspiring, Himmler once remarked to him that he knew of a revolt being planned. An outraged Hitler fired Canaris in 1943 when he was linked to the defection of key German spies to the Allies in Turkey. Canaris was involved with army conspirators in numerous assassination and coup attempts. He divulged a number of strategic secrets to the English. In March 1943 he flew to Smolensk to help plan the 20 July assassination attempt, but he was placed under house arrest before the conspirators' time came. The Nuremberg trials revealed Canaris's attempt to put a stop to genocide in occupied Russia.

Another candidate, and perhaps a likelier one, for Himmler's high-level courier of unquestionable integrity was Dr. Wilhelm Frick, Hitler's minister of the interior since January 1933. Frick had been with Hitler from the beginning, arrested along with Streicher and others in the Beer Hall Putsch and convicted then of high treason. Frick and Hitler together had originally appointed Himmler to his position of power. Frick has been connected to three confiscations of Hitler's health records: Spiethoff's records, Hoegner's records, and the Pasewalk documents. How much was Frick aware of Hitler's increasing mental instability? Frau Frick may have been expressing the family opinion when she responded to a comment that Hitler was leading the country headlong to disaster with the response: "Yes, the man is insane."[86]

DIAGNOSIS AND THE HITLER BIOGRAPHERS: OVERLOOKING SYPHILIS

When David Irving published *The Secret Diary of Hitler's Doctor* in 1983, he suggested that myths about Adolf Hitler having syphilis were "slain" by the negative results of blood tests sent anonymously to a laboratory in 1940 under the name of "Patient A" by Morell. But Irving was being hasty. The classic medical texts of syphilology warn against being misled by inaccurate blood tests. Stokes wrote: "A patient may have a negative Wassermann for years and still die of syphilis,"[87] especially in late, burned out, and partially treated cases. He cited numerous studies in which there were high percentages of false negatives in late syphilis. One study is of particular note with regard to Hitler. In a Mayo Clinic study of syphilis patients in 1920–1921, 56 percent had negative Wassermanns. This particular group had in common one key symptom of late syphilis: gastrointestinal pain. In 1936 the Cooperative Clinic Group found positive Wassermanns in only 52 percent of patients who had received previous treatment. The blood Wassermann was close to 100 percent accurate only in the brief window of time when a fresh syphilis lesion was teeming with spirochetes. Hitler would have been infected three decades before the blood work was done, with numerous opportunities for him to have received treatment in between. The original designers of the Tuskegee Syphilis Study questioned using the Wassermann as a screen for their subjects because they expected to lose 25 percent through false negatives, even though the men were young and the disease largely untreated. Even the Hestons, who, favoring a diagnosis of amphetamine toxicity, did not think Hitler had tertiary syphilis, noted that a negative Wassermann did not preclude a previous infection, and since syphilis was incurable, a previous infection meant a possible ongoing infection.

The negative Wassermann, misread as cast-iron proof, has been used retrospectively many times to deny other clues to syphilis in Hitler. If the Wassermann was negative, then there must never have been an episode with a prostitute in Vienna, Kersten must have made up his interview with Himmler, and Hitler must never have been tagged with syphilis in Pasewalk or treated for syphilis by Bodo Spiethoff or anyone else.

"The urinalysis established, as stated, that Hitler had never contracted syphilis,"[88] Irving added. But urinalysis is not used for diagnosing syphilis. Erroneous opinions about the syphilis tests

have kept subsequent biographers and medical scholars from seeing that Hitler's decline, both physical and mental, in the last years
of World War II was consistent with the ravages of tertiary syphilis.
Irving was optimistic when he claimed that with his publication
of the Morell diaries "the medical picture of the world's most famous dictator, Adolf Hitler, is now complete."[89]

The blood tests are not definitive. Hitler and Morell might not
be trusted to tell the truth even if the results had been positive.
And if they were covering up a case of rapidly progressing syphilis,
then we can't really trust that the blood of the anonymous "Patient A" even belonged to Hitler. Perhaps "Patient A" and his
Leibarzt were just splendidly successful in keeping their secret.

Ian Kershaw observed that despite the massive amount of research
done on Hitler, there is only a handful of "full, serious scholarly
biographies."[90] Of the serious, scholarly biographers, only Alan
Bullock considers syphilis, and he gives it one brief paragraph in
his 1953 biography, picking up Putzi Hanfstaengl's comment but
describing it as rumor instead of firsthand information. Bullock
wrote, "According to reports which Hanfstaengl, for example, re-
peats, Hitler contracted syphilis while he was a young man in Vienna. This may well be malicious gossip but it is worth adding that
more than one medical specialist has suggested that Hitler's later
symptoms—psychological as well as physical—could be those of a
man suffering from the tertiary stage of syphilis. Unless, however, a
medical report on Hitler should some day come to light this must
remain an open question."[91] Bullock concluded that Hitler suffered very little from ill health until 1943, and he saw that little as
psychosomatic.

The medical report on Hitler that Bullock hypothesized did
exist, at least in code, in Morell's papers, buried by a German officer at the end of the war. When these documents were found in
1959, they were shipped to the United States and microfilmed for
the National Archives in Washington, where the Hestons used
them (T253 reels 34–45) as a main source for their *Medical Casebook of Adolf Hitler.* Four years later David Irving published an ed-

ited version of the Morell diaries, using additional Morell material that had shown up at the National Archives "out of the blue" in 1981 (T253, reel 62).

As a professor of psychiatry, Leonard Heston concentrated on Hitler's mental condition and concluded that he was showing the signs of amphetamine abuse. Albert Speer, in an introduction to the Hestons' volume, agreed: "I drew up an account several hundred pages long of my observations of Hitler and my experiences with him as his close associate. The sections dealing with the changes in his character read like an anticipatory corroboration of the results of the Hestons' researches."[92]

The Hestons noted that Himmler had suggested central nervous system syphilis, entering on their calendar next to 1937: "Himmler: 'signs of neurosyphilis,' from the Kersten memoir." They observed: "Syphilis is protean in its manifestations, a notorious imitator of other diseases."[93] Yet they concluded that syphilis need not be considered further for two reasons. The first was that there was no dementia and, in particular, no loss of memory. "Dementia invariably occurs in neurosyphilis usually as a first manifestation, but if not initially, it appears within a few months. The second was that syphilis produces distinctive eye signs whereas a competent examination by Dr. Löhlein turned up no such abnormalities."[94] But character changes in neurosyphilis happen gradually; it can take many years for full-blown paresis with dementia to manifest. Hitler died before paresis or dementia was an issue. Many sources noted that Hitler's legendary memory was slipping. And although Löhlein did not find fixed and irregular pupils, he did find other signs of syphilis of the eye.

"While Dictator of Germany," the Hestons wrote, "Adolf Hitler had major illnesses of three organ systems: gastrointestinal, nervous, and vascular. That he was seriously ill is obvious from published descriptions of him but little attention has been paid to either the nature of the illnesses or their likely historical significance."[95] They ascribed this neglect to a lack of sufficient evidence such as they felt they had now amassed, both through the Morell papers and through their interviews with those who knew Hitler in his last days. Even though they dismissed syphilis in favor of their amphetamine theory to describe Hitler's late symptoms, they correctly noted that a negative Wassermann would not rule out earlier infection. And since there was no cure for syphilis, early infection meant continuing infection. They described the progression of Hitler's disease in language that suggests syphilis: "From at least mid-1942 until his suicide in April 1945 Hitler was intermittently incapacitated by organic brain disease with known signs, symptoms, and predictable effects on behavior."[96]

Fritz Redlich summarized previous medical biographers in a footnote, counting a mere handful of books and articles on Hitler's medical history. Each of his sources quickly and casually dismisses syphilis. For example, Anton Neumayr wrote: "Syphilis can be excluded with a probability bordering on certainty;"[97] Bert Edward Park concluded: "the absence of a profound dementia and the negative serology for syphilis documented in Morell's diary are evidence enough to discredit the possibility of this disease in Hitler's case."[98]

One person has considered that Hitler was a paretic: Alexander Kimel, a Holocaust survivor, has posted the information on his website. It is Kimmel's hypothesis that when Hitler disappeared from sight in 1908, inexplicably leaving no forwarding address, the reason may have been because he had contracted syphilis. Hitler had left his family home in Linz for Vienna in February 1908 (the year Putzi gave for infection). In his first months there, he dressed elegantly in a dark overcoat and carried an ivory-handled walking stick. He and Gustl, his friend from Linz and roommate in Vienna, attended the opera, especially Wagnerian opera. He saw *Tristan* more than thirty times. And then he disappeared, without a word to Gustl; when he surfaced again, he had undergone a transformation. By Christmas 1909 he was, in the words of Ian Kershaw, thin and bedraggled and lice-ridden; he had "reached rock bottom" and "joined the tramps, winos, and down-and-outs in society's basement."[99]

In 1998 Fritz Redlich, the retired dean of the Yale Department of Psychiatry, published *Hitler: Diagnosis of a Destructive Prophet,* the most complete study to date of Hitler's physical and mental ailments. Redlich wrote: "It is certain, however (and I rarely use this word) that Hitler did not suffer from general paresis, a severe meta-syphilitic illness with easily diagnosed signs and symptoms including rapid mental deterioration, psychotic and usually absurdly grandiose behavior, characteristic and easily recognized neurologic signs (such as irregular pupils that do not react to light), a severe dysarthria, and in untreated cases, positive tests for syphilis in serum and spinal fluid."[100] Redlich is correct: Hitler did not suffer from paresis, but again that doesn't mean that he was not in the warning stage.

There is no definitive proof that Adolf Hitler had syphilis, any more than there is undeniable evidence that he did not. A pattern of an ongoing syphilitic infection can be seen clearly enough in his life, however, to warrant reopening the file and posing some hard questions. What would be different if Hitler were infected in 1908 with a disease that he believed had a Jewish origin and tainted him sexually, that would have defined him from youth as an outsider, and that progressively ravaged his body and mind?

PART IV
Pox Gallery

A Gallery of Pox
The Myth of Syphilis

PHILIPPE RICORD, ACCUSED OF SEEING SYPHILIS EVERY-
where, retorted that he had not seen it nearly enough. Ellis H.
Hudson estimated an infection rate of 15 percent for treponemal
disease in an average untreated population. To get a full sense of
the enormity of the public health crisis, consider if 15 percent of a
population today were infected with a chronic, incurable, sexually
transmitted disease that could lead to dementia and death. Of
course, AIDS in some parts of the world today immediately comes
to mind.

The success with which syphilis was kept secret in individual
cases, the frequency of misdiagnoses, and the practice of failing to
record it on a death certificate all contributed to its being underestimated. Although the numbers would suggest that many well-
known people would have been infected prior to the use of penicillin in 1943, today even most historians can only recall a few
known syphilitics. Al Capone and Randolph Churchill seem to
have the highest name recognition.

Many people have been labeled, either casually or maliciously, as
having had syphilis, often with very little substantiation. Early in the
twentieth century, Iwan Bloch, the major proponent of the argument that syphilis came from Hispaniola, published an article suggesting that philosopher Arthur Schopenhauer was infected in
1813,[1] and this was the origin of his pessimism. Schopenhauer prac-

ticed one of the more fanciful prophylactics of the time: He bathed his penis in a glass of water to which a pinch of chloride of lime had been added. A smear campaign during his first election accused Franklin Delano Roosevelt of having syphilis; when his coffin was closed and no autopsy was performed, the rumor circulated again. According to Albert Speer, that was a story Hitler was fond of repeating. In *Einstein's Daughter: The Search for Lieserl*, Michele Zackheim dropped without further comment that Einstein may have infected Mileva Maric, the Serbian woman who was his first wife.

Suspected (or known) syphilitics include Idi Amin, Darwin, Donizetti, Dostoevsky, Dürer, Lenin, Meriwether Lewis, Mozart, Napoleon, Paganini, Edgar Allan Poe, Rabelais, Stalin, Tolstoi, and Woodrow Wilson. The list of syphilitics includes kings, queens, and emperors, popes and cardinals, sublime artists and vicious criminals. Cardinal Wolsey was accused of infecting Henry VIII by breathing into his ear. Bloody Mary had the signs of congenital syphilis. The painter of stylish café life and brothels, Henri Toulouse-Lautrec, died paralyzed in a sanatorium when he was thirty-five. The following vignettes tell of several well-known figures whose syphilis has not been questioned, except for Goya, about whom there is some debate.

IVAN THE TERRIBLE, 1530–1584

One of the most bloodthirsty syphilitics was Ivan IV of Russia, also known as the Terrible or the Awesome. At twenty-three, Ivan had a serious illness with a high fever that may have been the beginning of his disease. Later he ingested large quantities of mercury from a cauldron he kept bubbling in his bedroom. During his reign he had enemies flogged, hanged, burned, boiled, and variously mutilated. Vengeance for an alleged conspiracy in the town of Novgorod meant thousands were flogged to death, roasted over slow fires, and shoved under the ice. Corpses made the river overflow its banks. He was served by a corps of henchmen known as the Oprichniki, who dressed in black, rode black horses, and terrorized the countryside. Ivan led them in sacrilegious masses, after which they engaged in orgies of rape and torture. Ivan stabbed his son to death after they argued over Ivan's beating his pregnant daughter-in-law and causing her to miscarry. Ivan married eight times. When he discovered his seventh wife, Maria, was not a virgin on his wedding night, he had her drowned the next day. He claimed to have deflowered one thousand virgins. Ivan died of an apoplectic fit while preparing for a game of chess. In his last days, sleepless and terrified, he rubbed his hoard of jewels and claimed they had curative powers.

GOYA, 1746–1828

At age forty-six the painter Goya suffered for several months with an illness that caused deafness with tinnitus, blindness, disorientation, abdominal distress, weakness, and general malaise. His friend Zapater's comments that the illness was caused by improper behavior led to speculation about a venereal cause: "His lack of reflection has caught up with him, but now we must regard him with the compassion that his disgrace demands, and as a sick man, for whom all remedies must be procured."[2] Goya recuperated but remained deaf.

He first became ill on a trip to Andalusia. Too sick to continue traveling, he stopped in Cadiz at the home of his friend Sebastian Martinez, where he remained bedridden with colicky pains for two months. Zapater answered a letter from Martinez with worry about their friend Goya: "Since the nature of his malady is of the most fearful, I am forced to think with melancholy about his recuperation."[3] Goya was unable to write, Martinez said, because of trouble in his head, "where all the illness lies." He lost his appetite and had such vertigo that he could not walk up and down stairs. He experienced unusual moods, "raving with a humor that I myself cannot stand."[4]

Goya was never the same after that illness. In his painting brightly colored lyrical images gave way to a different style, with themes of insanity and witchcraft and titles such as *The Sleep of Reason Produces Monsters* and *Old Woman and Skeletal Figure Eating.* In 1819 he had another serious illness. When he developed urological problems in 1825, three physicians discovered paralysis and hardening of the bladder. Goya was eighty-two when he died in Bordeaux.

The authors of "What Ailed Goya" note that although several early investigators speculated that he had syphilis, they find the diagnosis unlikely because he lived thirty-six years after his initial illness and remained creative for the rest of his life. But four decades is not an unusual time for the progression of a case of syphilis; what is atypical is how late he was infected. They consider numerous other diagnoses including lead or quinine toxicity, malaria, measles, vogt-koyanagi–harada disease, Cogan's Syndrome, meningitis, encephalitis, and giant cell arteritis.

HEINRICH HEINE, 1797–1856

In "Five Illustrious Neuroluetics," MacDonald Critchley presents the following portrait of the German poet whom Nietzsche once described as his only equal in the German language. Heine's symptoms of tabes dorsalis began in 1837, with violent ocular pain, but he was not diagnosed until 1849, when he was treated by the Hungarian doctor David Gruby. Heine's physical degeneration was lyrically expressed throughout his poetry:

> *I am but cinder,*
> *Mere matter, rubbish, rotten tinder,*
> *Losing the shape we took at birth,*
> *Mouldering again to earth in earth*[5]

He spoke of paralysis like an iron band pressed into his chest. Sight failed in his left eye and he had to prop up his drooping eyelids with his fingers to be able to see, his insensitive lips could not feel his wife's kisses, and his food tasted like dirt. His legs had the texture of cotton wool. Eagerly he studied medical texts, jesting that he planned to lecture in heaven on earthly doctors' stupidity in dealing with spinal complaints. William Sharp's biography vividly describes his condition: "The frost of an undying fever scorched his veins, the frosts of a living death cramped his muscles, unborn agonies took possession of his wracked nerves."[6] When his poems were translated into Japanese, he bemoaned the futility of his spreading fame when his own circumstances were so pathetic. "What does it avail me that enthusiastic youths and maidens crown my marble busts with laurel wreaths, if meanwhile the shriveled fingers of an aged nurse press a blister of Spanish flies behind the ears of my actual body? Of what is it that all the roses of Shiraz so tenderly glow and bloom for me? When in the dreary solitude of my sickroom, I have nothing to smell, unless it be the perfume of warmed napkins?"[7] On his deathbed, he was asked if he had made peace with God. Don't bother yourself, Heine replied. God will forgive me; that is his job.

Heine wrote these words of misery that were set to music by Robert Schumann:

Madness churns in my soul and my heart is sick and sore
Blood pours from my eyes, runs from my body
Hot blood that records my suffering.[8]

JULES DE GONCOURT, 1830–1870

Edmund de Goncourt's portrait of his brother Jules's developing paresis also shows his own despair as he considered ending life for both of them. One of the first signs of mental degeneration happened in a restaurant when Jules emptied a saltshaker over his fish and clutched his fork violently with both hands. In social gatherings, he began to express himself without tact or propriety.

Jules had a premonition that his ability to work would not last much longer, and that was true. He observed that nervous disorders of the body destroy any sense of proportion in human joys and sorrows; they are experienced in extreme form. His brother noted that his face took on the "haggard mask of imbecility."[9] His speech degenerated to fragments of sentences. He cowered under the sheets in terror. Seizures convulsed his body, his arms jerked and twisted in their sockets, bloody foam oozed from his mouth. He died on 20 June 1870 after forty-eight hours in a coma.

EDOUARD MANET, 1832–1883

Auguste Manet thought he had rheumatism when the first signs of tabes dorsalis began causing a limp. He was partially paralyzed when his son Edouard painted *The Portrait of M. and Mme. Auguste Manet*. Like his father, Edouard Manet had tabes dorsalis. He first experienced pain in his left foot in 1878, developed a limp, and used a cane. When a Paris newspaper published a story that Manet was ill, he forced them to publish a retraction saying that his limp was merely the sign of a sprained ankle; thus, his secret was safe.

Manet died after amputation of a gangrenous leg, the result of taking ergot, a fungus from rye and other cereals that smoothes muscle tissue. His doctor had warned against overuse. On 14 August his leg turned black. Five days later it was amputated in the drawing room of his house, and in the general confusion thrown into the fireplace. He died in agony with fever and delirium.

LORD RANDOLPH CHURCHILL, 1849–1895

Frank Harris, teller of tall tales, tells this tale, tall or otherwise, about the experience that supposedly led to his friend Lord Randolph's infection. After a night of drinking, Randolph woke in a strange room with a dreadful taste in his mouth. He saw a strand of dirty gray hair on the pillow next to him. Horrified, he found his bed companion to be an old woman with one yellow tooth that waggled as she called him "Lovie." He threw all the money he had on the bed and ran in terror, with good reason: three weeks later he discovered a syphilitic sore for which he received mercury treatment.

Robert B. Greenblatt wrote of Winston Churchill's father: "It was not the capricious winds of political change that were Lord Randolph's undoing but the cunning spirochete that ravaged a daring and gifted soul, extinguishing his life at an age when his work was not yet done."[10] Elected to Parliament in 1874, Lord Randolph served for twenty years. Greenblatt summarized many manifestations of his disease: "signs of meningovascular syphilis—loss of mental astuteness, recurrent headaches, and bouts of extreme irritability; signs of tabes dorsalis—impotence, retention of urine . . . Charcot's joints, impaired gait and ataxia, and slapping of the feet; and the insidious onset of symptoms of general paresis—changes in personality, poor judgment, speech defects, and dementia leading to complete incapacitation."[11] He also had vertigo, numbness in the hands, increasing deafness, and trouble articulating. His handwriting became tremulous.

Lord Randolph, a stormy statesman who could be both brilliant and vicious, was one of the few syphilitics whose disease was publicly known during his lifetime. His speeches in Parliament were an embarrassment; once when "Randolph got up . . . his face prematurely aged, his hands shaking, his speech so garbled that it became unintelligible after the first sentence, members of the House fled to the lobby. . . . Randolph's face had a terrible mad look."[12]

More about Lord Randolph's decline comes from his wife, Jennie, who went on a world tour with him—bravely, since he was having increasing numbers of mad episodes. She disarmed him in their stateroom when he threatened her with a gun. When he went on berserk shopping sprees, Jennie would circumspectly follow him, returning his purchases. They traveled with a lead coffin since the doctors felt that Lord Randolph might die at any time.

ALPHONSE DAUDET, 1840–1897

Alphonse Daudet, novelist and short story writer, kept a diary entitled *La Doulou*,[13] a detailed chronicle of the excruciating pain that comes with tabes dorsalis, and a description of the horrors of treatment in a nineteenth-century spa. Julian Barnes discovered Daudet's painful odyssey when he was researching syphilis for *Flaubert's Parrot*, and was intrigued enough to translate it.

Daudet received his Pox from a high-ranking lady, a stenographer of the court, a woman of "the top drawer." Signs of tabes were first seen when he was forty-four; he died after thirteen years of illness. The description of his lightning pains is particularly vivid: "Great tracks of flame slashing and lighting up my carcass . . . all the pluckings of the strings of the human orchestra tuning its instruments . . . the human orchestra of pain. . . . tongues of burning coal, sharp as needles."[14] He felt, like the nymph of the Metamorphoses, that he was gradually turning into a tree, a rock. "What I suffered yesterday evening in the heel, in the sides! No words to describe it; one can only cry out."[15] He had trouble urinating, was hypersensitive to noise, complained of numbness, and was mortified by his unbalanced gait. Stomach crises with vomiting happened almost daily.

Daudet had as a friend and doctor the famous Jean-Martin Charcot, one of Freud's professors, the discoverer of Charcot's joint, and the first to describe gastric crises in tabes in 1874. Charcot diagnosed tabes in Daudet when another doctor missed it and sent him to a spa to undergo an experimental traction therapy used in Russia. Daudet was hung from a hook in the ceiling for several minutes, then suspended by his jaw alone for sixty long seconds. The omnipresent Edmond de Goncourt found the dimly lit scene quite indescribable: "a real Goya."[16]

Daudet consulted Alfred Fournier in 1884, eight years after Fournier had revealed the connection between tabes and a previous syphilitic infection, for a swelling of the scrotum. The visit was kept secret from Mme. Daudet. He had surgery and was treated with iodides. Charcot confirmed the seriousness of his condition:

"Long talk with Charcot. It is quite what I thought. I have it for life."[17] In the end the pain was so bad that only large quantities of drugs kept him from screaming.

Marcel Proust observed his friend's pain over ten years, and found him to be refined, and even purified, by his disease: "I saw this handsome invalid beautified by suffering, the poet whose approach turned pain into poetry, as iron is magnetized when brought near a magnet—this poet detached from himself and entirely devoted to us all, absorbed in *my* future and the future of other friends, smiting us and glorifying happiness and love."[18]

ARTHUR RIMBAUD, 1854–1891

Rimbaud wrote his last poem (with the exception of a few small *Illuminations*) when he was nineteen, and so he is one poet with syphilis whose work was not influenced by it, at least if biographer Enid Starkie is correct that he was not infected until 1887 when he traveled to the desert of Somali and in Harar was "less careful or more unlucky than others" and contracted the disease. In Harar he was careful not to use eating utensils used by others because of the open sores in his mouth. In April 1891 he left Harar in a litter with porters carrying him due to a tumor on his knee. His leg was amputated. He experienced progressive paralysis of internal organs as well as limbs. An attempt to revitalize his right arm was unsuccessful. He was hospitalized in November and died on 10 November 1891.

HUGO WOLF, 1860–1903

On 19 September 1897 Hugo Wolf shocked friends with the delusion that as the director of the Vienna opera he could dismiss Mahler. Later that evening he attacked the concierge. Realizing that there was something seriously wrong with their friend, they tricked him into thinking he was going to the opera to sign an agreement and took him to an asylum instead. There he continued to have delusions, thinking himself at various times to be Jupiter controlling the weather and the head of the asylum, planning to heal Nietzsche.

He improved enough to be released, but was unable to work. "The least mental occupation wearies me. I believe it is all over with me. I do not read, do not make music, do not think; in a word, I vegetate."[19] In October he threw himself in the river in a half-hearted suicide attempt but swam to shore. He was admitted to a different asylum, where on good days he could play the piano; other times he forgot his own identity and could not pronounce his friends' names when they visited. He experienced paralytic cramps and spreading paralysis. In August 1901 he was confined to a bed built like a cage, where he stayed until his death on 22 February 1903. His body was carried through the streets of Vienna during a carnival. He was buried near Beethoven and Schubert.

Some musicologists trace the agonized tone of his first important works, the songs of 1877–1878, to his infection. Ernest Newman felt that the supreme master of form in music was not Beethoven or Wagner, but Hugo Wolf. Perhaps this admiration is why Newman's 1906 biography of Wolf tells a story of progressive paralysis and brain disease, without mentioning the word that he knew applied to Wolf's condition, syphilis. According to Alma Mahler, Wolf had been infected in a brothel when he was seventeen. His friend Adalbert, the pianist, gave him as a gift his honorarium for an evening, time with a young woman—a poor gift since Hugo took home with him "the wound that will not heal."[20]

AL CAPONE, 1899–1947

Al Capone became a gangster because he had syphilis; that is the conclusion of his biographer, Laurence Bergreen. Young Al, quiet and withdrawn, turned into the brutal Al. "The Capone we remember was the creation of a disease that magnified his personality. Syphilis made Al Capone larger than life."[21] Mood swings became terrifying homicidal outbursts. He gambled away huge amounts of money with "infantile abandon" in the period before paresis when good judgment goes.

In prison, convict 40886 received bismuth therapy. When he was released, he became the patient of the well-known syphilologist Joseph Earle Moore of the Johns Hopkins Hospital. Not delighted at having the prospect of such notoriety for the hospital, Moore requested that Capone be admitted under an alias. It is from information Moore leaked to his friend H. L. Mencken that we know about Capone's medical history. According to what Mencken published, Capone's wife Mae escaped disease because Al was infected when he was very young.

Capone began to experience symptoms of paresis when in jail in Atlanta. In 1937, when he was transferred to Alcatraz, he had convulsions. He was treated with malaria therapy, but the convulsions returned after nine chills, and treatment was abandoned. Upon release, Capone went to Baltimore to consult Moore, who again tried malaria treatment, achieving a temperature of 106 degrees. Chills happened every other day; Moore planned fifteen of them. Mae, used to mob tactics, imagined that the malaria was meant to kill him. Capone eventually received penicillin, but too late to be of much use. He was a calm patient who usually seemed quite normal, until he began having delusions of grandeur, believing that he owned a factory with twenty-five thousand workers. After four months of treatment in Baltimore, he retired to Florida, where he played pinochle. When he lost, he ordered his opponent shot. Everyone laughed. They would not always have done so.

Epilogue

Pox began with my curiosity about syphilis in the lives of Baudelaire, Flaubert, and Maupassant as a way to learn more about Nietzsche's illnesses. But the project quickly expanded as I found one
reference after another to other cases—all hidden, mostly disputed—in the higher reaches of culture and politics.

Beethoven joined the list against current medical consensus
with William Osler's suggestion of a venereal cause for his typhus.
Van Gogh was added with Ken Wilkie's discovery of the Antwerp
doctor's diagnosis. Ashley Robins's discussion of Oscar Wilde's terminal surgery opened the dialogue in that touchy case. Kathleen
Ferris identified the theme in James Joyce's life and novels. After a
computer search on Constance Wilde's spinal paralysis turned up
Norbert Hirschhorn's article about tabes dorsalis in Mary Todd
Lincoln's medical history, I found that the spectre of syphilis
haunted her husband as well. And finally, Simon Wiesenthal's
search for rumors from Adolf Hitler's youth in Vienna sent me to
Nazi Germany for the longest and most challenging investigation
of all.

If I expected to come to grand philosophical conclusions
about how syphilis drastically changed culture, I was soon hum-
bled by realizing that the challenge of this project was not to speculate about the effect of syphilis on a life's work, or even to come
to a firm conclusion for or against a diagnosis in the contentious
cases (impossible anyway in the space of a short chapter). Instead
the task at hand was to assemble the clues into a recognizable, re-
peatable pattern that would open the question to debate. And so I
began to tell the story of syphilis in these lives by studying rumors

of infection, statements of friends, diagnoses of doctors, treatments prescribed, changing opinions of biographers and medical historians, and finally, the captivating wealth of forgotten information stored away in the old syphilis textbooks.

Looking at these stories today, I am struck by how often the dramatic insanity of late stage syphilis has eclipsed the decades of quiet misery, the exquisite chronicity, that preceded it. Syphilis as the Great Imitator was no abstraction. So many biographers have ignored the theme of syphilis and health in general as if it were irrelevant, or in order to avoid sullying a memory, or in deference to living family members, or because of the indelicacy of venereal disease, or out of a reluctance to confront the inner lives of their subjects.

Some will feel that this five-hundred-year-old shameful secret should remain shrouded in silence, the lid clamped shut on this Pandora's box. But today *T. pallidum*, the ancient, pale, twisted spirochete, still infects and silently reinfects new victims. Its interaction with the sexually transmitted killer HIV/AIDS continues to baffle scientists. Perhaps looking at the experience of those who left a literary archive recording the painful, debilitating, and sometimes euphoric progression of disease will remind us all of the long history that we have shared with this most devious parasite.

Ten Clues to Secret Syphilis

1. Indications of high-risk sexual behavior and infection:
   - Reports of visiting prostitutes
   - Letters revealing infection to close friends and family
   - Rumors spread by friends, often posthumously, about infection

2. A severe fever accompanied by extreme malaise:
   - A minor or severe rash, patchy baldness, mucous patches
   - A sudden change from good health to chronic relapsing illness
   - Self-definition as an outsider
   - Vows of chastity, fear of infecting others, decision not to have children

3. Medical treatment for syphilis, sometimes reported posthumously:
   - Consultation with a syphilologist
   - Treatment with mercury (blackened, rotten teeth), arsenic, or potassium iodide
   - Visits to many doctors and practitioners, unusual cures for a variety of mysterious ailments, spa regimens, and special diets

4. A long list of pains and ailments (progressing):
   Brain: severe headache, meningitis
   Bones: pain in the bones, joints, rheumatic complaints, arthritis
   Bowels: diarrhea, colitis
   Eyes: pain, inflammation, light sensitivity
   Ears: pain, tinnitus, partial or full deafness, vertigo
   Heart: pain in the chest, fear of heart attack

Liver: jaundice
Muscles: pain and episodic numbness or paralysis
Nerves: complaints of "nerves," seizures
Skin: localized rash, lesions
Stomach: acute gastrointestinal distress
Throat: pain, hoarseness, inability to speak

5. Emotional/behavioral warning signs of late syphilis:
   - Antisocial, bizarre, uncharacteristic, even criminal behavior
   - Mania, euphoria, grandiosity, electric excitement
   - Suicidal depression; suicide attempts
   - Irrational rage and/or violent behavior
   - Fear of madness and death, sense of impending disaster
   - Hypochondriasis, neurasthenia
   - Identification with emissary of God; hearing angels

6. Physical warning signs:
   - Changes in handwriting
   - Difficulty walking, paralysis
   - Sluggish, fixed, or unequal pupils
   - Tremors
   - Stolid face
   - Altered heart sounds

7. Insanity and paralysis:
   - Sudden or gradual dementia
   - Being committed to a mental institution
   - Diagnosis of paresis, GPI, dementia paralytica, or tabes dorsalis

8. Death:
   - Death by aneurysm or apoplexy
   - Autopsy report showing signs of syphilis

9. Posthumous diagnostic confusion:
   - Many diagnoses, many diagnostic loose ends
   - Syphilis considered and rejected for insufficient reason

10. Syphilis as a theme in creative work

Case Study from John H. Stokes,
Modern Clinical Syphilology (1926)

Fig. 703.

CUTANEOUS SIGNS OF SYPHILIS IN THE IDENTIFICATION OF EARLY VASCULAR LESIONS. THE PRESENTING SIGNS OF EARLY AORTITIS

A farmer's wife, aged forty-two, examined 1918.

Chief Complaint: Pressure in the chest. "Eczema" left forearm; desired general examination.

Her First Examiner Noted the Following: *Complaint of throbbing* at the back of the neck.

Tightness in chest at times amounting to pain on exertion.

Slight headache, slight *dyspnea,* cold numb arms.

Filled teeth, epigastric tenderness.

"Many reddened areas on left forearm."

Blood-pressure 146/78.

Heart Described as Negative: Noted, however, that second sound was somewhat accentuated.

Blood Wassermann Negative.

Dermatosyphilologic Examination: Patient would not undress, saying she came only for eczema on the arm.

The Lesion on the Forearm is Indurated, Arciform, and Leaves a Slight Atrophic Scar.

The patient denied infection with syphilis or gonorrhea.

"The Cutaneous Lesion is None the less Almost Certainly a Syphilid, in spite of the negative blood Wassermann."

Provocative Procedure: Negative throughout.

The Lesion, However, Vanished Within Eight Days.

On reconsideration and discussion, the patient admitted exposure at age eighteen.

Internist Asked to Reconsider General Findings: Consultant (Willius) reports: *Heart not enlarged.*

Accentuated second sound, especially at aortic area.

Low reverberant systolic murmur at aortic area, not transmitted.

"This, with the History of Retrosternal Pain, Make Aortitis Quite Definite."

Pupils reported very sluggish to light.

This Patient was Placed on Vigorous Treatment with Arsphenamin and Mercury and repeatedly studied during the next four years to watch the progress of the aortic lesion.

She Has Never Had a Positive Blood Wassermann Reaction, and the spinal fluid is normal.

The Valvular Lesion Passed Through a Stage of Accentuation (therapeutic paradox) in which the murmur became audible in the carotids, then much louder, always with accented second sound.

Diastolic Murmur was First Recognized Fourteen Months After Her First Examination: Pain in chest became more marked. For a short time the systolic murmur disappeared. Blood-pressure ranged from 146/66 to 160/86. Transient slight edema disappeared with tincture digitalis 10 minims t. i. d.

Then the Findings Became Stationary, and have remained so for four years, with the patient in excellent health.

x-Ray showed only slight enlargement. Electrocardiogram repeatedly negative. **This is the Stage at Which Syphilitic Aortitis Should Be Recognized** for satisfactory therapeutic results.

DISCUSSION

1. The cutaneous lesion in appearance and behavior under arsphenamin was, beyond reasonable doubt, a syphilid. Note how completely it was underestimated by the first medical examiner.

2. Note that dyspnea, precordial distress, slight hypertension, and accentuation of the aortic second sound were all significant points overlooked by the examiner when it came to interpretation, though he observed most of them.

3. The definite recognition of the early systolic murmur may have been the result of the action of treatment on the aorta or valve between first and second examinations, or have been identified by more expert auscultation.

4. The later appearance of the diastolic murmur marks the development of insufficiency probably from shrinkage of the cusps in healing, for there was no subsequent evidence of an advancing process instead of a healing one.

5. As the insufficiency developed, transient signs of a strain on compensation appeared, but were relieved by digitalis.

6. There is no evidence to date of an advance of the process either at the valve or in the myocardium as in some of the late cases here described.

7. The blood Wassermann reaction has played no part in the diagnosis. Serologic negativity in vascular syphilis is not rare. In late syphilis clinical signs, as here, take complete precedence over laboratory syphilology when they are present. It needs only that the physician shall recognize and correctly interpret them.

Notes

INTRODUCTION

1. Ronald Lehrer, *Nietzsche's Presence in Freud's Life and Thought* (Albany: State University of New York Press, 1995).

2. Deborah Hayden, "Nietzsche's Secrets," in *Nietzsche and Depth Psychology,* Jacob Golomb, Weaver Santaniello, and Ronald Lehrer, eds. (Albany: State University of New York Press, 1999), 295–315.

3. Ronald Hayman, *Nietzsche: A Critical Life* (New York: Penguin, 1982), 219.

4. Joseph Earle Moore, *The Modern Treatment of Syphilis* (Springfield, Ill.: Charles C. Thomas, 1943), 8.

CHAPTER I

1. David E. Stannard proposes these figures for pre-Columbian hemispheric population in *American Holocaust: The Conquest of the New World* (Oxford: Oxford University Press, 1992), 268.

2. Stannard, 70. According to Stannard (74–75), by 1496 the population of Hispaniola had fallen from eight million to less than five million; by 1518 it was less than twenty thousand; by 1535, the native population was virtually extinct through murder, disease, or the slave trade. Stannard's descriptions of the horrors are particularly graphic.

3. Kirkpatrick Sale, *The Conquest of Paradise: Christopher Columbus and the Columbian Legacy* (New York: Alfred A. Knopf, 1990), 148.

4. A. M. Fernandez de Ybarra, "The Medical History of Christopher Columbus," *JAMA* 22, no. 18 (5 May 1894): 649.

5. Sale, 174–175.

6. Samuel Eliot Morison, *Admiral of the Ocean Sea: A Life of Christopher Columbus* (Boston: Little, Brown, 1942), 564.

7. Philip Marshall Dale, *Medical Biographies* (Norman: University of Oklahoma Press, 1987), 18.

8. De Ybarra, 651.

9. Sale, 149.

10. De Ybarra, 651.

11. De Ybarra, 652.

12. Reiter's Syndrome includes arthritis, lower urogenital tract inflammation, eye infections, and skin and mucous membrane inflammatory lesions.

13. Thomas Parran, *Shadow on the Land* (New York: Reynal & Hitchcock, 1937), 33.

14. Christopher Wills, *Yellow Fever, Black Goddess: The Coevolution of People and Plagues* (Reading, Mass.: Addison-Wesley, 1996), 187.

15. Dale, 17.

16. Anton Luger, "The Origin of Syphilis: Clinical and Epidemiologic Considerations on the Columbian Theory," *Sexually Transmitted Diseases* (March-April 1993): 112.

17. De Ybarra, 648.

18. Sale uses the ambiguous phrase "retinal bleeding." De Ybarra downplayed the eye problems, noting only sties due to straining to see land in a diaphanous atmosphere.

CHAPTER 2

1. Ellis Herndon Hudson, *Treponematosis* (New York: Oxford University Press, 1946), 49.

2. Claude Quétel, *History of Syphilis* (Baltimore: Johns Hopkins University Press, 1990), 36. Diaz de Isla published his treatise in 1539.

3. Quétel, 36–37.

4. Quétel, 45.

5. Anton Luger argues that the sailors who returned in 1493 and fought in Naples in 1495 could not have been to blame, since two years and forty-seven days had passed since their return, and syphilis is only contagious for two years. This is not true, however; infectious relapses often occur for several years after the first two.

6. Quétel, 11.

7. According to H. S. Glasscheib, *The March of Medicine: The Emergence and Triumph of Modern Medicine* (New York: Putnam, 1963).

8. Quétel, 42. Note that Squillacio mentions that the disease only lasts a year, suggesting that he had seen cases in 1494, the year before the battle of Naples.

9. Quétel, 17. Grunpeck published in 1496.

10. Christopher Wills suggests that Oviedo may have taken the post to research native remedies for his own syphilis. Christopher Wills, *Yellow Fever, Black Goddess: The Coevolution of People and Plagues* (Reading, Mass.: Addison-Wesley, 1996), 194.

11. Quétel, 35.

12. Mary Spongberg, *Feminizing Venereal Disease: The Body of the Prostitute in Nineteenth-Century Medical Discourse* (New York: New York University Press, 1997), 18.

13. Quétel, 36–37.

14. From *The Encyclopedia Britannica*: Cortés sailed for Hispaniola in 1504 and contracted syphilis there. By 1511 he had recovered enough to take part in the conquest of Cuba and the fall of the Aztec empire. He was accused of poisoning Ponce de León and of murdering his first wife, Catalina.

15. Quétel, 36.

16. Erasmus wrote that "the welfare of the world would be preserved had the first syphilitics been burnt" and recommended that married men with syphilis should be castrated and their wives locked in chastity belts. Was he already infected when he wrote that harsh opinion? When the sarcophagus in the Basel Cathedral was opened for the installation of a new heating system, Erasmus's own bones were revealed to have strange thickenings that on histological investigation proved to have the unmistakable signs of syphilis. See also "Can a Diagnosis Be Made in Retrospect? The Case of Desiderius Erasmus," *Journal of Rheumatology* 13 (1986): 1181–1184.

17. C. J. Hackett proposed the mutation theory; Hudson countered (*Treponematosis,* 49).

18. E. H. Hudson, "Christopher Columbus and the History of Syphilis," *Acta Trop.* 25, no. 1 (1968): 1–16.

19. For a full discussion of the medical dispute at the Court of Ferrara, see Chapter 4 in Jon Arrizabalaga, John Henderson, and Roger French, *The Great Pox: The French Disease in Renaissance Europe* (New Haven: Yale University Press, 1997).

20. Hudson, *Treponematosis*, 39.

21. Loyd Thompson, *Syphilis* (Philadelphia: Lea & Febiger, 1916), 22.

22. For details of this theory, see Simon Wiesenthal, *Sails of Hope: The Secret Missions of Christopher Columbus* (New York: Macmillan, 1973).

23. Olivier Dutour et al., *The Origin of Syphilis in Europe: Before or After 1493?* (Paris: Editions Errance, 1993).

24. Those excavating at Blackfriars noted that the residents relished fish, which can skew carbon dating results.

25. *Secrets of the Dead: Part II: Unlocking the Syphilis Enigma*, directed by Christopher Salt, Public Broadcasting Service, 2000.

26. Bruce M. Rothschild, Fernando Luna Calderon, Alfredo Coppa, and Christine Rothschild, "First European Exposure to Syphilis: The Dominican Republic at the Time of Columbian Contact," *Clinical Infectious Diseases* 31 (October 2000): 936–941.

27. Today Hispaniola is divided into the Dominican Republic and Haiti. On July 9, 1982, a *New York Times* headline announced: "Five States Report Disorders in Haitians' Immune System." Thirty-four cases of a new and serious immune dis-

order had resulted in sixteen deaths among Haitian immigrants to the United States. As the debate continued about Hispaniola being the place of origin of syphilis, it was also being suspected of being the place of origin of the new sexually transmitted disease AIDS.

28. Rothschild bases his findings on distinctions between the way syphilis manifests in a population and the way yaws or bejel do. "Population frequency, absence of disease in subadults, absence of significant hand and foot involvement, and presence of unilateral tibial disease all contrast to findings in populations with yaws. Population frequency, juvenile sparing, unilateral disease, and extent of tibial remodeling also allow comparison with bejel." Rothschild et al., 938.

29. Rothschild et al., 939.

30. Rothschild et al., 936.

31. Personal communication.

CHAPTER 3

1. Lynn Margulis and Dorian Sagan, "The Beast with Five Genomes," *Natural History* (6 June 2001).

2. See E. H. Hudson, *Treponematosis* (New York: Oxford University Press, 1946), for a summary of various theories of the origin of the treponeme.

3. See Hudson, *Treponematosis.*

4. R. S. Morton, "Did Catherine the Great of Russia Have Syphilis?" *Genitourin Med* 67, no. 6 (December 1991): 498–502; from *Documents of Catherine the Great: Correspondence with Voltaire.*

5. "Can Genes Solve the Syphilis Mystery?" *Science* (11 May 2001).

6. For background on the controversy about the place of syphilis in the AIDS epidemic, see the four-part television series made by Canadian filmmaker and journalist Colman Jones, *The Cause of AIDS: Fact and Speculation*, at http://colman. net/aids/video.html. Jones provides film footage from early twentieth-century syphilology.

CHAPTER 4

1. Claude Quétel, *History of Syphilis* (Baltimore: Johns Hopkins University Press, 1990), 52.

2. Quétel, 123–124.

3. Quétel, 142.

4. Fournier was not the first to see this link, but he was the first to bring it to debate and finally to acceptance.

5. E. Hare. "The Origin and Spread of Dementia Paralytica." *Journal of Mental Science* 105 (1959): 594–626.

6. In *Henry IV,* Part I, Shakespeare gives these words to Falstaff: "A pox on this gout or a gout on this pox, for the one or the other plays the rogue with my great toe."

7. Harrison suggests that showers of treponemes in later years can render the blood infectious. *Harrison's Principles of Internal Medicine,* Vol. I, ed. Kurt J. Isselbacher et al. (New York: McGraw-Hill, 1998).

8. For example, a Johns Hopkins syphilis clinic study of 1,200 cases of early neurosyphilis compared Salvarsan, malaria, and a drug for tertiary syphilis, tryparsamide; a Cook County Hospital study counted the number of unnecessary surgeries in 1,000 tabes cases.

9. Jeffrey S. Sartin, and Harold O. Perry, "From Mercury to Malaria to Penicillin: The History of the Treatment of Syphilis at the Mayo Clinic—1916–1955," *Journal of the American Academy of Dermatology* 32, no. 2, pt. 1 (February 1995): 255–261.

10. Today some prefer to call it the "United States Public Health Study on the Natural History of Syphilis."

11. Joseph Earle Moore, *The Modern Treatment of Syphilis* (Springfield: Charles C. Thomas, 1943), 1933.

12. Eunice V. Rivers et al., "Twenty Years of Followup Experience in a Long-Range Medical Study," in *Tuskegee's Truths,* ed. Susan M. Reverby (Chapel Hill: University of North Carolina Press, 2000), 126–127.

13. James H. Jones, *Bad Blood: The Tuskegee Syphilis Experiment* (New York: Free Press, 1993), 134.

14. Peter Buxtun, personal communication, 25 August 2002.

15. Jones, 112.

16. Rudolph Kampmeier, "Final Report on the Tuskegee Syphilis Study," *Southern Medical Journal* 67 no. 110 (November 1974): 1349–1353.

17. Kampmeier, "Final Report," 1349.

18. Tom Junod, "Deadly Medicine," in Reverby, 523.

19. Junod, 515.

20. Those who had been treated for infection early in the disease had lesions and positive blood tests. Those never treated (or only later) had no lesions and negative blood tests upon reinfection. H. J. Magnuson et al., *Medicine* 35 (1956): 33–82.

21. Harris L. Coulter, *AIDS and Syphilis: The Hidden Link* (Berkeley: North Atlantic Books, 1987), 93–104.

22. Helen Dibble and Daniel Williams, "An Interview with Nurse Rivers," in Reverby, 337.

CHAPTER 5

1. Havelock Ellis, *Studies in the Psychology of Sex*, Vol. 6 (Philadelphia: F. A. Davis, 1910), 337, n. 1. Ellis reported hospitals full of children infected with syphilis due to this belief— "the victims not of disease but of superstition."

2. Burton Peter Thom, *Syphilis* (Philadelphia: Lea & Febiger, 1922), 202.

3. N. K. Banerjee, *Homeopathy in the Treatment of Gonorrhoea & Syphilis* (Delhi: B. Jain, 1995), 158.

4. John H. Stokes, *Modern Clinical Syphilology,* 3d ed. (Philadelphia: Saunders, 1944), 168.

5. In Germany, Adolf Hitler first heard about penicillin from one of his doctors, Karl Brandt. His private doctor, Theo Morell, attempted to develop penicillin and was credited by the German press with having done so, but his penicillin was ineffective.

6. Kurt J. Isselbacher et al., eds., *Harrison's Principles of Internal Medicine,* Vol. I, 13th ed. (New York: McGraw-Hill, 1994), 736.

CHAPTER 6

1. John H. Stokes, *Modern Clinical Syphilology*, 3d ed. (Philadelphia: Saunders, 1944), 26. The clinical picture in Stokes's eight stages: (1) inoculation; (2) primary chancre; (3) early secondary—skin lesions (first and second years); (4) late secondary—eruptions disappear but some symptoms persist (second to sixth years); (5) early recurrent—relapses of infectious lesions on mucous surfaces (second to sixth years); (6) latent and late recurrent—lesions are fewer in number but more destructive due to developing allergy and vascular change (fourth to tenth years); (7) late or tertiary—tumorlike masses; (8) late degenerative phase—lesions of cardiovascular and nervous systems.

2. Jonathan Hutchinson, *Syphilis* (New York: Cassell, 1909), 99.

3. Kurt J. Isselbacher et al., eds., *Harrison's Principles of Internal Medicine,* Vol. I (New York: McGraw-Hill, 1998), 731.

4. William Osler, *The Principles and Practice of Medicine*, 4th ed. (New York: Appleton, 1902), 961–962.

5. Stokes, *Syphilology*, 1017.

6. Stokes, *Syphilology*, 905.

CHAPTER 7

1. J. Hutchinson, cited in E. H. Hudson, *Treponematosis* (New York: Oxford University Press, 1946), 26.

2. Jonathan Hutchinson, *Syphilis* (New York: Cassell, 1909), 250.

3. John H. Stokes, *Modern Clinical Syphilology,* 3d ed. (Philadelphia: Saunders, 1944), 41.

4. Stokes, *MCS*, 3d ed., 34.

5. Stokes, *MCS*, 3d ed., 18.

6. Stokes, *MCS*, 3d ed., 38.

7. Mazzino Montinari, "Nietzsche and Wagner One Hundred Years Ago: 1980 Addendum," in *Nietzsche in Italy,* ed. Thomas Harrison (Saratoga, Calif.: ANMA Libri, 1988), 117.

8. N. K. Banerjee, *Homeopathy in the Treatment of Gonorrhoea & Syphilis* (Delhi: B. Jain, 1995), 212.

CHAPTER 8

1. Philip Weiss, "Beethoven's Hair Tells All," *New York Times Magazine* (30 November 1998).

2. Deborah Hayden, letter to the editor, *New York Times Magazine* (10 January 1999).

3. Russell Martin, *Beethoven's Hair* (New York: Broadway Books, 2000), 227.

4. Weiss, 108–110.

5. Edward Larkin, "Beethoven's Medical History," cited in Martin Cooper, *Beethoven: The Last Decade 1817–1827* (London: Oxford University Press, 1970), 451.

6. George R. Marek, *Beethoven: Biography of a Genius* (New York: Funk & Wagnalls, 1969), 312.

7. Marek, 12.

8. Marek, 312.

9. Dr. Elisabeth Prieger, a Bonn doctor and Beethoven enthusiast, concluded that the mercury prescriptions left "the presence of this disease in no doubt. These prescriptions the renowned otologist Politzer had had in his hands." Politzer's son-in-law assured her there was no doubt about these prescriptions. Politzer was known for observing eighth nerve damage early in the disease. Biographer Ernest Newman had no doubt either: "The fact of Beethoven's malady seems then to be beyond dispute" (Larkin, 450).

10. Larkin, 449.

11. Marek, 312: "As early as 1907 the famous physician William Osler thought that the symptoms of Beethoven's putative typhoid infection pointed rather to a venereal infection."

12. Maynard Solomon, *Beethoven* (New York: Schirmer, 1977), 220.

13. Anton Neumayr, *Music and Medicine: Haydn, Mozart, Beethoven, Schubert,* Vol. I, trans. Bruce Cooper Clarke (Bloomington, Ill.: Medi-Ed, 1994), 258.

14. Neumayr, Vol. I, 232.

15. Dr. Carl Smetana, not to be confused with Bedrich Smetana (1824–1884), the Czech composer who became deaf from syphilis and died in an insane asylum

in Prague. Musicologists wonder if the last movement of an 1876 String Quartet (*From My Life*) expresses the whistling of syphilitic tinnitus.

16. Neumayr, Vol. I, 274.

17. Neumayr, Vol. I, 274.

18. Elliot Forbes, ed., *Thayer's Life of Beethoven,* Vol. II (Princeton, N.J.: Princeton University Press, 1967), 779.

19. Neumayr, Vol. I, 240.

20. Neumayr, Vol. I, 242.

21. Neumayr, Vol. I, 244.

22. Marek, 216.

23. Philippe A. Autexier, *Beethoven: The Composer as Hero* (New York: Abrams, 1992), 104–106.

24. Neumayr, Vol. I, 320.

25. Neumayr, Vol. I, 320.

26. Larkin, 440.

27. Neumayr, Vol. I, 312.

28. Neumayr, Vol. I, 310.

29. Jonathan Hutchinson, *Syphilis* (New York: Cassell, 1909), 111.

30. From the autopsy report: "The facial nerves were of unusual thickness, the auditory nerves, on the contrary, were shriveled and destitute of neurina; the accompanying arteries were dilated to more than the size of a crow quill and cartilaginous. The left auditory nerve much the thinnest, arose by three very thin grayish striae, the right by one strong clearer white stria from the substance of the fourth ventricle." Adam K. Kubba and Madelaine Young noted that there was no indication of endarteritis obliterans, often associated with syphilis. "Ludwig van Beethoven: A Medical Biography," *The Lancet* 347, no. 8995 (20 January 1996): 167.

31. Neumayr, Vol. I, 310.

32. Sean Sellars, "Beethoven's Deafness," *South Africa Medical Journal* 48 (3 August 1974): 1585.

33. Solomon, 256.

34. Autexier, 117.

35. Larkin, 460.

36. Solomon, 262.

37. Neumayr, Vol. I, 301.

38. Neumayr, Vol. I, 301.

39. Larkin, 453.

40. Kubba and Young, 167.

41. Martin, 227.

42. Thomas G. Palferman, "Beethoven," *Journal of the Royal College of Physicians of London* 26 (1992): 112–114.

43. Palferman, 113.

44. Palferman, 114.

45. Marek, 6.

46. Larkin, 439.

47. Neumayr, Vol. I, 238.

48. Neumayr, Vol. I, 315.

49. Solomon, 263.

50. Marek, 313, 315.

51. Neumayr, Vol. I, 225.

52. Autexier, 111.

53. Autexier, 79.

54. Marek, 314.

CHAPTER 9

1. Brian Newbould, *Schubert: The Music and the Man* (Berkeley: University of California Press, 1997), 178.

2. Eric Sams, "Schubert's Illness Re-examined," *The Musical Times*, 112, no. 1643 (January 1980): 15–22.

3. Anton Neumayr, *Music and Medicine*, Vol. I, trans. Bruce Cooper Clarke (Bloomington, Ill.: Medi-Ed, 1994), 372.

4. Neumayr, Vol. I, 372.

5. Otto Erich Deutsch, *The Schubert Reader,* trans. Eric Blom (New York: Norton, 1947), 270.

6. Neumayr, Vol. I, 273.

7. Neumayr, Vol. I, 373.

8. Deutsch, 286.

9. Neumayr, Vol. I, 370.

10. Deutsch, 301.

11. Neumayr, Vol. I, 372.

12. Neumayr finds a diagnosis of syphilis to be straightforward, but he concludes that the arm pains were caused by too much piano playing and the headaches by eyestrain, because he assumed that the syphilis was healed from 1824 on. But there was no cure for syphilis then.

13. Deutsch, 363.

14. Neumayr, Vol. I, 377–378.

15. Neumayr, Vol. I, 379.

16. Neumayr, Vol. I, 382.

17. Neumayr, Vol. I, 386.

18. Elizabeth Normal McKay, *Franz Schubert: A Biography* (Oxford: Clarendon Press, 1996), 147.

19. Neumayr, Vol. I, 391.

20. Neumayr, Vol. I, 393.

21. Sams, "Schubert's Illness," 19.

22. Sams, "Schubert's Illness," 21.

CHAPTER 10

1. Anton Neumayr, *Music and Medicine: Hummel, Weber, Mendelssohn, Schumann, Brahms, Bruckner,* Vol. II (Bloomington, Ill.: Medi-Ed, 1995), 238.

2. Robert Schumann quoted in Franz Richarz's diary, in a document of The Foundation of the Archive of the Academy of the Arts, Berlin, 1994. Included in this document are Aribert Reimann, "The Last Years of Robert Schumann's Life: Record of an Illness" and Franz Hermann Franken, "Robert Schumann in the Mental Institution at Endenich."

3. Franken, 11.

4. Franken, 8.

5. Franken, 7.

6. Franken, 7.

7. Peter Ostwald, *Schumann: The Inner Voices of a Musical Genius* (Boston: Northeastern University Press, 1985), 298.

8. Neumayr, Vol. II, 242.

9. Neumayr, Vol. II, 252.

10. Neumayr, Vol. II, 256.

11. Ostwald, 76.

12. Ostwald, 78.

13. Ostwald, 78.

14. Ostwald, 21.

15. Ostwald, 21.

16. John H. Stokes, *Modern Clinical Syphilology,* 3d ed. (Philadelphia: Saunders, 1944), 1075.

17. Neumayr, Vol. II, 241.

18. Neumayr, Vol. II, 263.

19. Neumayr, Vol. II, 264.

20. John Davario, *Robert Schumann: Herald of a "New Poetic Age"* (Oxford: Oxford University Press, 1997), 79.

21. Ostwald, 97. Letter to his mother, 28 June 1833.

22. Neumayr, Vol. II, 266.

23. N. K. Banerjee, *Homeopathy in the Treatment of Gonorrhoea & Syphilis* (Delhi: B. Jain, 1995), 175.

24. Ostwald, 99–100.

25. Ostwald, 101.

26. Ostwald, 103.

27. Ostwald, 113.

28. Eliot Slater, "Schumann's Illness" in *Robert Schumann: The Man and His Music,* ed. Alan Walker (London: Barrie & Jenkins, 1972), 409.

29. Franken, 7.

30. Ostwald, 249.

31. Ostwald, 250.

32. Ostwald, 248.

33. Slater, 410.

34. Ostwald, 259.

35. Ostwald, 270.

36. Ostwald, 270.

37. Ostwald, 278.

38. Ostwald, 292.

39. Ostwald, 294.

40. Davario, 489.

41. Sams, "Schubert's Illness," 276.

42. Neumayr, Vol. II, 362.

43. Ostwald, xi.

44. Neumayr, Vol. II, 359.

45. Davario, 484.

CHAPTER II

1. Alex de Jonge, *Baudelaire: Prince of Clouds* (New York: Paddington, 1938), 55.

2. Roger L. Williams, *The Horror of Life* (Chicago: University of Chicago Press, 1980), 5.

3. Letter dated 10 February 1860, in Williams, 48.

4. Michael Lucey, *Gide's Bent: Sexuality, Politics, Writing* (New York: Oxford University Press, 1995), 9.

5. Williams, 43.

6. De Jonge, 58.

7. Williams, 10.

8. De Jonge, 180.

9. Williams, 30.

10. Williams, 52.

11. Joanna Richardson, *Baudelaire: A Biography* (New York: St. Martin's Press, 1994), 415. Richardson acknowledges that Baudelaire was suffering from the progression of syphilis, one of the few biographers to link his ongoing illness with the disease.

12. Richardson, 417.

13. Richardson, 432.

14. Richardson, 434.

15. Richardson, 434.

16. Richardson, 437.

17. Richardson, 443.

18. Richardson, 446.

19. Richardson, 446.

20. Richardson, 452.

21. Williams, 49.

CHAPTER 12

1. Jean H. Baker, *Mary Todd Lincoln* (New York, 1987), 330.

2. *Congressional Record*, 47th Cong., 1st sess., App. 430; No. 77; House 578, 652–653.

3. Norbert Hirschhorn and Robert G. Feldman, "Mary Lincoln's Final Illness: A Medical and Historical Reappraisal," *Journal of the History of Medicine*, 54 (October 1999): 315–332.

4. Hirschhorn and Feldman, "Mary Lincoln," 535.

5. A. McGehee Harvey and Victor A. McKusick, eds., *Osler's Textbook Revisited* (New York: Meredith, 1967), 342. From *The Principles and Practices of Medicine*, first published in 1892.

6. Hirschhorn and Feldman cite T. D. Pryce, "Diabetes with Ataxia," *British Medical Journal,* 1887, I, 883. See pages 535–536 of their article for more on this hypothesis.

7. Hirschhorn, "Mary Lincoln," 525.

8. Hirschhorn, "Mary Lincoln," 513.

9. Hirschhorn, "Mary Lincoln," 513.

10. Emanuel Hertz, *The Hidden Lincoln: From the Letters and Papers of William H. Herndon* (New York: Viking, 1938), 220.

11. Randolph Churchill was another compulsive shopper during the warning stage of paresis. When he and his wife, Jenny, went on his final European tour, she returned huge quantities of items he purchased.

12. John Stokes found 48 percent of neurosyphilis to be tabes dorsalis, 18.5 percent paresis, and 7.4 percent taboparesis. John H. Stokes, *Modern Clinical Syphilology,* 3d ed. (Philadelphia: Saunders, 1944), 976.

13. Hertz, 259. Douglas L. Wilson cites the letter dated January 1891 thus: "Now let me Explain the Matter in full which I have never done before. About the year 1835–36 Mr. Lincoln went to Beardstown and during a devilish passion had Connection with a girl and Caught the disease." *Honor's Voice* (New York: Alfred A. Knopf, 1998), 127. In a television interview with Brian Lamb (29 March 1998),

Wilson said: "We know that if we believe Herndon—and I do—that Lincoln told him that he thought he had syphilis at one time."

14. William H. Herndon and Jesse W. Weik, *Herndon's Life of Lincoln* (New York: De Capo Press, 1983, 173 n10).

15. Norbert Hirschhorn, Robert G. Feldman, and Ian A. Greaves, "Abraham Lincoln's Blue Pills," *Perspectives in Biology and Medicine* 44, no. 3 (Summer 2001): 323.

16. Herndon and Weik, 169.

17. Gore Vidal, *United States Essays: 1952–1992* (New York: Random House, 1993), 693.

18. Vidal, 667.

19. Vidal, 692.

20. See Hirschhorn and Feldman, "Mary Lincoln," 532, for details.

21. Vidal, 693.

22. Hirschhorn et al., "Blue Pills," 315–332.

23. Hertz, 199.

24. Hirschhorn et al., "Blue Pills," 328.

25. Hirschhorn et al., "Blue Pills," 318.

26. Hirschhorn et al., "Blue Pills," 319.

27. Jan Morris, *A Foreigner's Quest* (New York: DeCapo, 2000), 12.

CHAPTER 13

1. Julian Barnes, *Flaubert's Parrot* (New York: Vintage Random House, 1990), 24.

2. Enid Starkie, *Flaubert: The Making of the Master*, Vol. I (New York: Atheneum, 1967), 91.

3. Herbert Lottman, *Flaubert: A Biography* (Boston: Little, Brown, 1989), 57.

4. Lottman, 57.

5. Roger L. Williams, *The Horror of Life* (Chicago: University of Chicago Press, 1980), 127.

6. Robert Howland Chase, *General Paresis: Practical and Clinical* (Philadelphia: P. Blakiston's, 1902), 133; Jonathan Hutchinson, *Syphilis* (New York: Cassell, 1909): "Jackson distinguished epilepsy due to peripheral irritation, such as from syphilis, from the more typical kind. In Jacksonian epilepsy the spasms usually begin in one limb only and there is an interval before the patient loses consciousness"; Carl H. Browning and Ivy Mackenziem, *Recent Methods in the Diagnosis and Treatment of Syphilis* (London: Constable, 1924): "Epileptic or epileptiform convulsions may happen at various stages in the course of the disease. Exudative meningitis in the secondary stage may be heralded by epileptic seizures. Gummata, like tumors, may give rise to Jacksonian epilepsy with localized phenomena."

7. Lottman, 57.

8. For a summary of the various hypotheses about Flaubert's seizures, especially pro and con epilepsy, see Williams, 204–212. Syphilis has been overlooked in the diagnostic literature, in some cases because it was assumed that Flaubert was not infected until later, in others because of unfamiliarity with syphilitic epilepsy. Williams thought it "probable that Flaubert was not syphilitic by 1849 and was therefore susceptible to infection" (154). Julian Barnes, too, assumed later infection: "1850: In Egypt Gustave catches syphilis," 29.

9. John H. Stokes, *Modern Clinical Syphilology*, 3d ed. (Philadelphia: Saunders, 1944), 614.

10. John Stokes, *Modern Clinical Syphilology*, 1st ed. (Philadelphia: Saunders, 1926), 945.

11. Francis Steegmuller, ed. and trans., *The Letters of Gustave Flaubert 1830–1857* (Cambridge: Harvard University Press, 1980), 117.

12. Steegmuller, 129.

13. Steegmuller, 129.

14. Steegmuller, 135.

15. Benjamin Bart, *Flaubert* (Syracuse: Syracuse University Press, 1967), 221.

16. Barnes, 134.

17. Lottman, 94.

18. Henri Troyat, *Flaubert,* trans. Joan Pinkham (New York: Viking Penguin, 1992), 283.

19. Troyat, 282.

20. Troyat, 282.

21. Steegmuller, 239–240.

22. Troyat, 338.

23. M. Renault in *Le Concours Médical*, 22 January 1939, proposed syphilis as a cause of death. Jean-Maurienne was accused of tampering with Flaubert's reputation when he suggested that an aneurysm in the aorta ruptured forming the black collar, since aortic aneurysm was so often caused by syphilis.

24. Starkie, 305.

CHAPTER 14

1. Robert Sherard, *The Life, Work and Evil Fate of Guy de Maupassant* (New York: Brentano's, n.d.), 189.

2. Sherard, *Evil Fate*, ix.

3. Claude Quétel, *History of Syphilis* (Baltimore: Johns Hopkins University Press, 1990), 128–129. Recall Baudelaire's similar boasting: "Proud as a schoolboy who has just caught his first pox."

4. Guy de Maupassant, "Bed no. 29," in *The Complete Short Stories of Guy de Maupassant* (Garden City, N.Y.: Doubleday, 1955), 574.

5. Sherard, *Evil Fate*, 153.

6. Sherard, *Evil Fate*, 159.

7. Sherard, *Evil Fate*, 203.

8. Sherard, *Evil Fate*, 208. He cites this only as a "private letter."

9. Sherard, *Evil Fate*, 206.

10. Sherard, *Evil Fate*, 235.

11. Sherard, *Evil Fate*, 365.

12. Sherard, *Evil Fate*, 368.

13. Sherard, *Evil Fate*, 353.

14. Sherard, *Evil Fate*, 360.

15. Williams, *The Horror of Life* (Chicago: University of Chiacgo Press, 1980), 258.

16. Williams, 230.

17. Sherard, *Evil Fate*, 372.

18. Sherard, *Evil Fate*, 375.

19. Macdonald Critchley, *The Divine Banquet of the Brain* (New York: Raven, 1979), 213.

20. Sherard, *Evil Fate*, 378.

21. Sherard, *Evil Fate*, 382.

22. Robert Harborough Sherard, *Bernard Shaw, Frank Harris, and Oscar Wilde* (New York: Greystone, 1937), 259.

CHAPTER 15

1. Ken Wilkie, *In Search of van Gogh* (Rocklin, Calif.: Prima Publications, 1991), 146.

2. M. E. Tralbaut, *Vincent van Gogh* (New York: Alpine Fine Arts, 1981), 177–178.

3. Ronald de Leeuw, ed., *The Complete Letters of Vincent van Gogh,* Vols. I–III (Greenwich, Conn.: New York Graphic Society, 1958), Letter 448.

4. De Leeuw, Letter 158.

5. De Leeuw, Letter 164.

6. De Leeuw, Letter 172.

7. De Leeuw, Letter 173.

8. De Leeuw, Letter 200.

9. De Leeuw, Letter 178.

10. De Leeuw, Letter 21.

11. De Leeuw, Letter 195.

12. De Leeuw, Letter 198.

13. De Leeuw, Letter 206.

14. De Leeuw, Letter 209.

15. De Leeuw, Letter 208.

16. Pascal Bonafoux, *van Gogh* (New York: Henry Holt, 1990), 38.

17. De Leeuw, Letter 268a.

18. De Leeuw, Letter 268a.

19. De Leeuw, Letter 192.

20. De Leeuw, Letter 215.

21. De Leeuw, Letter 216.

22. De Leeuw, Letter 268a.

23. De Leeuw, Letter 217.

24. David Sweetman, *van Gogh: His Life and His Art* (New York: Crown, 1990), 158.

25. De Leeuw, Letter 564.

26. Tralbaut, 287.

27. John H. Stokes, *Modern Clinical Syphilology,* 3d ed. (Philadelphia: Saunders, 1944), 1128.

28. Karl Jaspers, *Strindberg and van Gogh: An Attempt at a Pathographic Analysis* (Tucson: University of Arizona Press, 1977), 187.

29. Tralbaut, 287. Tralbault also mentions Dupinet, who diagnosed "meningo-encephalitis luetica."

30. J. Hulsker, *Vincent and Theo van Gogh: A Dual Biography* (Ann Arbor, Mich.: Fuller Publications, 1990), 454.

31. David Sweetman, *Paul Gauguin: A Complete Life* (London: Hodder & Stoughton, 1995), 135.

32. Sweetman, *Gauguin,* 468.

33. For details about David Gruby, see John Thorne Crissey, and Lawrence Charles Parish, *The Dermatology and Syphilology of the Nineteenth Century* (New York: Praeger, 1981).

34. De Leeuw, Letter 481.

35. De Leeuw, Letter 481.

36. De Leeuw, Letter 489.

37. De Leeuw, Letter 574.

38. De Leeuw, Letter 434.

39. De Leeuw, Letter 592.

40. De Leeuw, Letter 589.

41. Jaspers, *Strindberg and van Gogh,* 166.

CHAPTER 16

1. Christopher Middleton found citizens of Turin who say that the horse incident may have happened several days before the collapse. In any case, the onset of

Nietzsche's insanity was sudden. Christopher Middleton, ed. and trans., *Selected Letters of Friedrich Nietzsche* (Chicago: University of Chicago Press, 1969), 352.

2. Middleton, 346.

3. Middleton, 353.

4. André Malraux, *Anti-Memoirs* (New York: Henry Holt, 1968), 23.

5. Graham Parkes, *Composing the Soul: Reaches of Nietzsche's Psychology* (Chicago: University of Chicago Press, 1994), 373.

6. Parkes, 373.

7. Claudia Crawford, "Nietzsche's Psychology and Rhetoric of World Redemption: Dionysus versus the Crucified," in *Nietzsche and Depth Psychology,* ed. Jacob Golomb et al. (Albany: State University of New York Press, 1999), 272.

8. Crawford, 272.

9. Middleton, 335.

10. Thomas Mann, "Nietzsche's Philosophy in the Light of Recent History," in *Last Essays,* trans. Richard Winston, Clara Winston et al. (New York: Alfred A. Knopf, 1959).

11. Karl Jaspers, *Nietzsche: An Introduction to the Understanding of His Philosophical Activity* (Tucson: University of Arizona Press, 1965), 95.

12. See William Schaberg, *The Nietzsche Canon* (Chicago: University of Chicago Press, 1995), for a summary of the number of copies of each book sold in Nietzsche's lifetime.

13. Herman Nunberg and Ernst Federn, eds., *Minutes of the Vienna Psychoanalytical Society,* Vol. II, 1908–1910 (New York: International Universities Press, 1967), 30.

14. Thomas Mann, *Last Essays,* 144.

15. Nunberg and Federn, Vol. II, 31–32.

16. Erich Podach, *The Madness of Nietzsche* (New York: Putnam, 1931), 236.

17. John H. Stokes, *Modern Clinical Syphilology,* 3d ed. (Philadelphia: Saunders, 1944), 479. Joseph Earle Moore included looking for a genital scar to confirm syphilis in his instructions for examinations of the prospective members of the Tuskegee Syphilis Study.

18. Stokes, *MCS,* 1002.

19. Stokes, *MCS,* 1002.

20. H. F. Peters, *Zarathustra's Sister* (New York: Marcus Wiener, 1985), 220.

21. Podach, 61.

22. Sandor L. Gilman, ed., *Conversations with Nietzsche* (New York: Oxford University Press, 1987), 258.

23. Gilman, 257.

24. Gilman, 257.

25. Gilman, 257–258.

26. Walter Kaufmann, entry on Nietzsche in *Encyclopedia of Philosophy*, Vol. V. (New York: Collier Macmillan, 1967).

27. R. J. Hollingdale, *Nietzsche: The Man and His Philosophy* (Boston: Ark Paperbacks, 1985), 33. Hollingdale refers to Blunck's *Friedrich Nietzsche: Kindheit und Jugend.*

28. Peters, 184–185.

29. Pia Daniela Volz, *Nietzsche im Labyrinth seiner Krankheit: Eine medizinisch-biographische Untersuchung* (Würzburg, Germany: Königshausen & Neumann, 1990), 227.

30. Podach, 58.

31. Hollingdale, *Nietzsche,* 33.

32. Gilman, 24.

33. Thomas Mann, *Dr. Faustus* (New York: Alfred A. Knopf, 1948), 155.

34. Mann, *Last Essays,* 145.

35. Angus Fletcher, "Music, Visconti, Mann, Nietzsche: *Death in Venice,*" in *Nietzsche in Italy,* ed. Thomas Harrison (Saratoga, Calif.: ANMA Libri, 1988), 303.

36. I am grateful to Dr. Joseph Henderson, a member of Jung's *Zarathustra* seminar group, for comments Jung made about Nietzsche in the seminar.

37. C. G. Jung, *Memories, Dreams, Reflections* (New York: Vintage, 1989), 101.

38. James L. Jarrett, ed., *Nietzsche's Zarathustra: Notes of the Seminar Given in 1934–1939 by C. G. Jung,* Vol. I (Princeton, N.J.: Princeton University Press, 1988), 637.

39. Jarrett, *Notes,* Vol. I, 609. Baudelaire wrote of the devil in *Flowers of Evil:* "Each day his flattery makes us eat a toad, and each step forward is a step to hell."

40. John Kerr, *A Most Dangerous Method: The Story of Jung, Freud, and Sabina Spielrein* (New York: Alfred A. Knopf, 1993), 175–176.

41. Jarrett, *Notes,* Vol. I, 635.

42. Jarrett, *Notes,* Vol. II, 1492.

43. Nunberg and Federn, Vol. I, 359.

44. Nunberg and Federn, Vol. II, 31.

45. Ernst L. Freud, ed., *The Letters of Sigmund Freud and Arnold Zweig* (New York: Harcout, Brace & world, 1970), 85.

46. Joachim Köhler, *Zarathustra's Secret* (New Haven, Conn.: Yale University Press, 2002).

47. See Rudolph Binion, *Frau Lou* (Princeton, N.J.: Princeton University Press, 1968), for more details about the alleged marriage proposal.

48. Ronald Hayman, *Nietzsche: A Critical Life* (New York: Penguin, 1982), 235.

49. Hayman, 235.

50. Hayman, 235.

51. Hayman, 232.

52. Volz, see 298–305.

53. Hayman, 24.

54. Hayman, 179.

55. Middleton, 146.

56. Middleon, 155.

57. Middleton, 156.

58. Hayman, 194.

59. Hayman, 195.

60. Middleton, 160.

61. According to Loyd Thompson: "There are at first yellowish patches of exudates scattered over the choroid. Later they may become white, due to atrophy of the choroids and be surrounded by a zone of pigment." Retinitis is usually an extension from disease of the choroid. *Syphilis* (Philadelphia: Lea & Febiger), 357.

62. Hayman, 206.

63. Hayman, 210.

64. Hayman, 211.

65. Hayman, 211.

66. Hayman, 212.

67. Hayman, 215.

68. Hayman, 219.

69. Middleton, 171.

70. Middleton, 179.

71. 22 February 1983.

72. Hayman, 261.

73. Middleton, 214.

74. Jaspers, 113.

CHAPTER 17

1. Merlin Holland and Rupert Hart-Davis, eds., *The Complete Letters of Oscar Wilde* (New York: Henry Holt, 2000), 1199.

2. Richard Ellmann, *Oscar Wilde* (New York: Alfred A. Knopf, 1988), 582. Ellmann misspelled the name as "Cleiss" due to the first signature being unclear. A French neurologist correctly identified Tucker's colleague as Paul Claisse.

3. Letter to Douglas William Gray, Esq., 3 December 1933, William Andrews Clark Memorial Library, University of California, Los Angeles.

4. Holland and Hart-Davis, 1228.

5. Letter to Robert Sherard, 3 January 1934, Clark Memorial Library.

6. Arthur Ransome, "Oscar Wilde: A Critical Study," in Melissa Knox, *Oscar Wilde: A Long and Lovely Suicide* (New Haven, Conn.: Yale University Press, 1994), xix.

7. Frank Harris, *Wilde: His Life and Confessions* (Garden City, N.Y.: Garden City Publications, 1930), 376.

8. Richard Ellmann, *Oscar Wilde*, 92 n. Melissa Knox agreed that syphilis was influential: "The impact of Wilde's syphilis on his development as a writer is hard to overestimate. His dread of the disease permeated every aspect of his work." Melissa Knox, *Oscar Wilde: A Long and Lovely Suicide* (New Haven: Yale University Press, 1994), 45.

9. Robert Harborough Sherard, *The Life, Work and Evil Fate of Guy de Maupassant* (New York: Brentano, n.d.), ix.

10. Robert Harborough Sherard, *Oscar Wilde: The Story of an Unhappy Friendship* (London: Greening, 1908), 17.

11. Sherard, *Unhappy Friendship*, 36.

12. Sherard, *Unhappy Friendship*, 14.

13. Sherard, *Unhappy Friendship*, prefatory note.

14. Robert Harborough Sherard, *Oscar Wilde Twice Defended from André Gide's Wicked Lies and Frank Harris's Vicious Libels* (Chicago: Argus Book Shop, 1934), 76.

15. André Gide, *If I Die: An Autobiography* (New York: Random House, 1935), 285.

16. Gide, 289.

17. Richard Ellmann told of Wilde's procuring of the young man for Gide, but delicately left out the part of the story that so incensed Robert Sherard.

18. Sherard, *Wicked*, 10.

19. May 1937, Clark Memorial Library.

20. Boris Brasol, *Oscar Wilde: The Man, the Artist, the Martyr* (New York: Octagon, 1975), 384. (Orig. pub. 1938.)

21. May 1937, Clark Memorial Library.

22. 13 May 1937, Clark Memorial Library.

23. Letter to Symons, 24 April 1935, Clark Memorial Library.

24. Merlin Holland, "Biography and the Art of Lying," in *The Cambridge Companion to Oscar Wilde* (Cambridge: Cambridge University Press, 1997), 14.

25. J. B. Lyons, "Did Arthur Symons Have G.P.I?" in *Thrust Syphilis Down to Hell* (Dublin: Glendale, 1988), 80.

26. Lyons, "Arthur Symons," 88.

27. Macdonald Critchley, "Medical Reflections on Oscar Wilde," *Mem Acad Chir* (Paris) 30 (1962): 73–84, mentions a letter in his private collection in which Sherard reveals this information. He does not name the recipient.

28. Ellmann, 92.

29. A. G. Gordon, "Diagnosis of Oscar Wilde," letter to *The Lancet* 357 (14 April 2001): 1, 209. Old Jess may be found in Robert Rhodes James's biography of Lord Randolph.

30. Ellmann, 94.

31. Barbara Belford, *Oscar Wilde: A Certain Genius* (New York: Random House, 2000), xii.

32. Ellmann, 218.

33. Belford, viii.

34. Ellmann, 265–266.

35. Ellmann, 245.

36. For more information about the legal issues, see Gary Schmidgall, *The Stranger Wilde: Interpreting Oscar* (New York: Dutton, 1994).

37. H. Montgomery Hyde, *Oscar Wilde: The Aftermath* (New York: Farrar, Straus, 1975) gives the sad details of Wilde's incarceration.

38. Anne Clark Amor, *Mrs. Oscar Wilde: A Woman of Some Importance* (New York: Sedgwick & Jackson, 1983), 215.

39. Amor, 224.

40. For a discussion of spinal paralysis from a fall compared with that of tabes dorsalis, see Norbert Hirschhorn and Robert G. Feldman, "Mary Lincoln's Final Illness: A Medical and Historical Reappraisal," *Journal of the History of Medicine* 54 (October 1999) 511–542.

41. Holland and Hart-Davis, 1174–1175.

42. Critchley, "Medical Reflections," 205.

43. Critchley, "Medical Reflections," 205.

44. Terence Cawthorne, "The Fatal Illness of Oscar Wilde," in *Ann Otol Rhonol Laryngol* 75 (1966): 664.

45. John H. Stokes, *Modern Clinical Syphilology*, 1st ed. (Philadelphia: Saunders, 1926), 581.

46. J. P. Nater, "Oscar Wilde's Skin Disease: Allergic Contact Dermatitis?" *Contact Dermatitis* 27, no. 1 (July 1992): 47–49. Belford notes, incorrectly, that a rash is characteristic only of secondary and not tertiary syphilis.

47. For example, George Clinton Andrews describes a syphilitic rash known as pityriasis rosea, a localized macular rash found on the chest, back, and arms (of note: not the face), most frequent in spring and autumn, with lesions that spread rapidly, disappearing spontaneously after a few weeks, only to recur. This condition is marked by a history of constitutional symptoms prior to onset, including malaise and sore throat. *Diseases of the Skin* (Philadelphia: Saunders, 1947).

48. Henry MacCormac, *Jacobi's Atlas of Dermocromes*, Vol. II, 4th ed. (London: William Heinemann Medical Books, 1926), 166.

49. Hyde, *Oscar Wilde: The Aftermath*, 74.

50. Ellmann, *Oscar Wilde*, 95.

51. Oscar Wilde, *The Picture of Dorian Gray* (Mattituck, N.Y.: Amsron House, 1982), 222–223.

52. Cawthorne, 657. Note that Harris did assume syphilis, as shown in a previous quotation.

53. J. B. Lyons, *What Did I Die Of? The Deaths of Parnell, Wilde, Synge, and Other Literary Pathologies* (Dublin: Lilliput Press, 1991), 123. J. G. O'Shea agreed: "Wilde's mental faculties were unimpaired—this is inconsistent with Ellman's diagnosis of neurosyphilis." "Unsullied Wilde," *Journal of the Royal College of Physicians of London* 24 no. 3 (July 1990).

54. Ross wrote that "Hobean, a well-known surgeon operated," but Wilde scholar Ashley Robins found no record of his name in the French medical registry for that year, nor did he find Hennion, Wilde's postoperative wound dresser. Wilde called Hennion a surgeon and he was also called "doctor" by those at the Alsace. Robins is sure, however, that Hennion was the male nurse/surgical dresser and that the surgery was performed by a leading Paris ear surgeon whose identity has still not been established.

55. Frank Harris assumed the operation Ross spoke of was for the excision of a tumor, guessing that it must have resulted from a sore place in Wilde's ear, the result of a fall while in prison.

56. BBC interview, 24 November 2000.

57. Ashley H. Robins and Sean L. Sellars, "Oscar Wilde's Terminal Illness: Reappraisal After a Century," *The Lancet* 356, no. 9244 (25 November 2000): 1841–1843.

58. Burton Peter Thom, *Syphilis* (Philadelphia: Lea & Febiger, 1922), 459–460. Other syphilologists have similar opinions. James Kirby Howles: "Gumma may simulate acute purulent otitis media," in *A Synopsis of Clinical Syphilis* (St. Louis: Mosby, 1943), 296. Joseph Earle Moore, writing on lesions of the ear in the tertiary phase of disease, noted association with an acute inflammatory process in the meninges.

59. William Allen Pusey, *Syphilis as a Modern Problem* (Chicago: American Medical Association, 1915), 88.

60. Clare Elfman, *The Case of the Pederast's Wife* (Chester Springs, Pa.: Dufour Editions, 2000), 182.

61. Holland, 13.

CHAPTER 18

1. Isak Dinesen, *Letters from Africa* (Chicago: University of Chicago Press, 1981), 281.

2. Dinesen, *Letters*, 127.

3. Dinesen, *Letters*, 165.

4. Dinesen, *Letters*, 151.

5. Dinesen, *Letters*, 221.

6. Dinesen, *Letters*, 213.

7. Dinesen, *Letters*, 214.

8. Blixen biographer Linda Donelson found Bror to be a good-hearted person whose "generosity spilled over in his being a womanizer. He shared his affections in every way. I found him a sympathetic figure." From an interview in *Scandanavian Press* 6, no. 1 (Winter 1999): 18–21.

9. John H. Stokes, *Modern Clinical Syphilology,* 3d ed. (Philadelphia: Saunders, 1944), 1012.

10. Rudolph H. Kampmeier, *Essentials of Syphilology* (Philadelphia: Lippincott, 1943), 365.

11. Stokes, *MCS,* 1015.

12. Isak Dinesen, *Out of Africa* (New York: Randon House, 1938), 379.

13. Kaare Weismann, "Neurosyphilis, or Chronic Heavy Metal Poisoning: Karen Blixen's Lifelong Disease," *Sexually Transmitted Disease* 22 (1995): 137–144.

14. Weismann, 142–42.

15. Kampmeier, 369. According to John Stokes, only 56 percent of tabes patients previously treated with arsenicals had both positive blood and spinal Wassermanns. Data from the Cooperative Clinical Studies.

16. Stokes, *MCS,* 1011.

17. Isak Dinesen, "The Third Cardinal's Tale," in *Last Tales* (New York: Vintage, 1957), 97–98.

CHAPTER 19

1. James Joyce, *Ulysses* (New York: Random House, 1986), 534.

2. Cornell University, Olin Library, Joyce Collection no. 31, in Kathleen Ferris, *James Joyce & the Burden of Disease* (Lexington: University Press of Kentucky, 1995), 26.

3. Cornell, no. 534.

4. Cornell, no. 536.

5. Brenda Maddox, *Nora: A Biography of Nora Joyce* (New York: Fawcett, 1989), 27.

6. Maddox, 141.

7. Richard Ellmann, *James Joyce* (New York: Oxford University Press, 1982), 150.

8. Kampmeier was the author of an article critiquing the press for the handling of the Tuskegee exposé.

9. Ferris, 5.

10. Hugh Kenner, "Review of *James Joyce and the Burden of Disease,*" *The Bulletin of the History of Medicine* 70, no. 2 (Summer 1996).

11. J. B. Lyons, *James Joyce and Medicine* (Dublin: Dolmen, 1973), 204.

12. Lyons, *Joyce,* 204.

13. John H. Stokes, *Modern Clinical Syphilology,* 3d ed. (Philadelphia: Saunders, 1944), 641.

14. J. D. Quin, "James Joyce: Seronegative Arthropathy or Syphilis?" *Journal of the History of Medicine and Allied Sciences* 46, no. 1 (January 1991): 86–88.

15. Burton A. Waisbren and Florence L. Walzl, "Paresis and the Priest: James Joyce's Symbolic Use of Syphilis in 'The Sisters,'" *Annals of Internal Medicine* 80 (1947): 758–762.

16. Waisbren and Walzl, 760.

17. Waisbren and Walzl, 761.

18. Stan Gêbler Davies, *James Joyce: A Portrait of the Artist* (London: Granada Publishing, 1982), 392.

19. Davies, 169.

20. Rheumatic fever has been given as the cause of this malaise, but Lyons (*Thrust Syphilis Down to Hell and Other Rejoyceana: Studies in the Border-Lands of Literature and Medicine* [Dublin: Glendale, 1988]) prefers to attribute the combination of rheumatic symptoms with iritis to either sarcoidosis or Reiter's syndrome.

21. Lyons, *Thrust Syphilis Down*, 26.

22. Maddox, 291.

23. Maddox, 301.

24. Ferris, 111. For a longer discussion of Lucia's illness related to syphilis, see pages 105–113.

25. Ellmann, *James Joyce*, 755.

26. Davies, *James Joyce*, 290.

CHAPTER 20

1. Simon Wiesenthal, "Did Hitler Have Syphilis?" in Simon Wiesenthal, *Justice Not Vengeance* (London: Weidenfeld & Nicolson, 1989), 132. See also Alan Levy, *The Wiesenthal File* (Grand Rapids, Mich.: William B. Eerdmans, 1999), 17–22.

2. Ernst Hanfstaengl, *Hitler: The Missing Years* (New York: Arcade, 1994), 123–124. (Orig. pub. 1957.)

3. Personal correspondence from Rudolph Binion, 3 August 2000.

4. Claude Quetél, *History of Syphilis* (Baltimore: Johns Hopkins University Press, 1990), 77.

5. Adolf Hitler, *Mein Kampf* (Boston: Houghton Mifflin, 1971), 257.

6. Ron Rosenbaum, *Explaining Hitler* (New York: Random House, 1998), 197.

7. Alan Wykes, *Hitler* (New York: Ballantine, 1970), 23.

8. Hitler, 247.

9. Alan Wykes, *The Doctor and His Enemy* (New York: Dutton, 1966), 40.

10. Wykes, *Hitler*, 98.

11. On 19 September 1994, *The New Yorker* published this hearsay in a review of Frederic Spotts's book *Bayreuth: The History of the Wagner Festival* (New Haven, Conn.: Yale University Press, 1994): "It seems that, besides putting the little Wag-

ners to bed, Hitler sexually abused Wieland. Spotts has revealed this incident—vouchsafed to him by one of Wieland's children—only since the publication of the book; he had omitted it as irrelevant," 110.

12. Ian Kershaw, *Hitler 1889–1936: Hubris* (New York: Norton, 1998), 44.

13. Robert G. L. Waite, *The Psychopathic God: Adolf Hitler* (New York: Basic Books, 1977), 410. Unfortunately, Waite gives no source here.

14. Joachim C. Fest, *Hitler* (New York: Harcourt Brace Jovanovich, 1974), 204.

15. Hitler, 257.

16. Hitler, 246.

17. Hitler, 59.

18. Hitler, 255–256.

19. Hitler, 256.

20. Hitler, 250.

21. Mary Spongberg, *Feminizing Venereal Disease* (New York: New York University Press, 1997), 160.

22. Hitler, 255.

23. Hitler, 249.

24. Hitler, 562.

25. John H. Stokes, *Modern Clinical Syphilology,* 3d ed. (Philadelphia: Saunders, 1944), 819. In a study of syphilis patients with intense stomach pain, 56 percent had negative Wassermanns.

26. Stokes, *MCS,* 1st ed., 938.

27. James Kirby Howles, *A Synopsis of Clinical Syphilis* (St. Louis: Mosby, 1943), 417.

28. John Toland, *Adolf Hitler* (Garden City, N.Y.: Doubleday, 1976), 824.

29. Leonard L. Heston and Renate Heston, *The Medical Casebook of Adolf Hitler: His Illnesses, Doctors and Drugs* (Briarcliff Manor, N.Y.: Stein & Day, 1979), 17.

30. David Irving, *The Secret Diaries of Hitler's Doctor* (New York: Macmillan, 1983), 87.

31. Irving, *Secret Diaries,* 97.

32. Irving, *Secret Diaries,* 51.

33. Fritz Redlich, *Hitler: Diagnosis of a Destructive Prophet* (New York: Oxford University Press, 1999), 234–235.

34. Stokes, *MCS,* 3d ed., 893.

35. Two American cardiologists recruited by the Hestons to review Hitler's records described the readings as nonspecific S-T changes with no specific pathology associated and concluded that the cardiac abnormalities were significant but of uncertain cause and prognosis. Fritz Redlich engaged four cardiologists to review the medical records; based on their reports, he concluded that the underlying cause of the vascular changes could not be determined. David Irving had Harley Street

specialists review the electrocardiograms; they found defects normal in a man of Hitler's age.

36. Stokes, *MCS*, 3d ed., 906.

37. Letter to Dr. Taliaferro Clark, Assistant Surgeon General, United Sates Public Health Service, 28 September 1932, in *Tuskegee's Truths,* ed. Susan Reverby (Chapel Hill: University of North Carolina Press, 2000), 79.

38. Irving, *Secret Diaries,* 27.

39. Irving, *Secret Diaries,* 50.

40. Heston and Heston, 56.

41. Irving, *Secret Diaries,* 292.

42. Irving, *Secret Diaries,* 300.

43. John H. Stokes, *Dermatology and Syphilology for Nurses* (Philadelphia: Saunders, 1937), 229.

44. Stokes, *MCS*, 3d ed., 959.

45. Stokes, *MCS*, 3d ed., 944. Rudolph Kampmeier agreed, saying that cardiovascular syphilis was the only form of progression or relapse whose incidence was not markedly reduced by Salvarsan treatment. R. H. Kampmeier, "Final Report on the Tuskegee Syphilis Study," *Southern Medical Journal* 67, no. 11 (November 1974): 1349–1353.

46. Stokes, *MCS,* 2d ed., 959.

47. Irving, *Secret Diaries,* entries beginning 7 August 1941.

48. Heston and Heston, 79–80.

49. Joseph Earle Moore suggested digitalis for ambulant cardiovascular patients troubled with moderate exertional dyspnea. *The Modern Treatment of Syphilis* (Springfield, Ill.: Charles C. Thomas, 1943), 290.

50. There is one report of night terror (called paroxysmal nocturnal dyspnea), which occurs with dramatic onset, like an asthmatic attack. Hermann Rauschning recalled: "Hitler wakes at night with convulsive shrieks. He shakes with fear. . . . He shouts confused, unintelligible phrases. He gasps, as if imagining himself to be suffocating. . . . [He] stood swaying in the room, looking wildly about him." Bert Edward Park, *The Impact of Illness on World Leaders* (Philadelphia: University of Pennsylvania Press, 1986), 163. This statement must be taken cautiously, since Rauschning was known to make up stories about Hitler. Park's theory was that the paroxysmal unexplained fear might have pointed to psychomotor epilepsy.

51. Stokes, *MCS*, 3d ed., 932.

52. Stokes, *MCS,* 1st ed., 826.

53. Heston and Heston, 50.

54. The Hestons mention four. Maser added that Stumpfegger voted against Parkinson's in Werner Maser, *Hitler: Legend, Myth and Reality* (New York: Harper & Row, 1971), 231.

55. Maser, 231.

56. Maser saw an assassination plot brewing when Crinis and Schellenberg were going to prepare some medication for Stumpfegger to administer, but he gives no background for this suspicion.

57. Redlich, 293.

58. For a list of the botched would-be assassinations, see Fest.

59. From an evening conference, 31 August 1944.

60. Introduction to Heston and Heston, 13.

61. Anton Neumayr, *Dictators in the Mirror of Medicine: Napoleon, Hitler, Stalin* (Bloomington, Ill.: Medi-Ed, 1995), 240.

62. Albert Speer, *Inside the Third Reich* (New York: Macmillan, 1970), 472.

63. H. R. Trevor-Roper, introduction to Felix Kersten, *The Kersten Memoirs: 1940–1945* (New York: Macmillan, 1957), 11.

64. Kersten, 165.

65. Kersten, 166.

66. Kersten, 166.

67. Kersten, 168.

68. Kersten, 166.

69. Kersten, 171.

70. Kersten, 171.

71. Kersten, 171.

72. Irving, *Secret Diaries,* 122.

73. Achim Besgin, *Der Stille Befehl: Medizinalrat Kersten, Himmler und das Dritte Reich* (München: Nymphenburger Verlagshandlung, 1960), 175.

74. Heston and Heston, 91.

75. "Hitler as Seen by His Doctors," 15 October 1945, from Consolidated Interrogation Report (Cir.) no. 2, Headquarters, United States Forces European Theater Military Intelligence Service Center APO 757, 2. Unpublished.

76. Hilter, 201–202.

77. Hitler, 204.

78. Ernst Weiss, *The Eyewitness* (1963; Boston: Houghton Mifflin, 1977), 95.

79. Weiss, 106.

80. Weiss, 139.

81. Weiss, 159.

82. Weiss, 184–185.

83. Rosenbaum, xlvi.

84. Rosenbaum, xlvi.

85. Rudolph Binion, *Hitler Among the Germans* (DeKalb: Northern Illinois University Press, 1976), 5.

86. Toland, 723.

87. Stokes, *Dermatology,* 202.

88. Irving, *Secret Diaries,* 40.

89. Irving, *Secret Diaries*, 8.

90. Kershaw himself accepts the Wassermann in a footnote: "Later rumours that he had himself been infected with syphilis by a Jewish prostitute were without foundation. Medical tests in 1940 showed that Hitler had not suffered from syphilis." *Hitler: 1889–1936*, 618 n.146.

91. Alan Bullock, *Hitler: A Study in Tyranny* (New York: Bantam Books, 1958), 392.

92. Albert Speer's introduction to Heston and Heston, 11.

93. Heston and Heston, 115.

94. Heston and Heston, 115.

95. Heston and Heston, 21.

96. Heston and Heston, 22.

97. Neumayr, *Dictators*, 280.

98. Park, 348.

99. Kershaw, *Hitler: 1889–1936*, 52.

100. Redlich, 231.

CHAPTER 21

1. Havelock Ellis, *Studies in the Psychology of Sex* (Philadelphia: F. A. Davis, 1910), 320. For details on Iwan Bloch's hypothesis about Schopenhauer, see *Medizinische Klinik*, nos. 25–26 (1906).

2. Ravin and Ravin, "What Ailed Goya?" *Survey of Ophthalmology* 44, no. 2 (September-October 1999): 166.

3. Ravin and Ravin, 166.

4. Ravin and Ravin, 166.

5. Critchley, *The Divine Banquet of the Brain* (New York: Raven, 1979), 205.

6. Critchley, *Divine Banquet*, 205.

7. Critchley, *Divine Banquet*, 205–206.

8. Peter Ostwald, *Schumann: The Inner Voice of a Musical Genius* (Boston: Northeastern University Press, 1985), 149.

9. Critchley, *Divine Banquet*, 207.

10. Robert B. Greenblatt, "The Humiliating Demise of Lord Randolph Churchill, 1849–1895," *Postgraduate Medicine* 75, no. 1 (January 1984): 134.

11. Greenblatt, 134.

12. Ralph G. Martin, *Jennie: The Life of Lady Randolph Churchill* (Englewood Cliffs, N.J.: Prentice Hall, 1969), 321.

13. Julian Barnes, who became interested in syphilis when he wrote *Flaubert's Parrot*, translated this book as *In the Land of Pain* (London: Jonathan Cape, 2002).

14. Critchley, *Divine Banquet*, 209.

15. Roger L. Williams, *The Horror of Life* (Chicago: University of Chicago Press, 1980), 293.

16. Critchley, *Divine Banquet*, 210.

17. Williams, 293.

18. Critchley, *Divine Banquet*, 211.

19. Ernest Newman, *Hugo Wolf* (New York: Dover, 1966), 146.

20. Newman, xii. Wolf's doctor was Joseph Breuer, whose children were taking piano lessons from Wolf at the time; he also was treated by Breuer's colleague, Sigmund Freud.

21. Laurence Bergreen, *Capone: The Man and the Era* (New York: Simon & Schuster, 1994), 46.

Bibliography

HISTORY

Arrizabalaga, Jon, John Henderson, and Roger French. *The Great Pox: The French Disease in Renaissance Europe.* New Haven, Conn.: Yale University Press, 1997.

Brandt, Alan M. *No Magic Bullet: A Social History of Venereal Disease in the United States Since 1880.* New York: Oxford University Press, expanded ed., 1987.

Cartwright, Frederick F., in collaboration with Michael D. Biddess. *Disease and History.* New York: Dorset, 1991.

Cleugh, James. *Secret Enemy: The Story of a Disease.* New York: Thomas Yoseloff, n.d.

Crissey, John Thorne, M.D., and Lawrence Charles Parish, M.D. *The Dermatology and Syphilology of the Nineteenth Century.* New York: Praeger, 1981.

Desowitz, Robert. *Tropical Diseases.* New York: HarperCollins, 1997.

Ellis, Havelock. *Studies in the Psychology of Sex,* Vol. VI. Philadelphia: F. A. Davis, 1910.

Glasscheib, H.S., M.D. *The March of Medicine: The Emergence and Triumph of Modern Medicine,* trans. Mervyn Savill. New York: Putnam, 1963.

Hare, E. "The Origin and Spread of Dementia Paralytica." *Journal of Mental Science* 105 (1959): 594–626.

Hudson, Ellis Herndon, M.D. *Treponematosis.* New York: Oxford University Press, 1946.

Jones, James H. *Bad Blood: The Tuskegee Syphilis Experiment.* New York: Free Press, 1993.

Karlen, Arno. *Napoleon's Glands and Other Ventures in Biohistory.* Boston: Little, Brown, 1984.

McNeill, William. *Plagues and Peoples.* New York: Doubleday, 1998.

Margulis, Lynn, and Dorian Sagan. "The Beast with Five Genomes." *Natural History* (6 June 2001).

Merians, Linda E., ed. *The Secret Malady: Venereal Disease in Eighteenth-Century Britain and France.* Lexington: University Press of Kentucky, 1996.

Morton, R.S. "Did Catherine the Great of Russia Have Syphilis?" *Genitourin Medicine* 67, no. 6 (December 1991): 498–502.

Osborne, Lawrence. *The Poisoned Embrace: A Brief History of Sexual Pessimism*. New York: Random House, 1994.

Parran, Thomas, M.D. *Shadow on the Land*. New York: Reynal & Hitchcock, 1937.

Quetél, Claude. *History of Syphilis*. Translated by Judith Braddock and Brian Pike. Baltimore: Johns Hopkins University Press, 1990.

Rosebury, Theodor. *Microbes and Morals: The Strange Story of Venereal Disease*. New York: Viking, 1971.

Sartin, Jeffrey S., M.D., and Harold O. Perry, M.D. "From Mercury to Malaria to Penicillin: The History of the Treatment of Syphilis at the Mayo Clinic—1916–1955." *Journal of the American Academy of Dermatology* 32, no. 2, pt. 1 (February 1995): 255–261.

Schiller, Francis. *A Möbius Strip*. Berkeley: University of California Press, 1982.

Spongberg, Mary. *Feminizing Venereal Disease: The Body of the Prostitute in Nineteenth-Century Medical Discourse*. New York: New York University, 1997.

Williams, Roger L. *The Horror of Life*. Chicago: University of Chicago Press, 1980.

Wills, Christopher. *Yellow Fever, Black Goddess: The Coevolution of People and Plagues*. Reading, Mass.: Addison-Wesley, 1996.

Zinsser, Hans. *Rats, Lice & History*. Boston: Little, Brown, 1963. (Orig. pub. 1934.)

MEDICAL

Andrews, George Clinton, M.D. *Diseases of the Skin*. Philadelphia: Saunders, 1947.

Banerjee, Dr. N.K., M.Sc., M.H.M.S. *Homeopathy in the Treatment of Gonorrhoea & Syphilis*. Delhi: B. Jain, 1995.

Brown, William J., M.D., et al. *Syphilis and Other Venereal Diseases*. Cambridge: Harvard University Press, 1970.

Browning, Carl H., M.D., and Ivy Mackenzie, M.D. *Recent Methods in the Diagnosis and Treatment of Syphilis*. London: Constable, 1924.

Chase, Robert Howland, M.D. *General Paresis*. Philadelphia: P. Blakiston's, 1902.

Cornil, V., M.D. *Syphilis*. Translated by J. Henry C. Simes, M.D., and J. William White, M.D. Philadelphia: Lea's Sons, 1882.

Dattner, Bernhard, M.D. *The Management of Neurosyphilis*. New York: Grune & Stratton, 1944.

Dennie, Charles C., M.D. *Syphilis: Acquired and Heredosyphilis*. New York: Harper, 1928.

Isselbacher, Kurt J., M.D., et al., eds. *Harrison's Principles of Internal Medicine*, Vol. I. New York: McGraw-Hill, 1998.

Harvey, A. McGehee, M.D., and Victor A. McKusick, M.D., eds. *Osler's Textbook Revisited*. New York: Meredith, 1967.

Howles, James Kirby, M.D. *A Synopsis of Clinical Syphilis*. St. Louis: Mosby, 1943.

Hutchinson, Jonathan. *Syphilis*. New York: Cassell, 1909. (Orig. pub. 1887.)

Kampmeier, Rudolph H., M.D. *Essentials of Syphilology.* Philadelphia: Lippincott, 1943.

_____. "Final Report on the Tuskegee Syphilis Study." *Southern Medical Journal* (November 1974):1349–1353.

Kolmer, John A., M.D. *Principles and Practice of Chemotherapy with Special Reference to the Treatment of Syphilis.* Philadelphia: Saunders, 1926.

MacCormac, Henry, M.D. *Jacobi's Atlas of Dermochromes,* Vol. II. 4th ed. London: William Heinemann Medical Books, 1926.

Moore, Joseph Earle, M.D.. *The Modern Treatment of Syphilis.* Springfield, Ill.: Charles C. Thomas, 1943.

Morton, Henry H., M.D. *Genitourinary Diseases and Syphilis.* 4th ed. St. Louis: Mosby, 1918.

Osler, William, M.D. *The Principles and Practice of Medicine.* 4th ed. New York: Appleton, 1902.

Pusey, William Allen, M.D., ed. *Dermatology and Syphilis.* Chicago: Year Book Publishers, 1930.

_____. *The History and Epidemiology of Syphilis.* Springfield, Ill.: Charles C. Thomas, 1933.

_____. *Syphilis as a Modern Problem.* Chicago: American Medical Association, 1915.

Ravogli, A., M.D. *Syphilis in Its Medical, Medico-Legal and Sociological Aspects.* New York: Grafton, 1907.

Schamberg, Jay F., M.D. *Treatment of Syphilis.* New York: Appleton, 1932.

Simons, Irving, M.D. *Unto the Fourth Generation.* New York: Dutton, 1940.

Stokes, John H., M.D., et al. *Dermatology and Syphilology for Nurses.* Philadelphia: Saunders, 1937.

_____. *Modern Clinical Syphilology.* Philadelphia: Saunders, 1st ed. 1926; 2d ed. 1934; 3d ed. 1944.

_____. *The Third Great Plague: A Discussion of Syphilis for Everyday People.* Philadelphia: Saunders, 1917.

Thom, Burton Peter, M.D. *Syphilis.* Philadelphia: Lea & Febiger, 1922.

Thomas, Evan W., M.D. *Syphilis: Its Course and Management.* New York: Macmillan, 1949.

Thompson, Loyd, M.D. *Syphilis.* Philadelphia: Lea & Febiger, 1916.

CHARLES BAUDELAIRE

De Jonge, Alex. *Baudelaire: Prince of Clouds.* New York: Paddington, 1938.

Hemmings, F. W. J. *Baudelaire the Damned.* New York: Scribner, 1982.

Richardson, Joanna. *Baudelaire: A Biography.* New York: St. Martin's Press, 1994.

Sartre, Jean-Paul. *Baudelaire.* Translated by Martin Turnell. New York: New Directions, 1950.

Starkie, Enid. *Baudelaire.* New York: New Directions, 1958.

LUDWIG VAN BEETHOVEN

Autexier, Philippe A. *Beethoven: The Composer as Hero.* New York: Abrams, 1992.

Cooper, Martin. *Beethoven: The Last Decade 1817–1827.* London: Oxford University Press, 1970.

Forbes, Elliot, ed. *Thayer's Life of Beethoven,* Vol II. Princeton, N.J.: Princeton University Press, 1967. (Orig. pub. 1921.)

Kubba, Adam K., and Madelaine Young. "Ludwig van Beethoven: A Medical Biography." *The Lancet* 347, no. 8995 (20 January 1996): 167.

Marek, George R. *Beethoven: Biography of a Genius.* New York: Funk & Wagnalls, 1969.

Martin, Russell. *Beethoven's Hair.* New York: Broadway Books, 2000.

Palferman, Thomas G. "Beethoven." *Journal of the Royal College of Physicians of London* 26 (1992): 112–114.

Sellars, S.L., M.D. "Beethoven's Deafness." *South Africa Medical Journal* 48 (3 August 1974): 1583–1587.

Solomon, Maynard. *Beethoven.* New York: Schirmer, 1977.

Sonneck, O. G., ed. *Beethoven: Impressions by His Contemporaries.* New York: Dover, 1967.

Weiss, Philip. "Beethoven's Hair Tells All." *New York Times Magazine* (30 November 1998): 108–139.

CHRISTOPHER COLUMBUS

Bradford, Ernle. *Christopher Columbus.* London: Park and Roche, 1973.

Crosby, Alfred, Jr. *The Columbian Exchange.* Westport, Conn.: Greenwood, 1972.

De Ybarra, A. M. Fernandez, M.D. "The Medical History of Christopher Columbus." *Journal of the American Medical Association* 22, no. 18 (5 May 1894).

Dutour, Olivier, et al. *The Origin of Syphilis in Europe: Before or After 1493?* Paris: Editions Errance, 1993.

Loewen, James W. *Lies My Teacher Told Me: Everything Your American History Textbook Got Wrong.* New York: Random House, n.d.

Luger, Anton, M.D. "The Origin of Syphilis: Clinical and Epidemiologic Considerations on the Columbian Theory." *Sexually Transmitted Diseases* (March–April 1993): 110–117.

Morison, Samuel Eliot. *Admiral of the Ocean Sea: A Life of Christopher Columbus.* Boston: Little, Brown, 1942.

Rothschild, Bruce M., Fernando Luna Calderon, Alfredo Coppa, and Christine Rothschild. "First European Exposure to Syphilis: The Dominican Republic at the Time of Columbian Contact." *Clinical Infectious Diseases* 31 (October 2000): 936–941.

Sale, Kirkpatrick. *The Conquest of Paradise: Christopher Columbus and the Columbian Legacy.* New York: Alfred A. Knopf, 1990.

Settipane, Guy A., M.D. *Columbus and the New World: Medical Implications.* Providence, R.I.: OceanSide Publications, 1995.

Stannard, David E. *American Holocaust: The Conquest of the New World.* Oxford: Oxford University Press, 1992.

Wiesenthal, Simon. *Sails of Hope: The Secret Missions of Christopher Columbus.* New York: Macmillan, 1973.

KAREN BLIXEN/ISAK DINESEN

Dinesen, Isak. *Last Tales.* New York: Vintage, 1975.

_____. *Letters from Africa, 1914–1931.* Translated by Anne Born. Chicago: University of Chicago Press, 1981.

_____. *Out of Africa.* New York: Random House, 1938.

Thurman, Judith. *Isak Dinesen: The Life of a Storyteller.* New York: St. Martin's Press, 1982.

Weismann, Kaare, M.D. "Neurosyphilis, or Chronic Heavy Metal Poisoning: Karen Blixen's Lifelong Disease." *Sexually Transmitted Disease* 22 (1995): 137–144.

GUSTAVE FLAUBERT

Barnes, Julian. *Flaubert's Parrot.* New York: Vintage Random House, 1990.

Bart, Benjamin F. *Flaubert.* Syracuse, N.Y.: Syracuse University Press, 1967.

Lottman, Herbert. *Flaubert: A Biography.* Boston: Little, Brown, 1989.

Starkie, Enid. *Flaubert: The Making of the Master,* Vol. I. New York: Atheneum, 1967.

_____. *Flaubert the Master: A Critical and Biographical Study (1856–1880).* New York: Atheneum, 1971.

Steegmuller, Francis, ed. and trans. *The Letters of Gustave Flaubert 1830–1857.* Cambridge, Mass.: Harvard University Press, 1980.

Troyat, Henri. *Flaubert.* Translated by Joan Pinkham. New York: Viking Penguin, 1992.

ADOLF HITLER

Besgin, Achim. *Der Stille Befehl: Medizinalrat Kersten, Himmler und das Dritte Reich.* München: Nymphenburger Verlagshandlung, 1960.

Binion, Rudolph. *Hitler Among the Germans.* DeKalb: Northern Illinois University Press, 1976. Reprint.

Bullock, Alan. *Hitler: A Study in Tyranny.* New York: Bantam Books, published by arrangement with Harper & Brothers, 1958. (Orig. pub. 1953.)

Bytwerk, Randall, L. *Julius Streicher: Nazi Editor of the Notorious Anti-Semitic Newspaper Der Stürmer.* New York: Cooper Square, 2001.

Fest, Joachim, C. *Hitler.* Translated by Richard Winston and Clara Winston. New York: Harcourt Brace Jovanovich, 1974.

Hanfstaengl, Ernst. *Hitler: The Missing Years.* New York: Arcade, 1994. (Orig. pub. 1957.)

Heston, Leonard L., M.D., and Renate Heston, R.N. *The Medical Casebook of Adolf Hitler: His Illnesses, Doctors and Drugs.* Briarcliff Manor, N.Y.: Stein & Day, 1979. Second edition published as *Adolph Hitler: His Drug Abuse, Doctors, Illnesses.* Portland, Oreg.: Baypoint Press, 1999.

Hitler, Adolf. *Mein Kampf.* Translated by Ralph Manheim. Boston: Houghton Mifflin, 1971. (Orig. pub. 1925.)

Irving, David. *Hitler's War and The War Path.* London: Focal Point, 2002.

————. *The Secret Diaries of Hitler's Doctor.* New York: Macmillan, 1983.

Kershaw, Ian. *Hitler: 1889–1936: Hubris.* New York: Norton, 1999.

————. *Hitler: 1936–1945: Nemesis.* New York: Norton, 2000.

Kersten, Felix. *The Kersten Memoirs 1940–1945.* Translated by Constantine Fitzgibbon and James Oliver; introduction by H. R. Trevor-Roper. New York: Macmillan, 1957.

Kubizek, August. *The Young Hitler I Knew.* Translated by E. V. Anderson. Boston: Houghton Mifflin, 1955.

Langer, Walter C. *The Mind of Adolph Hitler.* New York: Basic Books, 1972.

Levy, Alan. *The Wiesenthal File.* Grand Rapids, Mich.: William B. Eerdmans, 1994.

Maser, Werner. *Hitler: Legend, Myth and Reality.* Translated by Peter Ross and Betty Ross. New York: Harper & Row, 1971.

Manvell, Roger, and Heinrich Fraenkel. *Himmler.* New York: Putnam, 1965.

Moriarty, David M., M.D. *A Psychological Study of Adolf Hitler.* St. Louis: Warren H. Green, 1993.

Neumayr, Anton. *Dictators in the Mirror of Medicine: Napoleon, Hitler, Stalin.* Translated by David J. Parent. Bloomington, Ill.: Medi-Ed, 1995.

Park, Bert Edward. *The Impact of Illness on World Leaders.* Philadelphia: University of Pennsylvania Press, 1986.

Redlich, Fritz, M.D. *Hitler: Diagnosis of a Destructive Prophet.* New York: Oxford University Press, 1999.

Rosenbaum, Ron. *Explaining Hitler: The Search for the Origins of His Evil.* New York: Random House, 1998.

Speer, Albert. *Inside the Third Reich.* Translated by Richard Winston and Clara Winston. New York: Macmillan, 1970.

Toland, John. *Adolf Hitler.* Garden City, N.Y.: Doubleday, 1976.

Victor, George. *Hitler: The Pathology of Evil.* Washington, D.C.: Brassey's, 1998.

Waite, Robert G. L. *The Psychopathic God: Adolf Hitler.* New York: Basic Books, 1977. (Orig. pub. 1939.)

Weiss, Ernst. *The Eyewitness.* Translated by Ella R. W. McKee; foreword by Rudolph Binion. Boston: Houghton Mifflin, 1977. (Orig. pub. 1963.)

Wiesenthal, Simon. *Justice Not Vengeance.* Translated by Ewald Osers. London: Weidenfeld & Nicolson, 1989.

Wykes, Alan. *The Doctor and His Enemy.* New York: Dutton, 1966.

———. *Hitler: Ballantine's Illustrated History of World War II.* War Leader Book no. 3. New York: Ballantine, 1970.

JAMES JOYCE

Davies, Stan Gêbler. *James Joyce: A Portrait of the Artist.* London: Granada Publishing, 1982. (Orig. pub. 1975.)

Ellmann, Richard. *James Joyce.* New York: Oxford University Press, 1982.

Ferris, Kathleen. *James Joyce & the Burden of Disease.* Lexington: University Press of Kentucky, 1995.

Joyce, James. *Ulysses.* Edited by Hans Walter Gabler. New York: Random House, 1986.

Lyons, J. B. *James Joyce and Medicine.* Dublin: Dolmen, 1973.

———. *Thrust Syphilis Down to Hell and Other Rejoyceana: Studies in the Border-Lands of Literature and Medicine.* Dublin: Glendale, 1988.

Maddox, Brenda. *Nora: A Biography of Nora Joyce.* New York: Fawcett, 1989.

MARY TODD AND ABRAHAM LINCOLN

Baker, Jean H. *Mary Todd Lincoln.* New York: Norton, 1987.

Burlingame, Michael. *The Inner World of Abraham Lincoln.* Urbana: University of Illinois Press, 1994.

Herndon, William H., and Jesse W. Weik. *Herndon's Life of Lincoln.* New York: De Capo Press, 1983; reprint, Cleveland: World Publishing, 1942.

Hertz, Emanuel. *The Hidden Lincoln: From the Letters and Papers of William H. Herndon.* New York: Viking, 1938.

Hirschhorn, Norbert, and Robert G. Feldman. "Mary Lincoln's Final Illness: A Medical and Historical Reappraisal." *Journal of the History of Medicine* 54 (October 1999): 511–542.

Hirschhorn, Norbert, Robert G. Feldman, and Ian A. Greaves. "Abraham Lincoln's Blue Pills." *Perspectives in Biology and Medicine* 44, no. 3 (Summer 2001): 315–332.

Morris, Jan. *Lincoln: A Foreigner's Quest*. New York: De Capo Press, 2000.

Neely, Mark E., Jr., and R. Gerald McMurtry. *The Insanity File: The Case of Mary Todd Lincoln*. Carbondale: Southern Illinois University Press, 1986.

Turner, Justin G., and Linda Levitt Turner. *Mary Todd Lincoln: Her Life and Letters*. New York: Alfred A. Knopf, 1972.

Vidal, Gore. *United States Essays: 1952–1992*. New York: Random House, 1993.

Wilson, Douglas L. *Honor's Voice: The Transformation of Abraham Lincoln*. New York: Alfred A. Knopf, 1998.

GUY DE MAUPASSANT

De Maupassant, Guy. "Bed Number 29." In *The Complete Short Stories of Guy de Maupassant*. Garden City, N.Y.: Doubleday, 1955.

Lerner, Michael. *Maupassant*. New York: George Braziller, 1975.

Sherard, Robert Harborough. *The Life, Work and Evil Fate of Guy de Maupassant*. New York: Brentano's, n. d.

FRIEDRICH NIETZSCHE

Aldrich, Robert. *The Seduction of the Mediterranean: Writing, Art, and Homosexual Fantasy*. New York: Routledge, 1993.

Binion, Rudolph. *Frau Lou: Nietzsche's Wayward Disciple*. Princeton, N.J.: Princeton University Press, 1968.

Chamberlain, Lesley. *Nietzsche in Turin: The End of the Future*. London: Quartet Books, 1996.

Förster-Nietzsche, Elisabeth. *The Life of Nietzsche*. Vol. I, *The Young Nietzsche*, translated by A. M. Ludovici; Vol. II, *The Lonely Nietzsche*, translated by P. V. Cohn. New York: Sturgis & Walton, 1912–1915.

Freud, Ernst L., ed. *The Letters of Sigmund Freud and Arnold Zweig*. New York: Harcourt, Brace and World, 1970.

Gilman, Sandor, ed. *Conversations with Nietzsche: A Life in the Words of His Contemporaries*. Translated by David J. Parent. New York: Oxford University Press, 1987.

Golomb, Jacob, Weaver Santaniello, and Ronald Lehrer, eds. *Nietzsche and Depth Psychology*. Albany: State University of New York Press, 1999.

Harrison, Thomas, ed. *Nietzsche in Italy*. Saratoga, Calif.: ANMA Libri, 1988.

Hayman, Ronald. *Nietzsche: A Critical Life*. New York: Penguin, 1982.

Hollingdale, R. J. *Nietzsche: The Man and His Philosophy*. Baton Rouge: Louisiana State University Press, 1965.

Jarrett, James L., ed. *Nietzsche's* Zarathustra: *Notes of the Seminar Given in 1934–1939 by C.G. Jung,* Vols. I–II. Princeton, N.J.: Princeton University Press, 1988.

Jaspers, Karl. *Nietzsche: An Introduction to the Understanding of His Philosophical Activity*. Translated by Charles F. Wallraff and Frederick J. Schmitz. Tucson: University of Arizona Press, 1965.

Jung, C. G. *Memories, Dreams, Reflections*. Edited by Aniela Jaffe; translated by Richard Winston and Clara Winston. New York: Vintage, 1989.

Kaufmann, Walter. *Nietzsche: Philosopher, Psychologist, Antichrist*. Princeton, N.J.: Princeton University Press, 1978.

_____. "Nietzche." In *Encyclopedia of Philosophy*, Vol. 5. Edited by Paul Edwards. New York: Collier Macmillan, 1967.

Kerr, John. *A Most Dangerous Method: The Story of Jung, Freud, and Sabina Spielrein*. New York: Alfred A. Knopf, 1993.

Köhler, Joachim. *Zarathustra's Secret: The Interior of Friedrich Nietzsche*. New Haven, Conn.: Yale University Press, 2002.

Krell, David Farrell. *Infectious Nietzsche*. Bloomington: Indiana University Press, 1996.

Lehrer, Ronald. *Nietzsche's Presence in Freud's Life and Thought*. Albany: State University of New York Press, 1995.

Livingstone, Angela. *Salomé*. Mt. Kisco, N.Y.: Moyer Bell, 1984.

Macintyre, Ben. *Forgotten Fatherland: The Search for Elisabeth Nietzsche*. New York: Farrar Straus Giroux, 1992.

Malraux, André. *Anti-Memoirs*. Translated by Terence Kilmartin. New York: Henry Holt, 1968.

Mann, Thomas. *Dr. Faustus*. New York: Alfred A. Knopf, 1948.

_____. "Nietzsche's Philosophy in the Light of Recent History." In *Thomas Mann: Last Essays*. Translated by Richard Winston, Clara Winston et al. New York: Alfred A. Knopf, 1959.

Middleton, Christopher, ed. and trans. *Selected Letters of Friedrich Nietzsche*. Chicago: University of Chicago Press, 1969.

Nietzsche, Friedrich. *Ecce Homo*. Edited by R. J. Hollingdale. New York: Penguin, 1979.

Nunberg, Herman, and Ernst Federn, eds. *Minutes of the Vienna Psychoanalytical Society*, Vol. II, *1908–1910*. New York: International Universities Press, 1967.

Parkes, Graham. *Composing the Soul: Reaches of Nietzsche's Psychology*. Chicago: University of Chicago Press, 1994.

Peters, H. F. *My Sister, My Spouse: A Biography of Lou Andreas-Salomé*. New York: Norton, 1962.

―――――. *Zarathustra's Sister: The Case of Elisabeth and Friedrich*. New York: Marcus Wiener, 1985.

Pletsch, Carl. *Young Nietzsche: Becoming a Genius*. New York: Free Press, 1991.

Podach, Erich. *The Madness of Nietzsche*. Translated by F. A. Voigt. New York: Putnam, 1931.

Salomé, Lou. *Nietzsche*. Translated and edited by Siegfried Mandel. Redding Ridge, Conn.: Black Swan Books, 1988. (Orig. pub. 1894 as *Friedrich Nietzsche in seinen Werken*.)

Schaberg, William. *The Nietzsche Canon: A Publication History and Bibliography*. Chicago: University of Chicago Press, 1995.

Schain, Richard. *The Legend of Nietzsche's Syphilis*. Westport, Conn.: Greenwood, 2001.

Volz, Pia Daniela. *Nietzsche im Labyrinth seiner Krankheit: Eine medizinisch-biographische Untersuchung*. Würzburg, Germany: Königshausen and Neumann, 1990.

Zweig, Stefan. *Master Builders: A Typology of the Spirit*. Translated by Eden Paul and Cedar Paul. New York: Viking, 1939. (Orig. pub. 1925.)

FRANZ SCHUBERT

Deutsch, Otto Erich. *The Schubert Reader*. Translated by Eric Blom. New York: Norton, 1947.

McKay, Elizabeth Normal. *Franz Schubert: A Biography*. Oxford: Clarendon Press, 1996.

Newbould, Brian. *Schubert: The Music and the Man*. Berkeley: University of California Press, 1997.

Sams, Eric. "Schubert's Illness Re-examined." *Musical Times* 121, no. 1643 (January 1980): 15–22.

Woodford, Peggy. *Schubert: His Life and Times*. Neptune City, N.J.: Paganiniana Publishing, 1980.

ROBERT SCHUMANN

Davario, John. *Robert Schumann: Herald of a "New Poetic Age."* Oxford: Oxford University Press, 1997.

Neumayr, Anton. *Music & Medicine: Hummel, Weber, Mendelssohn, Schumann, Brahms, Bruckner*, Vol. II. Translated by Bruce Cooper Clarke. Bloomington, Ill.: Medi-Ed, 1995.

Ostwald, Peter. *Schumann: The Inner Voices of a Musical Genius*. Boston: Northeastern University Press, 1985.

Reich, Nancy B. *Clara Schumann: The Artist and the Woman*. Ithaca, N.Y.: Cornell University Press, 1985.

Sams, Eric. *The Songs of Robert Schumann*. Bloomington: Indiana University Press, 1993.

Taylor, Ronald. *Robert Schumann: His Life and Work*. London: Panther Books, 1985.

Walker, Alan, ed. *Robert Schumann: The Man and His Music*. London: Barrie & Jenkins, 1972.

VINCENT VAN GOGH

Arnold, Wilfred Niels. *Vincent van Gogh: Chemicals, Crises, and Creativity*. Boston: Birkhäuser, 1992.

Bonafoux, Pascal. *Van Gogh*. Translated by Alexandra Campbell. New York: Henry Holt, 1990.

De Leeuw, Ronald, ed. *The Complete Letters of Vincent van Gogh,* Vols. I.-III. Greenwich, Conn.: New York Graphic Society, 1958.

Edwards, Cliff. *Van Gogh and God*. Chicago: Loyola University Press, 1989.

Elgar, Frank. *Van Gogh: A Study of His Life and Work*. New York: Praeger, 1966.

Hulsker, J. *Vincent and Theo van Gogh: A Dual Biography*. Ann Arbor, Mich.: Fuller Publishing, 1990.

Jaspers, Karl. *Strindberg and van Gogh*. Translated by Oskar Grunow and David Woloshin. Tucson: University of Arizona Press, 1977.

Lubin, Albert J. *Stranger on the Earth: A Psychological Biography of Vincent van Gogh*. New York: Henry Holt, 1972.

Nagera, Humberto, M.D. *Vincent van Gogh: A Psychological Study*. London: George Allen & Unwin, 1967.

Sweetman, David. *Paul Gauguin: A Complete Life*. London: Hodder and Stoughton, 1995.

_____. *Van Gogh: His Life and His Art*. New York: Crown, 1990.

Tralbaut, M. E. *Vincent van Gogh*. New York: Alpine Fine Arts, 1981.

Wilkie, Ken. *In Search of van Gogh*. Rocklin, Calif.: Prima Publishing, 1991.

OSCAR WILDE

Aldington, Richard, and Stanley Weintraub, eds. *The Portable Oscar Wilde*. New York: Penguin Books, 1981.

Amor, Anne Clark. *Mrs. Oscar Wilde: A Woman of Some Importance*. London: Sedgwick & Jackson, 1983.

Belford, Barbara. *Oscar Wilde: A Certain Genius*. New York: Random House, 2000.

Brasol, Boris. *Oscar Wilde: The Man, the Artist, the Martyr*. New York: Octagon, 1975. (Orig. pub. 1938.)

Cawthorne, Terence. "The Fatal Illness of Oscar Wilde." *Annals of Otology, Rhonology, and Laryngology* 75 (1966): 657–666.

Critchley, Macdonald. "Medical Reflections on Oscar Wilde." *Mem Acad Chir* (Paris) 30 (1962): 73–84.

———. "Oscar Wilde's Fatal Illness: The Mystery Unshrouded." *Medical and Health Annual* (1990): 191–208.

Elfman, Clare. *The Case of the Pederast's Wife.* Chester Springs, Pa.: Dufour Editions, 2000.

Ellman, Richard. *Oscar Wilde.* New York: Alfred A. Knopf, 1988.

Fryer, Jonathan. *André & Oscar: The Literary Friendship of André Gide and Oscar Wilde.* New York: St. Martin's Press, 1998.

Gide, André. *If It Die: An Autobiography.* Translated by Dorothy Bussy. New York: Random House, 1935. (Orig. pub. as *Si le grain ne meurt,* 1920.)

Harris, Frank. *Oscar Wilde.* Introduction by Merlin Holland. New York: Carroll & Graf, 1997. (Orig. pub. 1916.)

———. *Oscar Wilde: His Life and Confessions.* Garden City, N.Y.: Garden City Publications, 1930.

Holland, Merlin. "Biography and the Art of Lying." In *The Cambridge Companion to Oscar Wilde,* edited by Peter Raby. Cambridge: Cambridge University Press, 1997.

———. *The Wilde Album.* New York: Henry Holt, 1997.

Holland, Merlin, and Rupert Hart-Davis. *The Complete Letters of Oscar Wilde.* New York: Henry Holt, 2000.

Holland, Vyvyan. *Son of Oscar Wilde.* New York: Carroll & Graf, 1999. (Orig. pub. 1954.)

Hyde, H. Montgomery. *Oscar Wilde: A Biography.* New York: Farrar, Straus & Giroux, 1975.

———. *Oscar Wilde: The Aftermath.* New York: Farrar, Straus, 1963.

Knox, Melissa. *Oscar Wilde: A Long and Lovely Suicide.* New Haven: Yale University Press, 1994.

Lyons, J. B. "Oscar Wilde's Final Illness." *Irish Studies Review* 11 (1995): 24–27.

———. *What Did I Die of?: The Deaths of Parnell, Wilde, Synge, and Other Literary Pathologies.* Dublin: Lilliput Press, 1991.

Pearce, Joseph. *The Unmasking of Oscar Wilde.* London: HarperCollins, 2000.

Pearson, Hesketh. *Oscar Wilde: His Life and Wit.* New York: Harper & Brothers, 1946.

Raby, Peter, ed. *The Cambridge Companion to Oscar Wilde.* Cambridge: Cambridge University Press, 1997.

Robins, Ashley H., and Sean L. Sellars. "Oscar Wilde's Terminal Illness: Reappraisal After a Century." *The Lancet* 356, no. 9244 (25 November 2000): 1841–1843.

Schmidgall, Gary. *The Stranger Wilde: Interpreting Oscar.* New York: Dutton, 1994.

Sedgwick, Eve Kosofsky. *Epistemology of the Closet*. Berkeley: University of California Press, 1990.

Sherard, Robert Harborough. *Bernard Shaw, Frank Harris & Oscar Wilde*. New York: Greystone, 1937.

_____. *The Life of Oscar Wilde*. New York: Dodd, Mead, 1928.

_____. *Oscar Wilde: The Story of an Unhappy Friendship*. London: Greening, 1908.

_____. *Oscar Wilde Twice Defended from André Gide's Wicked Lies and Frank Harris's Vicious Libels*. Chicago: Argus Book Shop, 1934.

Simmons, James C. *Star-Spangled Eden: 19th Century America Through the Eyes of Dickens, Wilde, Frances Trollope, Frank Harris, and Other British Travelers*. New York: Carroll & Graf, 2000.

Wilde, Oscar. *The Picture of Dorian Gray*. Mattituck, N.Y.: Ameron House, 1982.

GENERAL

Brombert, Beth Archer. *Edouard Manet: Rebel in a Frock Coat*. New York: Little, Brown, 1996.

Bergreen, Laurence. *Capone: The Man and the Era*. New York: Simon & Schuster, 1994.

Conrad, Barnaby, III. *Absinthe: History in a Bottle*. San Francisco: Chronicle Books, 1988.

Coulter, Harris L. *Aids and Syphilis: The Hidden Link*. Berkeley: North Atlantic Books, 1987.

Critchley, Macdonald. *The Divine Banquet of the Brain*. New York: Raven, 1979. (Includes the essay, "Five Illustrious Neuroluetics.")

Dale, Philip Marshall, M.D. *Medical Biographies*. Norman: University of Oklahoma Press, 1987. (Orig. pub. 1952.)

Daudet, Alphonse. *In the Land of Pain*. Translated and edited by Julian Barnes. London: Jonathan Cape, 2002.

Francis, Claude, and Fernande Gontier. *Creating Colette: Volume One: From Ingenue to Libertine, 1873–1913*. South Royalton, Vt.: Steerforth, 1999.

Gray, Fred D. *The Tuskegee Syphilis Study*. Montgomery, Ala.: Black Belt Press, 1998.

Jones, James H. *Bad Blood: The Tuskegee Syphilis Experiment*. New York: Free Press, 1993.

Lucey, Michael. *Gide's Bent: Sexuality, Politics, Writing*. New York: Oxford University Press, 1995.

Martin, Ralph G. *Jennie: The Life of Lady Randolph Churchill*. Englewood Cliffs, N.J.: Prentice Hall, 1969.

Mitchell, Robert Ben. *Syphilis as AIDS*. Austin, Tex.: Banned Books, 1958.

Neumayr, Anton. *Music & Medicine: Haydn, Mozart, Beethoven, Schubert*, Vol. I. Translated by Bruce Cooper Clarke. Bloomington, Ill.: Medi-Ed , 1994.

Newman, Ernest. *Hugo Wolf.* New York: Dover, 1966. (Orig. pub. 1907.)

Ober, William B., M.D. "To Cast a Pox: The Iconography of Syphilis." *American Journal Dermatopathology* 11, no. 1 (1989): 74–86.

Reverby, Susan M., ed. *Tuskegee's Truths: Rethinking the Tuskegee Syphilis Study.* Chapel Hill: University of North Carolina Press, 2000.

Sinclair, Upton. *Damaged Goods.* Glascow: Muir-Watson, n.d.

Thomson, Belinda. *Gauguin.* New York: Thames & Hudson, 1987.

Index